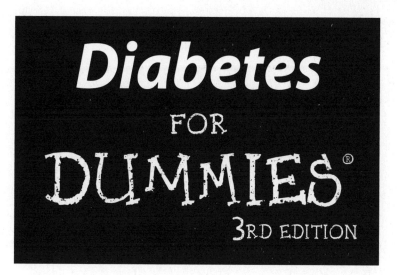

Diabetes
FOR
DUMMIES®
3RD EDITION

by Alan L. Rubin, MD

WILEY

Wiley Publishing, Inc.

Diabetes For Dummies®, 3rd Edition

Published by
Wiley Publishing, Inc.
111 River St.
Hoboken, NJ 07030-5774
www.wiley.com

Copyright © 2008 by Wiley Publishing, Inc., Indianapolis, Indiana

Published by Wiley Publishing, Inc., Indianapolis, Indiana

Published simultaneously in Canada

For general information on our other products and services or to obtain technical support, please contact our Customer Care Department within the U.S. at 800-762-2974, outside the U.S. at 317-572-3993, or fax 317-572-4002.

Wiley also publishes its books in a variety of electronic formats. Some content that appears in print may not be available in electronic books.

Library of Congress Control Number: 2008930526

ISBN: 978-0-470-27086-8

Manufactured in the United States of America

WILEY

Diabetes For Dummies, 3rd Edition

Cheat Sheet

Appropriate Standards for Continuing Diabetes Care

Following are guidelines for your diabetes care:

Frequency of visits:

- Daily if starting insulin
- Weekly for oral drugs
- Monthly if not stable
- Quarterly if stable

History at each visit:

- Frequency of hypoglycemia
- Results of blood glucose self-monitoring
- Changes in treatment
- Symptoms of complications
- Psychosocial issues
- New medications

Physical at each visit:

- Blood pressure
- Weight
- Foot exam if neuropathy is present

Physical at least annually:

- Dilated eye exam by eye doctor (Chapter 5)
- Filament test for foot sensation (Chapter 5)

Lab tests:

- Hemoglobin A1c every three months (Chapter 7)
- Fasting lipid profile yearly (Chapter 7)
- Microalbumin measurement yearly if urine protein negative (Chapter 7)

Frequency of blood glucose self-monitoring (Chapter 7):

- Before meals and bedtime for person with type 1 diabetes
- Before breakfast and supper for person with type 2 diabetes
- Once daily for person with stable diabetes
- Before and one hour after meals for pregnant woman with type 1 diabetes or gestational diabetes

Ten Commandments for Great Diabetes Control

Follow these commandments, and your problems should be few and far between:

- Major monitoring (see Chapter 7)
- Devout dieting (see Chapter 8)
- Tenacious testing (see Chapter 7)
- Enthusiastic exercising (see Chapter 9)
- Lifelong learning (see Chapter 12)
- Meticulous medicating (see Chapter 10)
- Appropriate attitude (see Chapter 1)
- Preventive planning (see Chapter 8)
- Fastidious foot care (see Chapter 5)
- Essential eye care (see Chapter 5)

For Dummies: Bestselling Book Series for Beginners

Diabetes For Dummies, 3rd Edition

Cheat Sheet

Oral Drugs for Diabetes

Your doctor may put you on one or another of these drugs Here you will find dosage and brand names so you can look up side effects and drug interactions in Chapter 10.

Class	Brand Name	Generic Name	Average Dose	Range
Sulfonylureas	Orinase	tolbutamide	1,500 mg	500–3,000 mg
	Tolinase	tolazamide	250 mg	100–1,000 mg
	Diabinase	chlorpropamide	250 mg	100–500 mg
	Dymelor	acetohexamide	500 mg	250–1,500 mg
	Glucotrol	glipazide	10 mg	2.5–40 mg
	DiaBeta, Glynase	glyburide	7.5 mg	1.25–20 mg
	Amaryl	glimepiride	4 mg	1–8 mg
Meglitinides	Prandin	repaglinide	1 mg	0.5–4 mg
	Starlix	nateglinide	180 mg	180–360 mg
Biguanides	Glucophage	metformin	1,000 mg	500–2,000 mg
Thiazolidinediones	Actos	pioglitazone	30 mg	15–45 mg
Alpha-glucosidase inhibitors	Precose	acarbose	100 mg	50–250 mg
	Glyset	miglitol	50 mg	25–75 mg
DPP-4 Inhibitors	Januvia	sitagliptin	100 mg	25–100 mg

Guidelines for Testing for Diabetes

These guidelines were developed by the American Diabetes Association to screen for diabetes at the earliest possible appropriate time:

✔ People with symptoms of thirst, frequent urination, and weight loss are tested immediately.

✔ People over age 45 should be tested every three years if normal.

✔ People should be tested at a younger age and more often if:

- They are obese.

- Their parent or siblings have diabetes.

- They are from a high-risk group, such as African American, Hispanic, or Native American.

- They have delivered a baby over nine pounds or had gestational diabetes.

- They have high blood pressure.

- They have low HDL cholesterol or high triglycerides.

For Dummies: Bestselling Book Series for Beginners

About the Author

Alan L. Rubin, M.D., is one of the nation's foremost experts on diabetes. He is a professional member of the American Diabetes Association and the Endocrine Society and has been in private practice specializing in diabetes and thyroid disease for more than 30 years. Dr. Rubin was Assistant Clinical Professor of Medicine at University of California Medical Center in San Francisco for 20 years. He has spoken about diabetes to professional medical audiences and non-medical audiences around the world. He has been a consultant to many pharmaceutical companies and companies that make diabetes products.

Dr. Rubin was one of the first specialists in his field to recognize the significance of patient self-testing of blood glucose, the major advance in diabetes care since the advent of insulin. As a result, he has been on numerous radio and television programs, talking about the cause, the prevention, and the treatment of diabetes and its complications.

Since publishing *Diabetes For Dummies,* Dr. Rubin has had four other bestselling For Dummies books — *Diabetes Cookbook For Dummies, Thyroid For Dummies, High Blood Pressure For Dummies,* and *Type 1 Diabetes For Dummies* — all published by Wiley Publishing. His five books cover the medical problems of 100 million Americans.

Dedication

This book is dedicated to my wife Enid and my children, Renee and Larry. Their patience, enthusiasm, and encouragement helped to make the writing a real pleasure.

This third edition is also dedicated to the thousands of people with diabetes who have written to thank me for helping them to understand what they are dealing with and for telling me where I need to provide more information and emphasis to make this an even better book.

Author's Acknowledgments

For this third edition, acquisitions editor Michael Lewis deserves major thanks. I have had the pleasure of working with him for several years. He is supportive, encouraging, and fun and I look forward to a long association with him. I am also blessed with another great project editor, Jennifer Connolly, who not only made sure that everything was readable and understandable, but offered excellent suggestions to improve the information. My thanks also to Dr. Seymour Levin for reviewing the book for scientific accuracy.

Ronnie and Michael Goldfield should definitely be considered the godparents of this book.

My friends in the Dawn Patrol, a group of guys with whom I play squash and solve the problems of the world thereafter, kept me laughing throughout the production of this book. Their willingness to follow me convinced me that others would be willing to read what I wrote.

My teachers are too numerous to mention, but one group deserves special attention. They are my patients over the last 35 years, the people whose trials and tribulations caused me to seek the knowledge that you will find in this book.

This book is written on the shoulders of thousands of men and women who made the discoveries and held the committee meetings. Their accomplishments cannot possibly be given adequate acclaim. We owe them big-time.

Publisher's Acknowledgments

We're proud of this book; please send us your comments through our Dummies online registration form located at www.dummies.com/register/.

Some of the people who helped bring this book to market include the following:

Acquisitions, Editorial, and Media Development

Project Editor: Jennifer Connolly

(Previous Edition: Joan Friedman)

Acquisitions Editor: Michael Lewis

(Previous Edition: Natasha Graf)

Technical Editor: Dr. Seymour Levin

(Previous Edition: Dr. Dawn Ayers)

Editorial Manager: Jennifer Ehrlich

Editorial Supervisor: Carmen Krikorian

Editorial Assistants: Jennette ElNaggar, David Lutton

Cover Photo: © Purestock

Cartoons: Rich Tennant, www.the5thwave.com

Illustrations: Kathryn Born, M.A.

Composition

Project Coordinator: Katie Key

Layout and Graphics: Carl Byers, Reuben W. Davis, Nikki Gately, Joyce Haughey, Ronald Terry

Proofreader: Sossity R. Smith

Indexer: Slivoskey Indexing Services

Publishing and Editorial for Consumer Dummies

Diane Graves Steele, Vice President and Publisher, Consumer Dummies

Joyce Pepple, Acquisitions Director, Consumer Dummies

Kristin A. Cocks, Product Development Director, Consumer Dummies

Michael Spring, Vice President and Publisher, Travel

Brice Gosnell, Associate Publisher, Travel

Kelly Regan, Editorial Director, Travel

Publishing for Technology Dummies

Andy Cummings, Vice President and Publisher, Dummies Technology/General User

Composition Services

Gerry Fahey, Vice President of Production Services

Debbie Stailey, Director of Composition Services

Contents at a Glance

Table of Contents

Introduction

A third edition: Wow, is it really necessary? You bet it is. So much has happened since the last edition. Doctors have learned so much more about the cause of the complications of diabetes, about new treatments for diabetes and, unfortunately, about the nature of diabetes — diabetes is not only not going away, but it is spreading almost like a contagious infection, especially in places where it was rarely seen before, places like China and India. As these places adopt a Western lifestyle, their people are developing Western diseases like diabetes, high blood pressure, and heart disease.

It is estimated that the current prevalence of diabetes throughout the world is 2.8 percent. By 2030 that figure is expected to go up to 4.4 percent. Put another way, there are currently 171 million people with diabetes in the world. By 2030 there will be 366 million, a little more than the current population of the United States.

The condition has gotten so prevalent that November is National Diabetes Awareness Month, and as I write this in November 2007 the world is about to "celebrate" World Diabetes Day. On World Diabetes Day, events take place like walks for diabetes, workshops for diabetes, and races for diabetes from Australia to Zagreb. In fact, the United Nations proclaims diabetes to be a worldwide, debilitating disease that is costly, has profound life-changing ramifications, and poses a risk to the entire world.

In the United States the situation is especially dire because large numbers of children are developing type 2 diabetes. It used to be rare in children. Because the long-term complications of diabetes, which you will learn about in Chapter 5, take 10 to 15 years of poor diabetic control to develop, the United States may soon begin to see a significant population of 25- to 30-year-old people with blindness, kidney failure, and painful nerve disease, not to mention amputations.

In a sense, a diagnosis of diabetes is both good news and bad news. It is bad news because you have a disease you'd happily do without. It is good news if you use it to make some changes in your lifestyle that can not only prevent complications but help you to live a longer and higher quality life.

As for laughing about it, at times you will feel like doing anything but laughing. But scientific studies are clear about the benefits of a positive attitude. In a very few words: He who laughs, lasts. Another point is that people learn more and retain more when humor is part of the process. If you have experienced something funny during the course of your diabetes care, I hope you share it with me. My goal is not to trivialize human suffering by being comic about it, but to lighten the burden of a chronic disease by showing that it is not all gloom and doom.

About This Book

As I said above, so much has changed in the four years since the second edition of *Diabetes For Dummies* was written that a third edition was clearly necessary. I need to tell you about new medicines (see Chapter 10), new glucose meters (Chapter 7), and new ideas about diet and exercise (Chapters 8 and 9). I also need to share new information about diabetes in certain ethnic groups (Chapter 2), diabetes in children (Chapter 13), and the occupational and insurance problems of people with diabetes (Chapter 15). Just about every chapter has something new, especially (obviously) Chapter 16, "What's New in Diabetes Care."

A new edition also gives me the opportunity to thank the thousands of people who have thanked me for *Diabetes For Dummies.* You have given me a sense of enormous gratification for writing this book. You have shared your stories with me, permitting me to laugh and cry with you. One of the best is the following from Andrea in Canada:

> *My 3-year-old daughter was recently diagnosed with diabetes type one. It has been a rough time. To help us out my brother and his wife bought us your book,* Diabetes For Dummies. *One day my daughter saw this bright yellow book and asked what I was reading. I told her* Diabetes For Dummies. *As soon as the words came out of my mouth, I regretted it. I didn't want her to think that dummies got diabetes so I quickly added, "I am the dummy." Without missing a beat, she then asked, "Am I the diabetes?"*
>
> *The story doesn't just end there. The other day she was relaxing on the couch. She looked at me and said, "I don't want to have diabetes anymore." Feeling terrible I responded, "I know sweetie; I don't want you to have it anymore either." I then explained that she would have diabetes for the rest of her life. With a very concerned look she then asked, "Will you be the dummy for the rest of your life?"*
>
> *As sad as it is, I guess you're right,* **one must look for humor in everything,** *otherwise we would have broken down by now.*

You're not required to read this book from cover to cover, although if you know nothing about diabetes, this may be a good approach. This book is designed to serve as a source for information about the problems that arise over the years. You can find the latest facts about diabetes and the best sources to discover any information that comes out after the publication of this edition.

Conventions Used in This Book

Throughout the book I use some specific conventions to make the text clearer, to highlight information, and to make your read as effortless as possible. These conventions are important to know so I list them below:

- ✔ **Sugar versus glucose:** Diabetes, as you know, is all about sugar. But sugars come in many types. So doctors avoid using the words *sugar* and *glucose* interchangeably. In this book (unless I slip up), I use the word *glucose* rather than *sugar.* (You might as well get used to it, sweetie.)

- ✔ **Emphasis on type 2 diabetes:** There are a number of different types of diabetes (see my explanation in Chapter 3), led by type 1 diabetes and type 2 diabetes. Because I recently published *Type 1 Diabetes For Dummies* (Wiley), most of what you read here will be about type 2 diabetes.

- ✔ *Diabetes Care:* You may often see me discuss findings from the journal, *Diabetes Care,* which is published by the ADA. This journal is the most widely read clinical diabetes journal by professionals around the world. Keep that in mind whenever you see me discuss its findings.

- ✔ **Abbreviations:** To save time, I use the following abbreviations:

    - • T1DM: Type 1 diabetes mellitus (formal name of type 1 diabetes)

    - • T2DM: Type 2 diabetes mellitus (formal name of type 1 diabetes)

What You're Not to Read

Throughout the book, you find shaded areas called *sidebars.* These sidebars contain material that is interesting but not essential. I hereby give you permission to skip them if the material inside them is of no particular interest to you. You will still understand everything else. In addition, I've noted some paragraphs that have a more technical nature with the Technical Stuff icon (see the section "Icons Used in This Book," later in this Introduction for more information on icons). Although these paragraphs both deepen your knowledge of diabetes as well as broaden your vocabulary, you can still understand the text without reading them. My feelings won't get hurt if you don't read these paragraphs, but these technical tidbits may come in handy during a high-stakes trivia game or at the very least can make you sound pretty smart in front of your doctor.

Foolish Assumptions

The book assumes that you know nothing about diabetes. So you will not suddenly have to face a term that is not explained and that you never heard of before. For those who already know a lot about diabetes, you can find more in-depth explanations. You can pick and choose how much you want to know about a subject, but the key points are clearly marked.

How This Book Is Organized

This book is divided into six parts to help you find out all you can about the topic of diabetes.

Part 1: Dealing with the Onset of Diabetes

To slay the dragon, you have to be able to identify it. This part explains the different types of diabetes, how you get them, and whether you can give them to others.

In this part, you find out how to deal with the emotional and psychological consequences of the diagnosis and what all those big words mean. You also find out how to prevent the complications of diabetes.

Part 11: How Diabetes Affects Your Body

In medical history, there have been a few diseases that seem to affect every part of the body. If you understand diabetes, you will have a pretty good grasp of how other illnesses can change the state of your health.

In this part, you find out what you need to know about both the short- and long-term complications of diabetes. You also find out about some sexual problems related to diabetes and the problems of a diabetic pregnancy.

Part 111: Managing Diabetes: The "Thriving with Diabetes" Lifestyle Plan

In this part, you discover all the tools available to treat diabetes. You find out about the kinds of tests that you should be doing on your own, as well as the tests your doctor should order to get a clear picture of the severity of your diabetes. I also show you what to do about your specific condition and how to follow the success of therapy.

You also discover the dietary changes that you need to make to control your blood glucose and how to get the most out of your exercise routine and medications.

Finally, you find out about the huge amount of help available to you and your family. It is yours for the taking, and you definitely should take advantage of it.

Part IV: Special Considerations for Living with Diabetes

The way that diabetes develops is different for each age group. In this part, you are shown those differences and how to manage them. I will have a lot more to say about children with type 2 diabetes mellitus (T2DM). You also find out about some of the special economic problems of people with diabetes, which relate to jobs and insurance.

Lastly, this part covers all the new developments in diagnosing, monitoring, and treating diabetes and helps correct a lot of misinformation about diabetes treatment.

Part V: The Part of Tens

This part presents some key suggestions: the stuff you most need to know, as well as the stuff you least want to know.

You discover the ten commandments of diabetes care and the myths that confuse many diabetic patients. You also find out how to get others to help you in your efforts to control your diabetes.

Part VI: Appendixes

Two special appendixes help you improve your diet by giving you recipes and diabetic exchanges. Another appendix points out hot spots to visit on the Internet. And in case you forget what a term means, you can quickly flip to the handy glossary in the back of this book.

Icons Used in This Book

The icons alert you to information you must know, information you should know, and information you may find interesting but can live without.

I use this icon whenever I tell a story about patients.

This icon gives you technical information or terminology that may be helpful, but not necessary, to your understanding of the topic.

When you see this icon, it means the information is essential and you should be aware of it.

This icon points out when you should see your doctor (for example, if your blood glucose level is too high or you need a particular test done).

This icon marks important information that can save you time and energy.

This icon warns against potential problems (for example, if you don't treat a complication of diabetes properly).

Where to Go from Here

Where you go from here depends upon your needs. If you already have a basic knowledge of diabetes and want to know more about complications, go to Chapter 3. If you are a novice, start at Chapter 1. If you want to know more about the medications you are taking, go to Chapter 10. Each chapter title clearly tells you what you will find there, so check the table of contents to find what you need rapidly.

Let's get started on this trip we are taking together. Welcome! I hope it will be as much fun and as enlightening for you as it was for me.

Part I
Dealing with the Onset of Diabetes

The 5th Wave   By Rich Tennant

"I call him 'Glucose,' because I need to keep him under control every day."

In this part . . .

You have found out that you or a loved one has diabetes. What do you do now? This part tells you about the emotional crisis that you may go through and emerge prepared to live with this chronic disease. I walk you through stages from wondering whether the diagnosis is correct to avoiding the complications associated with diabetes. You will discover the different kinds of diabetes and where you fit in. I explain the new concept of *prediabetes* and discuss how you can actually prevent diabetes.

Chapter 1

Dealing with Diabetes

As a person with diabetes, you're more than the sum of your blood glucose levels. You have feelings, and you have a history. The way that you respond to the challenges of diabetes determines whether the disease will be a moderate annoyance or the source of major sickness.

One of my patients told me about working at her first job out of college, where each employee birthday was celebrated with cake. She came to the first celebration and was urged to eat a slice. She refused and refused, until finally she had to say, "I can't eat the cake because I am diabetic." The woman urging her said, "Thank God. I thought you just had incredible willpower." Twenty years later, my patient clearly remembers being told that having diabetes is better than having willpower. Another patient told me the following: "The hardest thing about having diabetes is having to deal with doctors who do not respect me." Several times over the years, she had followed her doctor's recommendations exactly, but her glucose control had not been satisfactory. The doctor blamed her for this "failure."

Unless you live alone on a desert island (in which case I'm impressed that you got your hands on this book), your diabetes doesn't affect just you. How you deal with your diabetes affects your family, friends, and coworkers as they desire to help you. This chapter shows you how to cope with diabetes and how to understand its impact on your important relationships.

Achieving Anything . . . Or Everything!

Are you as pretty as Nicole Johnson, the 1999 Miss America? Are you as funny as Jackie Gleason or Jack Benny? Do you have the inventive powers of Thomas Alva Edison? You have at least one thing in common with all of these famous people — diabetes — and you may have even more. The fact is, many people — from athletes to actors and politicians to painters — have found success despite the fact that they have had diabetes. Just take a look at the following sections. Perhaps you can find not only inspiration from the names mentioned, but also the same greatness and strength that motivated these successful individuals even though they wrestled with diabetes.

Keeping good company

Diabetes is a common disease, so it's bound to occur in some very extraordinary people. The list of people with diabetes is long, and you may be amazed at the caliber of the company you keep. The point is that every one of these people lives or lived with this chronic illness, and every one of them was able to do something special with his or her life.

Many politicians have diabetes — perhaps the result of eating too many fundraising dinners full of alcohol, starchy foods, and calorie-rich desserts. (See Chapter 4 for the role diet plays in the onset of diabetes.) Mike Huckabee, former governor of Arkansas and recent presidential candidate is a prime example of an outstanding politician with type 2 diabetes (T2DM). Another former governor, Charles "Buddy" Roemer of Louisiana, also has T2DM. He has the distinction of being the first sitting governor in modern history to switch parties while in office. James Lloyd, who served in the U.S. Congress from 1975 to 1981 did not let his T2DM interfere with his political career. Marion Barry, who overcame not only T2DM but a drug habit, was mayor of Washington, D. C. for four separate terms.

Among actors and comedians with diabetes, Jackie Gleason is memorable for his motto, "How sweet it is!" (Could he have been referring to his diabetes or his blood glucose?) Jerry Lewis, who seems to go on and on, raising millions of dollars every year for children with muscular dystrophy, is another comedian who does not let diabetes ruin his sense of humor. Elizabeth Taylor, one of the most beautiful actresses in movies, never let her diabetes keep her from a great performance.

Walt Kelly, who drew the *Pogo* comic strip, joins Paul Cézanne in the category of artists with diabetes. Writers Mario Puzo, author of *The Godfather,* Ernest Hemingway, and H. G. Wells all made their marks despite their diabetes. In the business world, Ray Kroc founded the McDonald's chain while dealing with diabetes.

The list of singers and musicians with diabetes contains some of the greatest voices. Blues singer .B. B. King, soul singer Pattie Labelle, and jazz singer Peggy Lee are all great additions to the people with diabetes who are sterling entertainers. Neil Young is no slouch in the music department, either. His diabetes has not stopped him from recording some of the great albums of the last decades.

Diabetes doesn't prevent the achievement of great records in sports. Athletes tend to develop T2DM when they are no longer in great physical shape, but there are exceptions. Diabetes didn't stop Mike Sinclair from becoming a three-time Pro Bowler in the National Football League during eleven seasons. Joe Frazier could box like few others despite his diabetes mellitus. Billie Jean King put women's tennis on the map when she beat Bobby Riggs; diabetes certainly didn't slow her serve. (To read about the role of sports and exercise in your life, see Chapter 9.) Gary Hall is a swimmer with diabetes who won ten Olympic medals in 2000 and 2004. Adam Morrison is a professional basketball player with diabetes.

Realizing your potential

The names in the preceding paragraphs are just a few examples of people with diabetes who have achieved greatness. Here is my point: *Diabetes shouldn't stop you from doing what you want to do with your life.* You must follow the rules of good diabetic care, as I describe in Chapters 7 through 12. But if you follow these rules, you will actually be healthier than people without diabetes who smoke, overeat, and/or don't exercise enough.

Perhaps the many people with diabetes who have achieved greatness used the same personal strengths to overcome the difficulties associated with diabetes as they did to excel at their particular callings. Or maybe their diabetes forced them to be stronger and to persevere more, which contributed to their success. Chapter 15 shows you a few areas (such as piloting a commercial flight) in which certain people with diabetes can't participate — (due to the ignorance of some legislators). Those people with diabetes will achieve complete freedom of choice when they show that they can safely and competently do anything that a person without diabetes can do.

Reacting to Your Diagnosis

Do you remember what you were doing when you found out that you had diabetes? Unless you were too young to understand, the news was quite a shock. Suddenly you had a condition from which people can die. In fact, many of the feelings that you went through were exactly those of a person learning that he or she is dying. The following sections describe the normal stages of reacting to a diagnosis of a major medical condition, such as diabetes.

Experiencing denial

Your first response was probably to deny that you had diabetes, despite all of the evidence. Your denial mindset may have begun when your doctor tried to "sugarcoat" (forgive the pun) the news of your condition by telling you that you had just "a touch of diabetes," (an impossibility equivalent to "a touch of pregnancy"). You probably looked for any evidence that the whole thing was a mistake.

Perhaps you even neglected to take your medication, follow your diet, or perform the exercise that is so important to maintaining your body. Ultimately, you had to accept the diagnosis and begin to gather the information you needed to help yourself.

When you accepted the diabetes diagnosis, I hope you also shared the news with your family, friends, and people close to you. Having diabetes isn't something to be ashamed of, and you shouldn't hide it from anyone. You need the help of everyone in your community: your coworkers who need to know not to tempt you with treats that you can't eat; your friends who need to know how to give you *glucagon,* a treatment for low blood glucose, if you become unconscious from a severe insulin reaction (see Chapter 4); and your family who needs to know how to support and encourage you to keep going.

Your diabetes isn't your fault — nor is it a form of leprosy or some other disease that carries a social stigma. Diabetes also isn't contagious; no one can catch it from you.

When you're accepting and open about having diabetes, you'll find that you're far from alone in your situation. (If you don't believe me, read the section "Keeping good company," earlier in this chapter.) One of my patients told me about experiences she had that helped her feel part of a community. She arrived at work one morning and was very worried when she realized that she had forgotten her insulin. But she quickly found a source of comfort when she remembered that she could go to a diabetic coworker and ask to borrow some insulin. Another time, she was at a party and stepped into a friend's bedroom to take a shot of insulin, and she found a man there doing the same thing. Borrowing someone else's insulin is probably not a good idea because it may be contaminated, but you get the point.

Feeling anger

When you've passed the stage of denying that you have diabetes, you may become angry that you're saddled with this "terrible" diagnosis. But you'll quickly find that diabetes isn't so terrible and that you can't do anything to rid yourself of the disease. Anger only worsens your situation, and being angry about your diagnosis is detrimental in the following ways:

- If your anger becomes targeted at a person, he or she is hurt.

- You may feel guilty that your anger is harming you and those close to you.

- Anger can prevent you from successfully managing your diabetes.

As long as you're angry, you are not in a problem-solving mode. Diabetes requires your focus and attention. Use your energy positively to find creative ways to manage your diabetes. (For ways to manage your diabetes, see Part III.)

Bargaining for more time

The stage of anger often transitions into a stage when you become increasingly aware of your mortality and bargain for more time. Even though you probably realize that you have plenty of life ahead of you, you may feel overwhelmed by the talk of complications, blood tests, and pills or insulin. You may even experience depression, which makes good diabetic care all the more difficult.

Studies have shown that people with diabetes suffer from depression at a rate that is two to four times higher than the rate for the general population. Those with diabetes also experience anxiety at a rate three to five times higher than people without diabetes.

If you suffer from depression, you may feel that your diabetic situation creates problems for you that justify being depressed. You may rationalize your depression in the following ways:

- Diabetes hinders you as you try to make friends.

- You don't have the freedom to choose your leisure activities.

- You're too tired to overcome difficulties.

- You may dread the future and possible diabetic complications.

- You don't have the freedom to eat what you want.

- You are constantly annoyed with all of the minor inconveniences of dealing with diabetes.

All of the preceding concerns are legitimate, but they also are all surmountable. How do you handle your many concerns and fend off depression? The following are a few important methods:

- Try to achieve excellent blood glucose control (see Part III).

- Begin a regular exercise program (Chapter 9).

- Tell a friend or relative how you are feeling; get it off your chest (Chapter 20).

- Recognize that every abnormal blip in your blood glucose is not your fault (Chapter 7).

Moving on

If you can't overcome the depression brought on by your diabetic concerns, you may need to consider therapy or antidepressant drugs. But you probably won't reach that point. Or you may experience the various stages of reacting to your diabetes in a different order than I describe in the previous sections. Some stages may be more prominent, and others may be hardly noticeable.

Don't feel that any anger, denial, or depression is wrong. These are natural coping mechanisms that serve a psychological purpose for a brief time. Allow yourself to have these feelings — then drop them. Move on and learn to live normally with your diabetes.

Here are some key steps you can take to manage the emotional side of diabetes:

- ✔ **Focus on your successes.** Some things may go wrong as you find out all there is to know about managing diabetes, but most things will go right. As you concentrate on your successes, you will realize that you can cope with diabetes and not let it overwhelm you.

- ✔ **Involve the whole family in your diabetes.** A diabetic diet is a healthy diet for everyone. For instance, the exercise you do is good for the whole family. By doing it together, you strengthen the family ties while everyone benefits from a healthier lifestyle. Also, should you need your family to help you, for instance, during a particularly severe low blood glucose, their early involvement will give them the peace of mind to know they are helping, not hurting you (Chapter 20).

- ✔ **Develop a positive attitude.** A positive attitude gives you a can-do mind-set, whereas a negative attitude leads to low motivation preventing you from doing all that is necessary to manage your diabetes.

- ✔ **Find a great team, pinpoint problems, and set goals.** Determine the most difficult problems that you have with your diabetes and how to solve them by yourself or with the great team of supporting players like the diabetes specialist, the diabetes educator, the dietitian, the eye doctor, the foot doctor, and so forth. Set realistic goals to get you past your problems (Chapter 11).

- ✔ **Don't expect perfection.** Although you may feel that you're doing every-thing right, you may find that your blood glucose levels are off. This situation happens to every person with diabetes and this unpredictable, uncontrollable feature is one of the most frustrating of the disease. Don't beat yourself up over something you can't control. Keep doing the things I suggest in the treatment section and you will be very gratified at the end.

Maintaining a High Quality of Life

You may assume that a chronic disease like diabetes leads to a diminished quality of life. It's true that the percentage of people with diabetes who are depressed is greater than the percentage in the nondiabetic population. But do you have to settle for a lower quality of life just because you have diabetes? Of course not! A study reported in *Diabetes Care* in September 2007 showed that people with T2DM who were depressed adhered to their diet, exercise, and testing regimens far less often and missed medication much more often. However, those who were not depressed tended to act in the opposite way.

This study as well as several others have evaluated the quality of life question, and the following sections not only describe what these studies found, but they also describe the hope: that you can take control and ensure that you maintain a high quality of life.

The importance of regular exercise

Most of the other studies of quality of life for people with diabetes have been long-term studies. In one study of more than 2,000 people with diabetes receiving many different levels of intensity of treatment, the overall response was that quality of life was lower for the person with diabetes than for the general population. But several factors separated those with the lower quality of life from those who expressed more contentment with life.

One factor that contributed to a lower quality of life rating was a lack of physical activity, one negative factor that you can alter immediately. Physical activity is a habit that you must maintain on a lifelong basis. (See Chapter 9 for advice on exercise.) The problem is that making a long-term change to a more physically active lifestyle is difficult; most people become more active for a time but eventually fall back into inactive routines.

Another study demonstrated the tendency for people with diabetes (and for people in general) to abandon exercise programs after a certain period of time. This information was reported in the *New England Journal of Medicine* in July 1991. In this study, a group of people with diabetes received professional support for two years to encourage them to increase physical activity. For the first six months, the study participants responded well and exercised regularly resulting in improved blood glucose, weight management, and overall health. After that, participants began to drop out and not come to training sessions. At the end of the two-year study, most participants had regained their weight and slipped back into poor glucose control. However, it's noteworthy that the few who didn't stop their exercise maintained the benefits and continued to report an improved quality of life.

The (minimal) impact of insulin treatments

Perhaps you're afraid that intensified insulin treatment, which involves three or four daily shots of insulin and frequent testing of blood glucose, will keep you from doing the things that you want to do and will diminish your daily quality of life. (See Chapter 10 for more information about intensified insulin treatment.)

When you're having trouble coping

You wouldn't hesitate to seek help for your physical ailments associated with diabetes, but you may be reluctant to seek help when you can't adjust psychologically to diabetes. The problem is that sooner or later, your psychological maladjustment will ruin any control that you have over your diabetes. And, of course, you won't lead a very pleasant life if you're in a depressed or anxious state all the time. The following symptoms are indicators that you're past the point of handling your diabetes on your own and may be suffering from depression:

- You can't sleep.

- You have no energy when you're awake.

- You can't think clearly.

- You can't find activities that interest or amuse you.

- You feel worthless.

- You have frequent thoughts of suicide.

- You have no appetite.

- You find no humor in anything.

If you recognize several of these symptoms in your daily life, you need to get some help. Your sense of hopelessness may include the feeling that no one else can help you — simply not true. First, go to your primary physician or endocrinologist for advice. He or she may help you to see the need for some short-term or long-term therapy. Well-trained therapists — especially therapists trained to take care of people with diabetes — can see solutions that you can't see in your current state. You need to find a therapist whom you can trust, so that when you're feeling low you can talk to this person and feel assured that he or she is very interested in your welfare.

Your therapist may decide that you would benefit from medication to treat the anxiety or depression. Currently, many drugs are available that are proven safe and free of side effects. Sometimes a brief period of medication is enough to help you adjust to your diabetes.

You can also find help in a support group. The huge and continually growing number of support groups shows that positive things are happening in these groups. In most support groups, participants share their stories and problems, helping everyone involved cope with their own feelings of isolation, futility, or depression.

In *Diabetes Care* in November 1998 a study explored whether the extra effort and time consumed by such diabetes treatments had an adverse effect on people's quality of life. The study compared people with diabetes to people with other chronic diseases, such as gastrointestinal disease and hepatitis (liver infection), and then compared all of those groups to a group of people who had no disease. The diabetic group reported a higher quality of life than the other chronic illness groups. Interestingly, the people in the diabetic group were not so much concerned with the physical problems of diabetes, such as intense and time-consuming tests and treatments, as they were concerned with the social and psychological difficulties.

Other key quality of life factors

Many other studies have examined the different aspects of diabetes that affect quality of life. These studies show some useful information on the following topics:

- **Family support:** People with diabetes greatly benefit from their family's help in dealing with their disease. But do people with diabetes in a close family have better diabetic control? One study in *Diabetes Care* in February 1998 addressed this question and found some unexpected results. Having a supportive family didn't necessarily mean that the person with diabetes would maintain better glucose control. But a supportive family did make the person with diabetes feel more physically capable in general and much more comfortable with his or her place in society.

- **Insulin injections for adults:** Do adults with diabetes who require insulin shots experience a diminished quality of life? A report in *Diabetes Care* in June 1998 found that insulin injections don't reduce the quality of life; the person's sense of physical and emotional well-being remains the same after beginning insulin injections as it was before injections were necessary.

- **Insulin injections for teenagers:** Teenagers who require insulin injections don't always accept the treatment as well as adults do, so teenagers more often experience a diminished quality of life. However, a study of more than 2,000 such teenagers in *Diabetes Care* in November 2001 showed that as their diabetic control improved, they felt like they were in better health, experienced greater satisfaction with their lives, and therefore believed themselves to be less of a burden to their families.

- **Stress management:** A study described in *Diabetes Care* in January 2002 showed that lowering stress lowers blood glucose. Patients were divided into two groups, one of which received diabetes education alone and the other diabetes education plus five sessions of stress management. The latter group showed significant improvement in diabetic control versus the former group, who received only diabetes education.

✔ **Quality of life over the long term:** How does a person's perception of quality of life change over time? As they age, do most people with diabetes feel that their quality of life increases, decreases, or persists at a steady level? The consensus of several studies is that most people with diabetes experience an increasing quality of life as they get older. People feel better about themselves and their diabetes after dealing with the disease for a decade or more. This report shows the healing property of time.

The bottom line

So what can you do to maintain a high quality of life with diabetes? Here are the steps that accomplish the most for you:

✔ Keep your blood glucose as normal as possible (see Part III).

✔ Make exercise a regular part of your lifestyle (Chapter 9).

✔ Get plenty of support from family, friends, and medical resources Chapter 20).

✔ Stay aware of the latest developments in diabetes care.

✔ Maintain a healthy attitude. Remember that someday you will laugh about things that bug you now, so why wait?

Chapter 2

It's the Glucose

*T*he Greeks and Romans knew about diabetes. The way they tested for the condition was — prepare yourself — by tasting people's urine. In this way, the Romans discovered that the urine of certain people was *mellitus,* the Latin word for *sweet.* (They got their honey from the island of Malta, which they called *Mellita.*) In addition, the Greeks noticed that when people with sweet urine drank, the fluids came out in the urine almost as fast as they went in the mouth, like a siphon. The Greek word for *siphon* is *diabetes.* Thus we have the origins of the modern name for the disease, *diabetes mellitus.*

In this chapter, I cover some not-so-fun stuff about diabetes — the big words, the definitions, and so on. But if you really want to understand what's happening to your body when you have diabetes — and I know I would — then you won't want to skip this chapter.

Detecting Prediabetes

Diabetes does not suddenly appear one day without previous notification from your body. For a period of time, which may last up to ten years, you may not quite achieve the criteria for a diagnosis of diabetes, but you aren't quite normal either. During this time, you have what's called *prediabetes.*

A person with prediabetes does not usually develop eye disease, kidney disease, or nerve damage (all potential complications of diabetes, which I discuss in Chapter 5). However, a person with prediabetes has a much greater risk of developing heart disease and brain attacks than someone with entirely normal blood glucose levels. Prediabetes has a lot in common with insulin resistance syndrome, also known as the *metabolic syndrome,* which I discuss in Chapter 5. The following two sections take the mystery out of whether you may have prediabetes by giving you some guidelines on when to get tested as well as what testing for prediabetes involves.

Knowing whether you should get tested

Approximately 54 million people in the United States have prediabetes, although most don't know it. Testing for prediabetes is a good idea for everyone over the age of 45. I also recommend testing for people who are under 45 if they are overweight and have one or more of the following risk factors:

- ✔ A high-risk ethnic group: African American, Hispanic, Asian, or Native American
- ✔ High blood pressure
- ✔ Low HDL or "good" cholesterol
- ✔ High triglycerides
- ✔ A family history of diabetes
- ✔ Diabetes during a pregnancy or having a newborn who weighed more than nine pounds

A study in the journal *Diabetes Care* in November 2007 showed that testing for prediabetes in overweight or obese people over age 45 is highly cost effective if they then undergo lifestyle modification (see Chapters 7 through 12) or take medication if necessary.

Testing for prediabetes

Testing for prediabetes involves finding out your blood glucose level , the level of sugar in your blood. Prediabetes exists when the body's blood glucose level is higher than normal, but not high enough to meet the standard definition of diabetes mellitus (which I discuss in the section "Testing for diabetes," later in this chapter). Testing is done by measuring a random capillary blood glucose. If the level is greater than 100 mg/dl, a fasting plasma glucose or oral glucose tolerance test is performed. Table 2-1 shows the glucose levels that indicate prediabetes:

- ✔ If the glucose before the test (the fasting plasma glucose) is between 100 and 125 mg/dl, the person has impaired fasting glucose, the glucose before eating (see Table 2-1). The glucose in the fasting (no food for 8 hours) state is not normal but not high enough to diagnose diabetes.
- ✔ If the glucose is between 140 and 199 mg/dl at one hour after eating, the person has impaired glucose tolerance. Both impaired fasting glucose and impaired glucose tolerance may be present.

Table 2-1	Diagnosing Prediabetes	
Condition	*Glucose Before Eating*	*Glucose One Hour After Eating*
Normal	Less than 100 mg/dl (5.5 mmol/L)	Less than 140 mg/dl (7.8 mmol/L)
Prediabetes	100–125 mg/dl (5.5–7 mmol/L)	140–199 mg/dl (7.8–11.1 mmol/L)

Diagnosing prediabetes can be the best thing that ever happened to a person! It could be the wake up call that he or she needs. The diagnosis may motivate a person to make crucial lifestyle changes, especially diet and exercise, which have been shown to prevent the onset of diabetes in people with prediabetes. And for those who don't respond to lifestyle changes, medication may accomplish the same thing.

After a diagnosis of prediabetes is made, all the techniques described in Chapters 7 through 12 can help prevent the onset of clinical diabetes. If patients with prediabetes are left untreated, large numbers of these patients will develop diabetes over time. Preventing diabetes saves almost ten thousand dollars of costs for the treatment of diabetes. And it prevented almost 20 percent of those with prediabetes from becoming diabetic.

Understanding What Diabetes Does

When prediabetes becomes diabetes, the body's blood glucose level registers even higher. In this section, I discuss the role of glucose in your body, the evidence for diabetes, and the symptoms you may experience with diabetes.

Realizing the role of glucose

The body has three sources of energy: protein, fat, and carbohydrates. I discuss the first two sources in greater detail in Chapter 8, but I'll tackle the third one now. Sugar is a carbohydrate. Many different kinds of sugars exist in nature, but glucose, the sugar that has the starring role in the body, provides a source of instant energy so that muscles can move and important chemical reactions can take place. Table sugar, or *sucrose*, is actually two different kinds of sugar — glucose and fructose — linked together. Fructose is the type of sugar found in fruits and vegetables. Because fructose is sweeter than glucose, sucrose, a combination of fructose and glucose, is sweeter than glucose alone as well. Therefore, your taste buds don't need as much sucrose or fructose to get the same sweet taste of glucose.

Frequent thirst and urination are the most commonly recognized symptoms of diabetes, but diabetes mellitus is not the only condition that causes these symptoms. Another condition in which fluids go in and out of the body like a siphon is called *diabetes insipidus.* With this condition, the urine is not sweet. Diabetes insipidus is an entirely different disease that you should not mistake for diabetes mellitus. Diabetes insipidus results when a hormone in the brain called *antidiuretic hormone* is missing. This hormone normally helps the kidneys prevent the loss of a lot of the water in the body. Other than the name *diabetes,* this condition has nothing to do with diabetes mellitus.

Testing for diabetes

The standard definition of diabetes mellitus is *excessive glucose in a blood sample.* For years, doctors set this level fairly high. The standard level for normal glucose was lowered in 1997 because too many people were experiencing complications of diabetes even though they did not have the disease by the then-current standard. In November 2003, the standard level was modified again.

After much discussion, many meetings, and the usual deliberations that surround a momentous decision, the American Diabetes Association published the new standard for diagnosis, which includes any one of the following three criteria:

✔ **Casual plasma glucose** concentration greater than or equal to 200 mg/dl, along with symptoms of diabetes (which I discuss in the section "Losing control of glucose" later in this chapter). *Casual plasma glucose* refers to the glucose level when the patient eats normally prior to the test.

Mg/dl stands for *milligrams per deciliter.* The rest of the world uses the International System (SI), where the units are mmol/L, which means *millimoles per liter.* To get mmol/L, you divide mg/dl by 18. Therefore, 200 mg/dl equals 11.1 mmol/L.

✔ **Fasting plasma glucose (FPG)** of greater than or equal to 126 mg/dl or 7 mmol/L. *Fasting* means that the patient has consumed no food for eight hours prior to the test.

✔ **Blood glucose** of greater than or equal to 200 mg/dl (11.1 mmol/L) when tested two hours (2-h PG) after ingesting 75 grams of glucose by mouth. This test has long been known as the *Oral Glucose Tolerance Test.* Although this time-consuming, cumbersome test is rarely done, it remains the gold standard for the diagnosis of diabetes.

Putting the criteria for diagnosis another way:

✔ FPG less than 100 mg/dl (5.5 mmol/L) is a normal fasting glucose.

✔ FPG greater than or equal to 100 mg/dl but less than 126 mg/dl (7.0 mmol/L) is impaired fasting glucose (indicating prediabetes).

✔ FPG equal to or greater than 126 mg/dl (7.0 mmol/L) gives a provisional diagnosis of diabetes.

✔ 2-h PG less than 140 mg/dl (7.8 mmol/L) is normal glucose tolerance.

✔ 2-h PG greater than or equal to 140 mg/dl but less than 200 mg/dl (11.1 mmol/L) is impaired glucose tolerance.

✔ 2-h PG equal to or greater than 200 mg/ dl gives a provisional diagnosis of diabetes.

If you test positive for diabetes one time, that is not enough to confirm a diagnosis. Any one of the tests must be positive on another occasion to make a diagnosis of diabetes. I've had patients come to me with a diagnosis of diabetes after being tested only once, and a second test has shown the initial diagnosis to be incorrect.

Controlling glucose

In order to understand the symptoms of diabetes, you need to know a little about the way the body normally handles glucose and what happens when things go wrong.

A hormone called *insulin* finely controls the level of glucose in your blood. A *hormone* is a chemical substance made in one part of the body that travels (usually through the bloodstream) to a distant part of the body where it performs its work. In the case of insulin, that work is to act like a key to open a cell (such as a muscle, fat, or liver cell) so that glucose can enter. If glucose can't enter the cell, it can provide no energy to the body.

Insulin is essential for growth. In addition to providing the key to entry of glucose into the cell, insulin is considered the *builder hormone* because it enables fat and muscle to form. It promotes the storage of glucose in a form called *glycogen* for use when fuel is not coming in. It also blocks the breakdown of protein. Without insulin, you do not survive for long.

With this fine-tuning, your body keeps the level of glucose pretty steady at about 60 to 100 mg/dl (3.3 to 6.4 mmol/L) all the time.

Losing control of glucose

Your glucose starts to rise in your blood when you don't have a sufficient amount of insulin or when your insulin is not working effectively. When your glucose rises above 180 mg/dl (10.0 mmol/L), glucose begins to spill into the urine and make it sweet. Up to that point, the kidney, the filter for the blood, is able to extract the glucose before it enters your urine. The loss of glucose into the urine leads to many of the short-term complications of diabetes. (See Chapter 4 for more on short-term complications.)

The following list contains the most common early symptoms of diabetes and how they occur. One or more of the following symptoms may be present when diabetes is diagnosed:

- **Frequent urination and thirst:** The glucose in the urine draws more water out of your blood, so more urine forms. More urine in your bladder makes you feel the need to urinate more frequently, day and night. As the amount of water in your blood declines, you feel thirsty and drink much more frequently.

- **Blurry vision:** As the glucose level shifts from normal to very high, the lens of the eye swells due to water intake. This swelling prevents the eye from focusing light at the correct place and blurring occurs.

- **Extreme hunger:** Inability to get energy in the form of glucose into the muscle cells that need it leads to a feeling of hunger despite all the glucose that is floating in the blood stream. Such hunger is called "starvation in the midst of plenty."

- **Fatigue:** Without sufficient insulin, or with ineffective insulin, glucose can't enter cells (such as muscle and fat cells) that depend on insulin to act as a key. (The most important exception here is the brain, which does not need insulin.) As a result, glucose can't be used as a fuel to move muscles or to facilitate the many other chemical reactions that have to take place to produce energy. A person with diabetes often complains of fatigue and feels much stronger after treatment allows glucose to enter his or her cells again.

- **Weight loss:** Weight loss occurs among some people with diabetes because they lack insulin, the builder hormone. When the body lacks insulin for any reason, the body begins to break down. You lose muscle tissue. Some of the muscle converts into glucose even though the glucose cannot get into cells. It passes out of your body in the urine. Fat tissue breaks down into small fat particles that can provide an alternate source of energy. As your body breaks down and you lose glucose in the urine, you often experience weight loss. However, most people with diabetes are heavy rather than skinny. (I explain why in Chapter 3.)

> ✔ **Persistent vaginal infection among women:** As blood glucose rises, all the fluids in your body contain higher levels of glucose, including the sweat and body secretions such as semen in men and vaginal secretions in women. Many bugs, such as bacteria and fungi, thrive in the high glucose environment. Women begin to complain of itching or burning, an abnormal discharge from the vagina, and sometimes an odor.

A study in the November 2007 issue of *Diabetes Care,* however, showed that in a group of over 15,000 people being treated for diabetes, 44 percent of them reported not one of the symptoms above in the previous year when given a questionnaire. It is no wonder that a third of people with diabetes do not know they have it.

Tracing the History of Diabetes Treatment

More than 2,000 years ago, people writing in China and India described a condition that must have been diabetes mellitus. The description is the same one that the Greeks and Romans reported — urine that tasted sweet. Scholars from India and China were the first to describe frequent urination. But not until 1776 did researchers discover the cause of the sweetness — glucose. And it wasn't until the nineteenth century that doctors developed a new chemical test to actually measure glucose in the urine.

Later discoveries showed that the pancreas produces a crucial substance that controls the glucose in the blood: insulin. Since that discovery was made, scientists have found ways to extract insulin and purify it so it can be given to people whose insulin levels are too low.

After insulin was discovered, diabetes specialists, led by Elliot Joslin and others, recommended three basic treatments for diabetes that are as valuable today as they were in 1921:

> ✔ Diet (see Chapter 8)
>
> ✔ Exercise (see Chapter 9)
>
> ✔ Medication (see Chapter 10)

Although the discovery of insulin immediately saved the lives of thousands of very sick individuals for whom the only treatment had been starvation, it did not solve the problem of diabetes. As these people aged, they were found to have unexpected complications in the eyes, the kidneys, and the nervous system (see Chapter 5). And insulin did not address the problem of the much larger group of people with diabetes now known as type 2 (see Chapter 3). Their problem was not lack of insulin but resistance to its actions. (Fortunately, doctors do have the tools now to bring the disease under control.)

Tracking diabetes around the world

Diabetes is a global health problem. A 2004 study in *Diabetes Care* in October estimated that approximately 171 million people around the world had diabetes in 2000 and that by the year 2030, the number would rise to more than 366 million.

Diabetes is most concentrated in areas where large food supplies allow people to eat more calories than they need so that they develop *obesity,* a condition of excessive fat. Several different types of diabetes exist, but the type usually associated with obesity, called *type 2 diabetes* (see Chapter 3), is far more prevalent than the other types.

Another reason diabetes cases have continued to grow in number throughout the world is that the lifespan of the population is increasing. What's the connection? Well, as a person ages, his or her chances of developing diabetes increases greatly. Along with obesity, age is a major risk factor for diabetes. (See Chapter 3 for more risk factors.) So, as other diseases are controlled and the population in general gets older, more diabetes is being diagnosed.

One very interesting study traced people of Japanese ancestry as they went from living in Japan to living in Hawaii to living in the United States mainland. In Japan, where people customarily maintain a normal weight, they tended to have a very low incidence of diabetes. As they moved to Hawaii, the incidence of diabetes began to rise along with their average weight. On the U.S. mainland, where food is most available, these Japanese had the highest rate of diabetes of all.

In general, as people migrate, not only the number of calories they consume but the composition of their diets changes. Before they migrate, they tend to consume a low-fat, high-fiber diet. After they reach their destination, they adopt the local diet, which tends to be higher in fat and lower in fiber. The carbohydrates in the new diet are from high-energy foods, which do not tend to be filling, promoting more caloric intake.

The Japanese provide another interesting lesson about the place of obesity as a factor in the onset of diabetes. Japanese Sumo wrestlers have to gain enormous quantities of weight in order to fight in a certain weight class. Even while they are still fighting, they demonstrate a high frequency of diabetes. After they become more sedentary, the frequency goes up to 40 percent, a huge prevalence.

The North American Indian, another group, shows the consequences of switching from a moderate calorie, relatively nutritious diet to a higher calorie diet. Some tribes, such as the Pima Indians, have a prevalence of diabetes as high as one out of two people. In contrast, the presence of diabetes in South American Indian tribes, such as in Chile where they have maintained a more traditional diet, is extremely rare.

In China, as the country becomes more affluent, doctors are seeing a significant increase in the incidence of diabetes. Migrant Chinese populations show even higher rates, especially where the environment allows them to gain more weight and be more sedentary.

In the United States in the year 2005, about 20.8 million people had diabetes. This number represents about 7 to 8 percent of the population. Currently only two thirds of the people with diabetes are aware that they have the condition. The big project is to get people to know their blood glucose level just like they know their cholesterol, and to seek treatment.

The next major leap in the effort to treat diabetes, occurring in 1955, was the discovery of the group of drugs called *sulfonylureas* (see Chapter 10), the first drugs that could be taken by mouth to lower blood glucose levels. But even as those drugs were improving patient care, the only way to know if someone's blood glucose level was high was to test the urine, which was entirely inadequate for good diabetic control (see Chapter 7).

diabetes 1997 after

Around 1980, the first portable meters for blood glucose testing became available. It became possible, for the first time, to relate treatment to a measurable outcome. This development has led, in turn, to the discovery of other great drugs for diabetes like metformin, pioglitazone, and others yet to come.

If you are not using these wonderful tools for your diabetes, you are missing the boat. You can find out exactly how to use portable meters in Part III.

Sharing Some Real Patient Stories

The numbers that are used to diagnose diabetes don't begin to reflect the human dimensions of the disease. People end up with test results after days, months, or even years of minor discomforts that reach the point where they can no longer be tolerated. The next few stories of real (though renamed) patients can help you understand that diabetes is a disease that happens to real people — people who are working, relaxing, traveling, sleeping, and doing many other things that make life so complex.

Jane Fein was a forty-six-year-old woman who worked in a computer company and had to do a lot of standing. She noticed that she had been having some tingling in her feet but thought it was due to all the standing. However, she had gained 22 pounds in the last six years and couldn't seem to shed them. She was beginning to wake up a few times at night to go to the bathroom. She thought these symptoms might be associated with her menopause, which was just beginning. She decided to see her gynecologist, who told her everything was fine but suggested a urinalysis because she was waking up so much. To everyone's surprise, glucose was present in her urine, and the gynecologist sent her to an internist. The internist did a random (casual) glucose test in the lab. It was 225 mg/dl (12.5 mmol/L). He did a fasting blood glucose test the next morning, and it was 163 mg/dl (9.0 mmol/L). He made a diagnosis of type 2 diabetes (see Chapter 3) and started Jane on a program of diet and exercise.

Leslie Law was a 28-year-old woman who had just started a new job. She ate well but was losing weight. She noticed increased thirst and urination, which caused her boss to comment upon her frequent absences in the middle of work. She decided to stop drinking so many beverages, but the urination continued, and she began to feel very weak. One afternoon, she fainted at the office and was taken to the hospital. Her blood glucose was found to be 683 mg/dl (37.9 mmol/L). She was given fluids because she was very dehydrated, and a repeat blood glucose test came back at 592 mg/dl (32.9 mmol/L). Leslie began insulin treatment, rapidly regained her weight and her strength, and returned to work after a few days.

Sal Renolo was a 46-year-old black belt judo instructor. Despite his very active lifestyle, he was not careful about his diet and had gained 16 pounds in the last few years. He was more fatigued than he had been in the past but blamed this fatigue on his increasing age. His mother had diabetes, but he assumed that his physical fitness would protect him from this condition. However, he could barely get through a one-hour class without excusing himself for a bathroom break. One of his new students had diabetes, and he suggested to Sal that he ought to have the problem checked, but Sal insisted that he could not possibly have diabetes with all his activity. The symptoms of fatigue and frequent urination got worse, and Sal finally made an appointment with the doctor. Blood tests revealed a random blood glucose level of 264 mg/dl (14.7 mmol/L). The following week, another random blood glucose was 289 (16.0 mmol/L). The doctor told Sal he had diabetes, but Sal refused to believe it. He left the doctor's office angry but vowed to lose weight and did so successfully. On a repeat visit to the doctor, a random glucose was 167 mg/dl (9.3 mmol/L). Sal told the doctor that he knew he did not have diabetes, but the resolve to eat carefully did not last, and he was back six weeks later with a glucose of 302 mg/dl (16.8 mmol/L). Finally, Sal accepted the diagnosis and started treatment. He rapidly returned to his usual state of health, and the fatigue disappeared.

Debby O'Leary's active sex life with her husband was continually being interrupted by vaginal yeast infections, which resulted in an unpleasant odor and redness and itching. Over-the-counter preparations promptly cured the condition, but it always rapidly returned. Finally, after three of these infections in two months, she decided to see her gynecologist. The gynecologist told her she needed a prescription drug. The cure lasted a little longer this time, but the infection promptly returned. On a return visit, the gynecologist did a urinalysis and found glucose in her urine. A random blood test showed a glucose of 243 mg/dl (13.5 mmol/L). He sent her to an internist, who ordered a variety of tests including a fasting blood glucose, which was 149 mg/dl (8.3 mmol/L). The doctor told her she had diabetes and recommended exercise and diet to start with. She followed his advice and as a result she not only lowered her blood glucose to the point that she no longer developed yeast infections, but also her resulting weight loss and increase of energy made her sex life with her husband even more satisfying.

Chapter 3

What Type of Diabetes Do You Have?

*L*adies and gentlemen, I'd like to introduce you to your pancreas. This shy little organ — to which you've probably never given a moment's attention — can rear its lovely head at entirely unexpected moments. (You probably didn't even know that your pancreas has a head and a tail, but it does. Now you've broken the ice!) Most of the time, your pancreas hides behind your stomach quietly doing its work, assisting with digestion first and then helping to make use of the digested food. The information in this chapter should put you on closer terms with your pancreas, which is good, because you need your pancreas as much as it needs you. In one way or another, the pancreas plays a role in all of the various types of diabetes.

Here's the good news: You can prevent diabetes. Here's the bad news: You can't do so quite as easily as you may like. Your best method for preventing diabetes is to pick your parents carefully, but that method is slightly impractical, even with modern technology.

In general, you can prevent a disease if it meets two requirements. First, you have to be able to identify if you are at high risk for getting the disease. Second, some treatments or actions must exist that can definitely reduce the occurrence of the disease. This chapter shows you how to identify whether you're at risk for type 1 or type 2 diabetes, and it covers definite actions that you can take to prevent both of these types of diabetes.

This chapter also helps you get a clear understanding of your type of diabetes, how it relates to the other types of diabetes, and how the failure of your friendly pancreas to do its assigned job can lead to a host of unfortunate consequences. (I cover these consequences in detail in Part II.)

Getting to Know Your Pancreas

You don't see your pancreas very often, but you hear from it all the time. It has two major functions. One is to produce *digestive enzymes,* which are the chemicals in your small intestine that help to break down food. The digestive enzymes don't have much relation to diabetes, so I won't spend much time talking about them. Your pancreas's other function is to produce and secrete directly into the blood a hormone of major importance, *insulin.* The following sections explore the ins and outs of your pancreas and insulin so that you're well acquainted with both.

Examining your pancreas

Figure 3-1 shows the microscopic appearance of the pancreas. The following list explains the different cells found in the pancreas as well as their functions:

- **B cells:** The insulin-producing pancreas cells (also called *beta* cells) are found in groups called *Islets of Langerhans.*

- **A cells:** These *glucagon*-producing cells (a hormone that is very important to people with diabetes because it raises blood glucose when the glucose level gets too low) are present in the Islets of Langerhans.

- **D cells:** These cells make *somatostatin* (a hormone that blocks the secretion of other hormones but doesn't have a use in diabetes because it causes high blood sugar and increased ketones by blocking insulin as well) and like the cells described above, are also found in the Islets of Langerhans.

Understanding insulin

If you understand only one hormone in your body, insulin should be that hormone (especially if you want to understand diabetes). Over the course of your life, the insulin that your body produces or the insulin that you inject into your body (as I describe in Chapter 10) affects whether or not you control the glucose levels in your blood and avoid the complications of the disease.

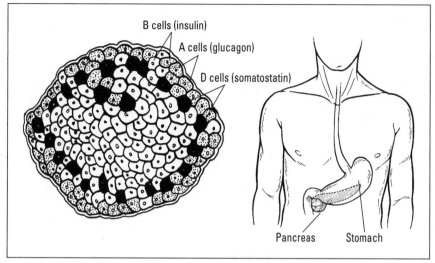

Figure 3-1:
The pancreas and its parts.

Think of your insulin as an insurance agent, who lives in San Francisco (which is your pancreas) but travels from there to do business in Seattle (your muscles), Denver (your fat tissue), Los Angeles (your liver), and other places. This insulin insurance agent is insuring your good health.

Wherever insulin travels in your body, it opens up the cells so that glucose can enter them. After glucose enters, the cells can immediately use it for energy, store it in a storage form of glucose (called *glycogen*) for rapid use later on, or convert it to fat for use even later as energy.

After glucose leaves your blood and enters your cells, your blood glucose level falls. Your pancreas can tell when your glucose is falling, and it turns off the release of insulin to prevent unhealthy low levels of blood glucose called *hypoglycemia* (see Chapter 4). At the same time, your liver begins to release glucose from storage and makes new glucose from amino acids in your blood.

If your insurance agent (insulin, remember? — stick with me here!) doesn't show up when you need him (meaning that you have an absence of insulin, as in type 1 diabetes) or he does a poor job when he shows up (such as when you have a resistance to insulin, as in type 2 diabetes), your insurance coverage may be very poor (in which case your blood glucose starts to climb). High blood glucose is the beginning of all your problems.

Doctors have proven that high blood glucose is bad for you and that keeping the blood glucose as normal as possible prevents the complications of diabetes (which I explain in Part II). Most treatments for diabetes are directed at restoring the blood glucose to normal.

Type 1 Diabetes and You

John Phillips, a 6-year-old boy, was always very active, and his parents became concerned when the counselors at summer camp told them that he seemed to not have much energy. When he got home from camp, John's parents noticed that he was thirsty all the time and running to the bathroom. He was very hungry but seemed to be losing weight, despite eating more than enough. John's parents took him to the pediatrician, who did several blood glucose tests and told them that their son has *type 1 diabetes mellitus* (T1DM), which used to be called *juvenile diabetes* or *insulin-dependent diabetes.*

This story has a happy ending because John's parents were willing to do the necessary things to bring John's glucose under control. John is just as energetic as ever, but he has had to get used to a few inconveniences in his daily routine. (I cover such daily lifestyle changes in Part III.) The following sections detail the symptoms and causes of this type of diabetes.

Identifying symptoms of type 1 diabetes

Following are some of the major signs and symptoms of type 1 diabetes. If you experience the following symptoms, ask your doctor about the possibility that you have diabetes:

- ✔ **Frequent urination:** You experience frequent urination because your kidneys can't return all the glucose to your bloodstream when your blood glucose level is greater than 180 mg/dl (10 mmol/L). (See Chapter 7 for all the details on blood glucose level testing.) The large amount of glucose in your urine makes the urine very concentrated. As a result, your body draws water out of your blood and into the urine to reduce that high concentration of glucose. This water and glucose fill up the bladder repeatedly.

- ✔ **Increase in thirst:** Your thirst increases as you experience frequent urination, because you lose so much water in the urine that your body begins to dehydrate.

- ✔ **Weight loss:** You lose weight as your body loses glucose in the urine and your body breaks down muscle and fat looking for energy.

- ✔ **Increase in hunger:** Your body has plenty of extra glucose in the blood, but your cells become malnourished because you lack insulin to allow the glucose to enter your cells. As a result, you become increasingly hungry. Your body goes through "hunger in the midst of plenty."

- ✔ **Weakness:** You feel weak because your muscle cells and other tissues do not get the energy that they require from glucose.

Type 1 diabetes used to be called *juvenile diabetes* because it occurs most frequently in children. However, so many cases are found in adults that doctors don't use the term *juvenile* any more. Some children are diagnosed early in life, and other children have a more severe onset of the disease as they get a little older.

With children over age ten, the early signs and symptoms of diabetes may have been missed by parents, counselors, or teachers. These kids have a great deal of fat breakdown in their bodies to provide energy, and this fat breakdown creates other problems. *Ketone bodies,* products of the breakdown of fats, begin to accumulate in the blood and spill into the urine. Ketone bodies are acidic and lead to nausea, abdominal pain, and sometimes vomiting.

At the same time as fat is breaking down, the child's blood glucose rises higher. Dangerous levels as high as 400 to 600 mg/dl (22.2 to 33.3 mmol/L) are not uncommon, but levels as low as 300 (16.6 mmol/L), not quite as dangerous are possible. The child's blood is like thick maple syrup and doesn't circulate as freely as normal. The large amount of water leaving the body with the glucose depletes important substances such as sodium and potassium. The vomiting causes the child to lose more fluids and body substances. All these abnormalities cause the child to become very drowsy and possibly lose consciousness. This situation is called *diabetic ketoacidosis,* and if it isn't identified and corrected quickly, the child can die. (See Chapter 4 for more details on the symptoms, causes, and treatments of ketoacidosis.)

A few special circumstances affect the symptoms that you may see in persons with type 1 diabetes. Remember the following factors:

- ✔ **The "honeymoon" period** is a time after the diagnosis of diabetes when the person's insulin needs decline for one to six months and the disease seems to get milder. The honeymoon period is longer when a child is older at the time of diagnosis, but the apparent diminishing of the disease is always temporary.

- ✔ **Males and females** get type 1 diabetes to an equal degree.

- ✔ **Warm summer months** are associated with a decrease in the occurrence of diabetes compared to the winter months, particularly in older children over ten. The probable reason for this occurrence is that a virus is involved in bringing on diabetes (which I discuss in the next section), and viruses spread much more when children are learning and playing together inside in the winter.

Investigating the causes of type 1 diabetes

When your doctor diagnoses you with type 1 diabetes, you almost certainly will wonder what could have caused you to acquire the disease. Did someone with diabetes sneeze on you? Did you eat so much sugary food that your body reacted by giving you diabetes? Rest assured that the causes of diabetes aren't so simple.

Type 1 diabetes is an *autoimmune disease,* meaning that your body is unkind enough to react against — and, in this case, destroy — a vital part of itself, namely the insulin-producing beta (B) cells of the pancreas. One way that doctors discovered that type 1 diabetes is an autoimmune disease is by measuring proteins in the blood, called *antibodies,* which are literally substances directed against your body — and, in particular, against your islet cells. (These specific antibodies are called *islet cell antibodies and GAD antibodies.*) Doctors find islet cell antibodies and GAD antibodies in relatives of people who have type 1 diabetes and in the people with diabetes themselves for a few years before the disease begins.

Another clue that type 1 diabetes is an autoimmune disease is that drugs that reduce autoimmunity, also delay the onset of type 1 diabetes. Also, type 1 diabetes tends to occur in people who have other known autoimmune diseases.

You may wonder how doctors can know in advance that certain people will develop diabetes. The method of predicting isn't 100 percent accurate, but people who get type 1 diabetes more often have certain abnormal characteristics on their genetic material, their *chromosomes,* that are not present in people who don't get diabetes. Doctors can look for these abnormal characteristics on your DNA. But having these abnormal characteristics doesn't guarantee that you'll get diabetes.

Another essential factor in predicting whether you will develop diabetes is your exposure to something in the environment, most likely a virus. I discuss this factor in detail in the next section.

Getting type 1 diabetes

To develop diabetes, most people also have to come in contact with something in the environment that triggers the destruction of their *beta cells,* the cells that make insulin. Doctors think that this environmental trigger is probably a virus, and they've identified several viruses that may be to blame.

Doctors think they are the same viruses that cause the common cold. Persons with type 1 diabetes probably get the virus just like any cold virus — from someone else who has the virus who sneezes on them. But because they also have the genetic tendency, they get type 1 diabetes.

This type of virus can cause diabetes by attacking your pancreas directly and diminishing your ability to produce insulin, which quickly creates the diabetic condition in your body. The virus can also cause diabetes if it is made up of a substance that is also naturally present in your pancreas. If the virus and your pancreas possess the same substance, the antibodies that your body produces to fight off the virus will also attack the shared substance in your pancreas, leaving you in the same condition as if the virus itself attacked your pancreas.

A small number (about 10 percent) of patients who develop type 1 diabetes don't seem to need an environmental factor to trigger the diabetes. In them, the disease is entirely an autoimmune destruction of the beta cells. If you fall into this category of people with diabetes, you may have other autoimmune diseases, such as autoimmune thyroid disease.

You may be curious about how likely you are to get type 1 diabetes if someone in your immediate family has it. Studies of many families have provided fairly good answers to this question. Here are some facts about the genetics of diabetes:

- ✔ You get half of your total genetic material from each parent, but if one of your parents has type 1 diabetes, the odds are only 3 to 4 percent that you will get it.

- ✔ If you and your sibling are identical twins (meaning that you have *exactly* the same genetic material), you have about a 20 percent chance of getting type 1 diabetes if your sibling develops the disease.

- ✔ If you have only half of your genetic material in common with your sibling who has type 1 diabetes (meaning you are a fraternal twin rather than an identical twin), your chance of getting type 1 diabetes drops to 5 percent.

- ✔ If none of the genetic material associated with diabetes is the same as your sibling with type 1 diabetes, your chance of developing type 1 diabetes is less than 1 percent.

These relatively low chances of both siblings getting diabetes clearly show that more factors than your genetic inheritance from your parents are involved in acquiring type 1 diabetes. Otherwise, identical twins would both have type 1 diabetes almost 100 percent of the time.

Preventing type 1 diabetes

Type 1 diabetes is an excellent candidate for two types of preventative treatments that should be available to patients in the not-too-distant future:

- ✔ In order to prevent diabetes, you will be able to undergo treatments before the disease starts, which is a method called *primary prevention.* Possible candidates for primary prevention are people with family histories of type 1 diabetes. If you fall into that category, your doctor can analyze your DNA to see whether you have the genetic material most often found in people who have diabetes. If you do, you could receive primary prevention to block the disease.

- ✔ *Secondary prevention* is treatment that is given to a person with diabetes after the disease is triggered but before the person becomes sick. In order to try secondary prevention, your doctor must be able to recognize that diabetes has begun, even though you aren't sick. And months to years must pass between diagnosis and the onset of symptoms in order to have enough time for the treatment to prevent sickness.

An example of primary prevention for type 1 diabetes would be vaccination against the viruses that may be associated with diabetes. Unfortunately, doctors haven't yet pinpointed the exact virus or viruses, so vaccinations aren't yet practical. Doctors have tried vaccinations in countries (such as Finland) where type 1 diabetes occurs most often, but the vaccinations didn't stop the number of new cases of type 1 diabetes from rising. Doctors also have considered giving antiviral agents to people who are at high risk of acquiring diabetes, but this approach, although successful, has been tested only in animals so far.

You may think that all the recent scientific advances in gene research would enable doctors to change people's genetic material to prevent the onset of type 1 diabetes. Although scientists have made great strides in identifying the genes associated with diabetes, they haven't quite reached the point where they can change those genes. Such methods for primary prevention of type 1 diabetes are something for the future.

Some doctors believe that certain chemicals in cow's milk bring on type 1 diabetes. Researchers are comparing breastfed babies who are susceptible to type 1 diabetes to susceptible babies who are given cow's milk. They haven't yet determined whether cow's milk is a factor that causes type 1 diabetes. If cow's milk turns out to be the culprit, type 1 diabetes could be prevented by using only breast milk up to a certain age.

Lots of trials of secondary prevention are underway, though most show only partial success. Most of these trials make use of doctors' knowledge that patients whose bodies produce autoantibodies have type 1 diabetes and that the antibodies are gradually destroying their insulin-producing beta cells. Therefore, the treatment is aimed at preventing the production of antibodies. In these patients, full-blown type 1 diabetes may take a couple of years to appear and create major problems, so the doctor has time to intervene.

The most prevalent methods of secondary prevention for type 1 diabetes attempt to block the autoimmune disease from destroying all of your pancreas's beta cells. The following list shows some of the more promising secondary prevention trials and techniques:

- **Steroid drugs:** You can take steroid drugs, such as prednisone, to block autoimmune conditions. When doctors find islet cell antibodies in a person with type 1 diabetes, they give the person these steroids, which reduce the amount of islet cell antibodies and seem to prolong the period between the development of the antibodies and the onset of symptoms, such as excessive thirst and urination.

  But this approach isn't 100 percent successful, and it could have many side effects — especially in children under ten. Small children who use steroids suffer from growth problems, infections, and other unwanted side effects. If diabetes becomes active, the reason may be the failure of the steroid to prevent the autoimmune destruction of the pancreas, as well as the glucose abnormalities caused by the steroid itself.

- **Cytotoxic drugs:** C*cytotoxic drugs,* another group of drugs used to increase the time between antibodies and diseases, act against the cells that may participate in the destruction of the pancreatic beta cells. Again, studies have shown only a slowing down of the time between antibodies and symptoms. Cytotoxic drugs destroy various types of cells — and not just the bad cells. Studies of cytotoxic drugs have all been complicated by side effects that were severe and damaging to some of the patients.

- **Nicotinamide:** In animal studies, nicotinamide (a B vitamin) protects the beta cells of mice that are diabetes-prone. A similar trial in humans was somewhat successful, showing that 20 percent of patients using nicotinamide didn't develop symptoms of diabetes and didn't lose as many beta cells. Doctors are surprised that a drug known to raise plasma glucose (see Chapter 2) could prevent diabetes.

- **Insulin:** In another study, small amounts of insulin were given to people who have islet cell antibodies, in an attempt to prolong the time between antibodies and symptoms. This approach initially showed some promise, but further into the study, there has been no difference in the development of diabetes between those given insulin and those who did not receive it.

The most important study of prevention ever done for type 1 diabetes is called the Diabetes Control and Complications Trial (DCCT), published in 1993. The DCCT showed that keeping very tight control over your blood glucose is possible but difficult. The difficult part of keeping your blood glucose close to normal is that you increase your risk of having low blood glucose, or hypoglycemia (see Chapter 4). The DCCT study showed that you can prevent the complications of diabetes — including eye, kidney, and nerve disease — by keeping your blood glucose as close to normal as possible. If you already suffer from such complications, improving your blood glucose control very significantly slows the progression of the complications. Since the DCCT, doctors generally treat type 1 diabetes by keeping the patient's blood glucose as close to normal as is possible and as is practical.

If you would like to read much more on the subject of type 1 diabetes, please see my book *Type 1 Diabetes For Dummies* (Wiley).

Having Type 2 Diabetes

Edythe Fokel, a 46-year-old woman, has gained about 10 pounds in the last year, so that her 5-foot 5-inch body now weighs about 155 pounds. Edythe doesn't do much exercise. She has felt somewhat fatigued recently, but she blames her age and approaching menopause. She also blames the fact that she now gets up several times a night to urinate, which she didn't used to do. She is disturbed because her vision is blurry, and her job requires working on a computer. Finally, Edythe goes to her gynecologist after developing a rash and discharge in her vagina. When Edythe describes her symptoms, her gynecologist decides to do a blood glucose test. He refers her back to her primary physician when Edythe's blood glucose level registers at 220 mg/dl (12.2 mmol/L).

Edythe's primary doctor asks her whether other members of her family have had diabetes, and she replies that her mother and a sister are both being treated for it. The doctor also asks Edythe about any tingling in her feet, and she admits that she has noticed some tingling for the past few months but didn't think it was important. The primary doctor repeats the random blood glucose test, which comes back at 260 mg/dl (14.4 mmol/L). He informs Edythe that she has type 2 diabetes.

The signs and symptoms that Edythe manifests in this scenario, along with the results of the two blood glucose tests, provide a textbook picture of type 2 diabetes. (Type 2 diabetes used to be known as *adult onset diabetes* or *non-insulin dependent diabetes.*) But be aware that people with type 2 diabetes may have few or none of these symptoms. Because of the varying symptoms it is important for your doctor to check your blood glucose level on a regular basis. (I discuss how often you should do this test in Chapter 7.)

Most people with type 2 diabetes are over the age of forty. Your chances of getting type 2 diabetes increase as you get older. Because the symptoms are so mild at first, you may not notice them. You may ignore these symptoms for years before they become bothersome enough to consult your doctor. So type 2 diabetes is a disease of gradual onset rather than the severe emergency that can herald type 1 diabetes. No autoimmunity is involved in type 2 diabetes, so no antibodies are found. Doctors believe that no virus is involved in the onset of type 2 diabetes.

Recent statistics show that worldwide, ten times more people have type 2 diabetes than type 1 diabetes. Although type 2 is the much more prevalent type of diabetes, those with type 2 diabetes seem to have milder severity of complications (such as eye disease and kidney disease) from diabetes. (See Part II for details about the possible complications of diabetes. See Part III for treatments that can help you prevent these complications.)

Identifying symptoms of type 2 diabetes

A fairly large percentage of the U.S. population (approximately 20 million people) has type 2 diabetes. The numbers are on the rise, and one reason is an increase in the incidence of obesity, a major risk factor for type 2 diabetes. If you're obese, you are considerably more likely to acquire type 2 diabetes than you would be if you maintained your ideal weight. (See Chapter 8 for the details on how to figure out your weight classification.)

The following signs and symptoms are good indicators that you have type 2 diabetes. If you experience two or more of these symptoms, call your doctor:

- ✔ **Fatigue:** Type 2 diabetes makes you tired because your body's cells aren't getting the glucose fuel that they need. Even though there is plenty of insulin in your blood, your body is resistant to its actions. (See the "Getting to Know Your Pancreas" section for more explanation.)

- ✔ **Frequent urination and thirst:** As with type 1 diabetes, you find yourself urinating more frequently than usual, which dehydrates your body and leaves you thirsty.

- ✔ **Blurred vision:** The lenses of your eyes swell and shrink as your blood glucose levels rise and fall. Your vision blurs because your eyes can't adjust quickly enough to these lens changes.

- ✔ **Slow healing of skin, gum, and urinary infections:** Your white blood cells, which help with healing and defend your body against infections, don't function correctly in the high-glucose environment present in your body when it has diabetes. Unfortunately, the bugs that cause infections thrive in the same high-glucose environment. So diabetes leaves your body especially susceptible to infections.

- ✔ **Genital itching:** Yeast infections also love a high-glucose environment. So diabetes is often accompanied by the itching and discomfort of yeast infections.

- ✔ **Numbness in the feet or legs:** You experience numbness because of a common long-term complication of diabetes called *neuropathy*. (I explain the details of neuropathy in Chapter 5.) If you notice numbness and neuropathy along with the other symptoms of diabetes, you probably have had the disease for quite a while, because neuropathy takes more than five years to develop in a diabetic environment. Occasionally numbness occurs earlier when there are extreme elevations of the glucose.

- ✔ **Heart disease, stroke, and peripheral vascular disease:** Heart disease, stroke, and peripheral vascular disease (blockage of arteries in the legs) occur much more often in type 2s than in the nondiabetic population. But these complications may appear when you are merely glucose-intolerant (which I explain in the next section), before you actually have diagnosable diabetes.

The signs and symptoms of type 2 diabetes are similar in some cases to the symptoms of type 1 diabetes (which I cover in the "Identifying symptoms of type 1 diabetes" section, earlier in this chapter), but in many ways they are different. The following list shows some of the differences between symptoms in type 1 and type 2 diabetes:

- ✔ **Age of onset:** People with type 1 diabetes are usually younger than those with type 2 diabetes. However, the increasing incidence of type 2 diabetes in overweight children is making this difference less useful for separating type 1 and type 2 diabetes.

- ✔ **Body weight:** Those with type 1 diabetes are usually thin or normal in weight, but obesity is a common characteristic of people with type 2 diabetes.

- ✔ **Level of glucose:** People with type 1 diabetes have higher glucose levels at the onset of the disease. Those with type 1 diabetes usually have blood glucose levels of 300 to 400 mg/dl (16.6 to 22.2 mmol/L), and those with type 2 diabetes usually have blood glucose levels of 200 to 250 mg/dl (11.1 to 13.9 mmol/L).

- ✔ **Severity of onset:** Type 1 diabetes usually has a much more severe onset, but type 2 diabetes gradually shows its symptoms.

Investigating the causes of type 2 diabetes

If you've been diagnosed with type 2 diabetes, you're probably shocked and curious about why you developed the disease. Doctors have learned quite a bit about the causes of type 2 diabetes. For example, they know that type 2 diabetes runs in families.

Usually, people with type 2 diabetes can find a relative who has had the disease. Therefore, doctors consider type 2 diabetes to be much more of a genetic disease than type 1 diabetes. In studies of identical twins, when one twin has type 2 diabetes, the likelihood that type 2 diabetes will develop in the other twin is nearly 100 percent.

Insulin resistance

People with type 2 diabetes have plenty of insulin in their bodies (unlike people with type 1 diabetes), but their bodies respond to the insulin in abnormal ways. Those with type 2 diabetes are *insulin-resistant,* meaning that their bodies resist the normal, healthy functioning of insulin. This resistance, combined with not having enough insulin to overcome the insulin resistance, causes type 2 diabetes.

Before obesity or lack of exercise (or diabetes for that matter) is present, future type 2 patients already show signs of insulin resistance. First, the amount of insulin in their blood is elevated compared to normal people. Second, a shot of insulin doesn't reduce the blood glucose in these insulin-resistant people nearly as much as it does in people without insulin resistance. (See Chapter 10 to find out more about insulin shots in diabetes.)

When your body needs to make extra insulin just to keep your blood glucose normal, your insulin is, obviously, less effective than it should be — which means that you have *impaired glucose tolerance.* Your body goes through impaired glucose tolerance before you actually have diabetes, because your blood glucose is still lower than the levels needed for a diagnosis of diabetes (see Chapter 2). When you have impaired glucose tolerance and you add other factors such as weight gain, a sedentary lifestyle, and aging, your pancreas can't keep up with your insulin demands, and you develop diabetes.

Another factor that comes into play when doctors make a diagnosis of type 2 diabetes is the release of sugar from the glycogen stored in your liver, known as your *hepatic glucose output.* People with type 2 diabetes have high glucose levels in the morning after having fasted all night. You would think that your glucose would be low in the morning if you haven't eaten any sugar. But your liver is a storage bank for a lot of glucose, and it can make even more from other substances in the body. As your insulin resistance increases, your liver begins to release glucose inappropriately, and your fasting blood glucose level rises.

Mistaken beliefs about type 2

People often think that the following factors cause type 2 diabetes, but they actually have nothing to do with the onset of the disease:

✔ **Sugar:** Eating excessive amounts of sugar does not cause diabetes, but it may bring out the disease to the extent that it makes you fat. Eating too much protein or fat will do the same thing.

✔ **Emotions:** Changes in your emotions do not play a large role in the development of type 2 diabetes, but they may be very important in dealing with diabetes mellitus and subsequent control.

✔ **Stress:** Too much stress isn't a major factor that causes diabetes.

✔ **Antibodies:** Antibodies against islet cells are not a major factor in type 2 diabetes (see the section "Investigating the causes of type 1 diabetes," earlier in this chapter). Type 2 diabetes isn't an autoimmune disease like type 1.

✔ **Gender:** Males and females are equally as likely to develop type 2 diabetes. Gender doesn't play a role in the onset of this disease.

✔ **Diabetic ketoacidosis:** Type 2 diabetes isn't generally associated with diabetic ketoacidosis (see Chapter 4). People with type 2 diabetes are ketosis resistant, except under extremely severe stress caused by infections or trauma. (See Chapter 4 for a discussion of *hyperosmolar syndrome,* a related condition in which people with type 2 diabetes have extremely high glucose but don't have the fat breakdown that leads to acidosis.)

Getting type 2 diabetes

Genetic inheritance is necessary in type 2 diabetes, but environmental factors such as obesity and lack of exercise trigger the disease. People with type 2 diabetes are insulin-resistant before they become obese or sedentary. Aging, poor eating habits, obesity, and failure to exercise combine to bring out the disease.

Inheritance seems to be a much stronger factor in type 2 diabetes than in type 1 diabetes. Consider the following:

✔ If your father has type 2 diabetes but your mother doesn't, you have about a 4 percent chance of getting the disease.

✔ If your mother has type 2 diabetes but your father doesn't, your chances of getting it leap to about 10 percent.

✔ Nearly 100 percent of the time, an identical twin of a person with type 2 diabetes eventually gets the disease.

✔ If your brother or sister (*not* an identical twin) gets type 2, you have about a 40 percent chance of doing the same.

TIP

Here's an interesting fact: Spouses of people with type 2 diabetes are at higher risk of developing diabetes and should be screened just like relatives of people with diabetes. Why? Because they share the environmental risk factors for diabetes, such as poor diet and a sedentary lifestyle. If your wife is a good cook and you have a big-screen TV, watch out!

Some early warning signs appear in the population that is most at risk to develop type 2 diabetes. People with type 2 diabetes often have a history of malnutrition at a young age. Perhaps these people didn't make enough insulin-producing cells when they were young, because they didn't need them for their reduced food intake. When someone like this is presented with ample supplies of food at an older age, his or her pancreas may not have enough insulin-producing cells to handle the load.

In developing countries, where people often don't get enough food, those whose genetic makeup enables their bodies to use carbohydrates in a very efficient manner have an advantage over the rest of the population because they can survive on the low food and calorie supplies. However, if these people later receive ample supplies of food, their bodies are overwhelmed and they're likely to become fat and sedentary and develop diabetes. This fact may explain why people in developing countries are the most at risk to develop type 2 diabetes. Population studies show that the incidence of diabetes is greatest in developing countries such as China and India.

Preventing type 2 diabetes

Doctors can predict type 2 diabetes years in advance of its actual diagnosis by studying the close relatives of people who have the condition. This early warning period offers plenty of time to try techniques of primary prevention (which I explain in the "Preventing type 1 diabetes" section, earlier in this chapter). After a doctor discovers that someone's blood glucose levels are high and diagnoses type 2 diabetes, complications such as eye disease and kidney disease (see Chapter 5) usually take ten or more years to develop in that person. During this time, doctors can apply secondary prevention techniques (the various treatments I discuss in Part III).

Because so many people suffer from type 2 diabetes, doctors have had a wealth of people to study in order to determine the most important environmental factors that turn a genetic predisposition to type 2 diabetes into a clinical disease. The following are the major environmental factors:

- ✔ **High body mass index:** The *body mass index (BMI)* is the way that doctors look at weight in relation to height. BMI is a better indicator of a healthy weight than just weight alone, because, for instance, a person who weighs 150 pounds and is 62 inches tall is overweight, but a person who weighs 150 pounds and is 70 inches tall is thin.

You can easily determine your BMI by using the following formula: Multiply your weight (in pounds) by 703, then divide that number by your height (in inches). Divide that result by your height (in inches) again. If you use the metric system, divide your weight in kilograms by your height in meters and divide that result by your height in meters again. Using this formula, the 150-pound person with a height of 62 inches has a BMI of 27.5, while the person with the height of 70 inches has a BMI of 21.6. The result is expressed in kilograms per meter squared (kg/m^2).

Current guidelines state that a person with a BMI from 25 to 29.9 is overweight, and a person with a BMI of 30 or greater is obese. A BMI between 20 and 25 is considered normal. A person with a BMI of 40 or higher has morbid obesity.

Many studies have verified the great importance of the BMI level in determining who gets diabetes. For example, a large study of thousands of nurses in the United States showed that nurses with a BMI greater than 35 had diabetes almost 100 times more often than nurses with a BMI less than 22. Even among the women in this study considered to be lean, those with the higher BMI, though still in the category of lean, had three times the prevalence of diabetes compared to those with lower BMI. Another large study of U.S. physicians found the same relationship of high BMI to high levels of type 2 diabetes. The same study showed that the length of time that you're obese is important; participants who were obese ten years earlier were more likely to have diabetes than those who had become obese more recently.

✔ **Physical inactivity:** Physical inactivity has a high association with diabetes, as evidenced in many studies. Former athletes have diabetes less often than nonathletes. The same study of nurses' health that I cite in the preceding bullet showed that women who were physically active on a regular basis had diabetes only two-thirds as often as the couch potatoes. A study conducted in Hawaii, which did not include any obese people, showed that the occurrence of diabetes was greatest for people who don't exercise.

✔ **Central distribution of fat:** When people with diabetes become fat, they tend to carry the extra weight as centrally distributed fat, also known as *visceral fat.* You check your visceral fat when you measure your waistline, because this type of fat stays around your midsection. So a person with visceral fat is more apple-shaped than pear-shaped. Visceral fat also happens to be the type of fat that probably comes and goes most easily on your body, and it is relatively easy to lose when you diet. Visceral fat seems to cause more insulin resistance than fat in other areas, and it is also correlated with the occurrence of coronary artery disease. If you have a lot of visceral fat, losing just 5 to 10 percent of your weight may very dramatically reduce your chance of diabetes or a heart attack.

If you are 40 or younger and your waistline measures 39.5 inches (100 centimeters) or greater, or you are between the ages of 40 and 60 and your waistline measures 35.5 inches (90 centimeters) or more, you have a significantly increased risk of a heart attack.

Asians tend to develop visceral fat at a lower weight than non-Asians and are therefore more prone to type 2 diabetes at a lower weight. Asian Indians are particularly susceptible, developing diabetes up to ten years earlier than Chinese and Japanese.

✓ **Low intake of dietary fiber:** Populations with a high prevalence of diabetes tend to eat a diet that is low in fiber. Dietary fiber seems to be protective against diabetes, because it slows down the rate at which glucose enters the bloodstream.

If you recognize any of the preceding factors in your body or lifestyle, you can correct them in time to prevent diabetes. Type 2 diabetes allows the high-risk individual or the diagnosed person the time to work toward prevention or control of the disease. In Part III, I show you specific ways to reduce your weight, increase your exercise, improve your diet, and prevent or reverse diabetes and diabetic complications.

Recognizing a variant of type 2 diabetes

As many as 10 percent of people diagnosed with type 2 diabetes do not respond well to medications that stimulate the pancreas to release more insulin like the sulfonylurea class of drugs (see Chapter 10). When they are tested they are found to have GAD antibodies similar to those found in T1DM. This condition is really adult-onset T1DM rather than T2DM. The treatment is similar to that for T1DM.

These patients are divided by their level of GAD antibodies into two groups. The ones who are higher than 32 GAD units have more severe diabetes that is harder to control. Those with lower levels of GAD have milder diabetes, suggesting they have some remaining pancreatic ability to make and release insulin.

If you are having trouble with controlling your diabetes with oral drugs that work by causing more insulin release, ask your doctor to test you for GAD antibodies.

Possibilities for future prevention of diabetes

Researchers have performed many valuable studies on the prevention of type 2 diabetes. The results of these studies suggest that you can prevent diabetes, but probably only by making major lifestyle changes and sticking to them over a long period of time. Here are some important conclusions based on prevention research:

✔ Taking drugs that don't treat your insulin resistance doesn't help to prevent your diabetes or its complications.

✔ If you exercise regularly, you may delay the onset of diabetes.

✔ If you maintain a proper diet and exercise regularly, you can delay the onset of diabetes and slow the complications that may occur.

✔ Controlling both your blood pressure and your blood glucose has substantial benefits for preventing the complications of diabetes.

A study reported in the *New England Journal of Medicine* in July 1991 confirmed the preceding conclusions by looking at obese people who had close relatives with type 2 diabetes — which meant that these people were highly likely to develop diabetes. For six months, the researchers gave the participants extensive training in exercise routines and maintaining proper diet. Many of the participants lost significant amounts of weight, improved their overall health, and staved off the development of diabetes. But after six months, many of the people being studied were no longer participating as fully and sticking as closely to the diet and exercise regimens. By the time twelve months of the study had passed, more of the participants were straying farther from the diet and exercise that they needed, and they were regaining some of the weight they had lost. The researchers found that the people who were able to maintain the proper diet and exercise — which helped them not to gain weight — were least likely to develop diabetes. The main point I want to make is that this study proves the importance (and, for many people, the difficulty) of maintaining a program of diet and exercise for a long period of time.

The results of the Diabetes Prevention Program, a study of more than 3,000 people, were published in the *New England Journal of Medicine* in February 2002. They clearly showed that diet and exercise are effective in preventing type 2 diabetes. Participants who successfully modified their diet and exercise routines reduced their chances of developing type 2 diabetes by 58 percent. They generally did thirty minutes of moderate exercise (like walking) every day and lost between 5 and 7 percent of their body weight during the three-year study period. In contrast, patients who used a drug called *metformin* (see Chapter 10) without modifying their diet and exercise reduced their risk of developing type 2 diabetes by only 31 percent.

Another recent study, the Finnish Diabetes Prevention Study (reported in *Diabetes Care* in December 2003), shows that lifestyle changes can be accomplished and sustained not only in a research setting (like that of the Diabetes Prevention Program) but in a community setting as well, where patients are taken care of by their own doctors. Study participants worked with a nutritionist to improve their diets and received some advice on exercise. They continue to be successful after three years, with the same 58 percent reduction in the onset of diabetes.

Restoring insulin sensitivity in people at risk for prediabetes (see Chapter 2) was the focus of another recent study, published in *Diabetes Care* in March 2002. This study compared intensive lifestyle change, both diet and exercise, with moderate lifestyle change. The intensive group ate less fat and did more vigorous exercise than the moderate group, and every member of the intensive group increased his or her insulin sensitivity, which resulted in holding off the development of diabetes.

Having Gestational Diabetes

If you're pregnant (yes, that excludes you men) and you've never had diabetes before, during your pregnancy you could acquire a form of diabetes called *gestational diabetes.* If you already have diabetes when you become pregnant, that is called *pregestational diabetes.* As I discuss in Chapter 6, the difference between pregestational diabetes and gestational diabetes is very important in terms of the consequences for both mother and baby. Gestational diabetes occurs in about 2 percent of all pregnancies.

During your pregnancy, you can acquire gestational diabetes because the growing fetus and the placenta create various hormones to help the fetus grow and develop properly. Some of these hormones have other characteristics, such as anti-insulin properties, that decrease your body's sensitivity to insulin, increase glucose production, and can cause diabetes.

At approximately your 20th week of pregnancy, your body produces enough of these hormones to block your insulin's normal actions and cause diabetes. After you give birth, when the fetus and placenta are no longer in your body, their anti-insulin hormones are gone and your diabetes disappears.

Even though gestational diabetes subsides after you give birth, more than half of the women who experience gestational diabetes develop type 2 diabetes within fifteen years after the pregnancy. This high likelihood of type 2 diabetes probably results from a genetic susceptibility to diabetes in these women, which is magnified by the large amount of anti-insulin hormones in their bodies during pregnancy.

Your obstetrician should do a test for gestational diabetes around the 24th to 28th week of your pregnancy.

Recognizing Other Types of Diabetes

Cases of diabetes other than type 1, type 2, or gestational are rare and usually don't cause severe diabetes in the people who have them. But occasionally one of these other types is responsible for a more severe case of diabetes, so you should know that they exist. The following list gives you a brief rundown of the symptoms and causes for other types of diabetes:

- **Diabetes due to loss or disease of pancreatic tissue:** If you have a disease, such as cancer, that necessitates the removal of some of your pancreas, you lose your pancreas's valuable insulin-producing beta cells, and your body becomes diabetic. This form of diabetes isn't always severe because you lose glucagon, another hormone found in your pancreas, after your pancreatic surgery. Glucagon blocks insulin action in your body, so when your body has less glucagon, it can function with less insulin, leaving you with a milder case of diabetes.

✔ **Diabetes due to iron overload:** Another disease that damages the pancreas, as well as the liver, the heart, the joints, and the nervous system, is *hemochromatosis.* This condition results from excessive absorption of iron into the blood. When the blood deposits too much iron into these organs, damage can occur. This hereditary condition is present in 1 of every 200 people in the United States; half of those who have it develop a clinical disease, sometimes diabetes.

Hemochromatosis is less common in younger women, who are protected by the monthly loss of iron that occurs with menstrual bleeding. This finding has led to the current treatment for hemochromatosis, which is removing blood from the patient regularly until the blood iron returns to normal, then repeating the procedure occasionally to keep iron levels normal. If treatment is done early enough (before organs are damaged), complications, such as diabetes, are avoidable.

✔ **Diabetes due to other diseases:** Your body contains a number of hormones that block insulin action or have actions that are opposed to insulin's actions. You produce these hormones in glands other than your pancreas. If you get a tumor on one of these hormone-producing glands, the gland sometimes produces excessive levels of the hormones that act in opposition to insulin. Usually, this condition gives you simple glucose intolerance rather than diabetes, because your pancreas makes extra insulin to combat the hormones. But if you have a genetic tendency to develop diabetes, you may develop diabetes in this case.

✔ **Diabetes due to hormone treatments for other diseases:** If you take hormones to treat a disease other than diabetes, those hormones could cause diabetes in your body. The hormone that is most likely to cause diabetes in this situation is *hydrocortisone,* an anti-inflammatory agent used in diseases of inflammation, such as arthritis. (Similar drugs are prednisone and dexamethasone.) If you take hydrocortisone and you have the symptoms of diabetes listed in earlier sections of this chapter, talk to your doctor.

✔ **Diabetes due to other drugs:** If you're taking other commonly used drugs, be aware that some of them raise your blood glucose as a side effect. Some antihypertensive drugs, especially hydrochlorothiazide, raise your blood glucose level. Niacin, a drug commonly used for lowering cholesterol, also raises your blood glucose. If you have a genetic tendency toward diabetes, taking these drugs may be enough to give you the disease.

Conditions and hormones that can lead to diabetes

The following is a partial list of hormones caused by tumors and their associated conditions:

✔ Excessive adrenal gland hormone (hydrocortisone) is present in **Cushing's Syndrome.** Hydrocortisone stimulates the liver to put out more glucose while it blocks the uptake of glucose by muscle tissue.

✔ Excessive prolactin is present in a **prolactin secreting tumor of the pituitary gland.** It blocks insulin action, and glucose intolerance results.

✔ Excessive growth hormone is made by a tumor of the pituitary gland resulting in **acromegaly.** Growth hormone reduces insulin sensitivity and forces the pancreas to make much more insulin.

✔ Excessive epinephrine is made by a **pheochromocytoma** (a tumor of another part of the adrenal gland). It causes increased liver production of glucose, while it blocks insulin secretion.

✔ Excessive aldosterone is made by still another part of the adrenal gland in a condition called **primary hyperaldosteronism.** This condition causes glucose intolerance in a different way — by facilitating the loss of body potassium, which has a negative effect on insulin production.

✔ Excessive thyroid hormone found in **hyperthyroidism** causes the liver and other organs to produce excessive quantities of glucose. Hyperthyroidism is also a disease of autoimmunity, which may play a role in the loss of glucose tolerance.

✔ A **glucagon secreting tumor of the pancreas** can create excessive glucagon. Glucagon has many properties that are opposite to insulin. This condition is rare; only around 100 cases of it have been described in medical literature, so don't lose sleep over this one.

✔ A **somatostatin secreting tumor of the pancreas** can create excessive somatostatin. Somatostatin is another hormone made in a cell present in the Islets of Langerhans. Somatostatin actually blocks insulin from leaving the beta cell, but it also blocks glucagon and other hormones, so the diabetes is very mild. This condition occurs even less often than the glucagon secreting tumor.

Part II
How Diabetes Affects Your Body

The 5th Wave   By Rich Tennant

"Oh dear, it's Troy's Harpo-glycemia. I can always tell — fatigue, confusion, the compulsion to play the harp in a trench coat and fright-wig...."

In this part . . .

Diabetes can affect every part of your body, but especially the eyes, the kidneys, the nervous system, and the heart. None of this need ever happen. This part explains these effects, how they occur, the kinds of symptoms they produce, and what you and your doctor need to do to treat them. Remember that everything I describe in this part is preventable, and even if you have not been able to prevent them, they're very treatable.

The effects mentioned above are due to hyperglycemia or high blood glucose and occur only after years. This part has lots of information about hypoglycemia or low blood glucose that often occurs at the beginning of treatment and is usually due to over-treatment. I discuss at length a condition called the *metabolic syndrome* that predates diabetes but can cause heart disease. And speaking of length, I also describe in detail the new drugs available to treat erection problems resulting from diabetes. It is important that you know about the effects and respond to them appropriately.

Chapter 4

Battling Short-Term Complications

. . . .

In This Chapter

▶ Defining short-term complications

▶ Dealing with low blood glucose

▶ Handling very high blood glucose

. . . .

C hapters 2 and 3 tell you all about how doctors make a diagnosis of dia-betes and how they determine which type of diabetes you have. But you need to understand how diabetes can affect you. The previous chapters cover some of the signs and symptoms of diabetes, which you could consider to be the shortest of the short-term complications of the disease because they're generally mild and begin to subside when you start treatment. This chapter covers the more serious forms of short-term complications of dia-betes, which occur when your blood glucose is out of control — reaching dangerously high or low levels.

With the exception of mild *hypoglycemia* (low blood glucose where you can manage it yourself), you should treat all the complications in this chapter as medical emergencies. Don't try to treat these complications at home. Keep in touch with your doctor and go to the hospital promptly if your blood glucose is uncontrollably high or you're unable to hold down food. You may need a few hours in the emergency room or a day or two in the hospital to reverse your problems.

Solving Short-Term Complications

Although the complications that I cover in this chapter are called *short-term,* you may experience them at any time during the course of your diabetes. *Short-term* simply means that these complications arise rapidly in your body, as opposed to the long-term complications that take ten or more years to develop. (See Chapter 5 for all the details about long-term complications.) Short-term complications develop in days or even hours, and fortunately they respond to treatment just as rapidly.

Generally, you experience the severe short-term complications associated with high blood glucose when you aren't monitoring your blood glucose levels. Small children and older folks who live alone or have illnesses are most susceptible to lapses in glucose monitoring and, therefore, to short-term complications. If you suffer an acute illness or trauma, you should monitor your glucose even more frequently than usual because you're more vulnerable to short-term complications.

The short-term complications of diabetes affect your ability to function normally. For example, if you're a student, you may have difficulty studying or taking tests. Or you may have trouble driving your car properly. For this reason, you may find that the Bureau of Motor Vehicles and the Federal Aviation Association are extra careful about giving you, and all people with diabetes, a driver's license or a pilot's license. Potential employers may question your ability to perform certain jobs. But most companies and government agencies are very enlightened about diabetes and do everything possible to accommodate you in these situations. (Chapter 15 shows you how to overcome some challenges that you may face with employment and insurance.)

You don't have to feel limited in what you can do. You can control your diabetes, and all of the short-term complications are avoidable. If you take your medication at the appropriate time, eat the proper foods at the proper times, and monitor your blood glucose regularly, you're unlikely to suffer from any severe short-term complications. As you closely monitor and control your blood glucose, it may drop to lower than normal levels, but monitoring quickly alerts you to the drop so you can treat it before it affects your mental and physical functioning. (See Chapter 7 for all the details on glucose monitoring and other testing.)

Understanding Hypoglycemia

The condition of having low blood glucose is known as *hypoglycemia.* If you have diabetes, you can get hypoglycemia only as a consequence of your diabetes treatment.

As a person with diabetes, you're in constant combat with high blood glucose, which is responsible for most of the long-term and short-term complications of the disease. Your doctor prescribes drugs and other treatments in an effort to fine-tune your blood glucose as it would be in the body of a person who does not have diabetes. (Part III explains many techniques that help you control your blood glucose levels.) But, unfortunately, these drugs and treatments aren't always perfect. If you take too much of a drug, exercise too much, or eat too little, your blood glucose can drop to the low levels at which symptoms develop. The following sections explain more about the seriousness of hypoglycemia as well as its symptoms, causes, and treatment.

The seriousness of hypoglycemia

One of the readers who wrote to thank me for the first edition of this book told me how her son had once gone on a blind date. He and his date went to a bar where they had a drink before dinner. As he sat there, he began to say, "Sugar, baby, sugar, baby, sugar, baby." At first his date was offended until she realized that he had a glazed look in his eyes and found that he was wearing a bracelet identifying him as a person with diabetes. He was suffering from hypoglycemia and needed glucose.

This story is amusing, but the subject is very serious. Hypoglycemia can ruin your day and leave you feeling dazed and exhausted afterwards. You also run the risk of overtreating it, leaving yourself with a very high blood glucose.

Hypoglycemia is a barrier that prevents most patients with diabetes from achieving normal blood glucose levels. They can lower their blood glucose enough to prevent long-term complications such as eye disease, kidney disease, and nerve disease, but preventing heart disease requires a lower glucose level that is difficult to sustain because of the threat of hypoglycemia, particularly for people with type 1 diabetes. A normal blood glucose is between 80 and 140 mg/dl. Hypoglycemia begins below 80 mg/dl but you may not feel symptoms until it goes below 60 mg/dl.

The positive news is that most patients experience complete recovery from the effects of hypoglycemia.

Symptoms of hypoglycemia

Your body doesn't function well when you have too little glucose in your blood. Your brain needs glucose to run the rest of your body, as well as to function intellectually. Your muscles need the energy that glucose provides in much the same way that your car needs gasoline. So, when your body detects that it has low blood glucose, it sends out a group of hormones that rapidly raise your glucose. But those hormones have to fight the strength of the diabetes medication that has been pushing down your glucose levels.

At what level of blood glucose do you develop hypoglycemia? Unfortunately, the level varies for different individuals, particularly depending on the length of time that the person has had diabetes. But most experts agree that a blood glucose of 60 mg/dl (3.3 mmol/L) or less is associated with signs and symptoms of hypoglycemia in most people.

Doctors traditionally put the symptoms of hypoglycemia into two major categories:

✔ **Symptoms due to the side effects of the hormones (especially epinephrine) that your body sends out to counter the glucose-lowering effect of insulin:** This category of symptoms is called *adrenergic* symptoms, because epinephrine comes from your adrenal gland.

✔ **Symptoms that are due to your brain not receiving enough fuel so that your intellectual function suffers:** This category of symptoms is called *neuroglycopenic* symptoms, which is medicalese for "not enough (*penic*) glucose (*glyco*) in the brain (*neuro*)." (If your brain could speak, it would just say, "Whew, I'm ready for a meal!")

Adrenergic symptoms occur most often when your blood glucose falls rapidly. The following adrenergic symptoms may tip you off that you're hypoglycemic:

✔ Whiteness, or pallor, of your skin

✔ Sweating

✔ Rapid heartbeat

✔ Palpitations, or the feeling that your heart is beating too fast

✔ Anxiety

✔ Numbness in the lips, fingers or toes

✔ Irritability

✔ Sensation of hunger

Neuroglycopenic symptoms occur most often when your hypoglycemia takes longer to develop. The symptoms become more severe as your blood glucose drops lower. The following neuroglycopenic symptoms are often signs that you're becoming (or already are) hypoglycemic:

✔ Headache

✔ Loss of concentration

✔ Visual disorders, such as double vision or blurred vision

✔ Fatigue

✔ Confusion and trouble concentrating

✔ Trouble hearing

✔ Poor color vision

✔ Feeling of warmth

✔ Slurred speech

✔ Convulsions

✔ Coma, or an inability to be awakened

Intelligent people lose their ability to think clearly when they become hypoglycemic. They make simple mistakes, and other people often assume that they are drunk.

One of my patients was driving on a highway when another driver noticed that she was weaving back and forth in her lane and reported her to the highway patrol. A patrolman stopped her, concluded that she was drunk, and took her to jail. Fortunately, someone noticed that she was wearing a diabetic medical bracelet. After promptly receiving the nutrition that she needed, she rapidly recovered. No charges were filed, but clearly this situation is one that you want to avoid. Always test your blood glucose level to make sure that it's satisfactory before driving your car. Should you be low, a couple of glucose tablets will solve the problem.

If you take insulin or a *sulfonylurea drug,* which squeezes more insulin out of your reluctant pancreas, for your own safety you need to wear or carry with you some form of identification, in case you unexpectedly develop hypoglycemia. (See Chapter 10 for a full explanation of insulin and the sulfonylurea medications.) You can find a simple bracelet at the Medicalert Foundation at `www.medicalert.org`. If you prefer something a little sexier that you will be proud to wear as jewelry, try `www.mylifewear.com`.

Causes of hypoglycemia

Hypoglycemia results from elevated amounts of insulin driving down your blood glucose to low levels, but an extra high dose of insulin or sulfonylurea medication isn't always the culprit that elevates your insulin level. The amount of food you take in, the amount of fuel (glucose) that you burn for energy, the amount of insulin circulating in your body, and your body's ability to raise glucose by releasing it from the liver or making it from other body substances all affect your blood glucose level.

On average, hypoglycemia occurs about 10 percent of the time in people with type 1 diabetes, but it causes noticeable symptoms only about twice a week and is severe perhaps once a year. In people with type 2 diabetes, severe hypoglycemia occurs only one-tenth as often. The medications described in the next section are part of the reason that people with type 1 diabetes have to deal with hypoglycemia more often.

Insulin and sulfonylurea medications

Many people with type 1 diabetes (and some with type 2) rely on insulin injections or sulfonylurea medications to control the disease. When you take insulin shots, you have to time your food intake to raise your blood glucose as the insulin is taking effect. Chapter 10 explains the different kinds of insulin and the proper methods for administering them. But remember that the different types of insulin are most potent at differing amounts of time (minutes or hours) after you inject them. If you skip a meal or take your insulin too early or too late, your glucose and insulin levels won't be in sync and you'll develop hypoglycemia. If you go on a diet and don't adjust your medication, the same thing happens.

If you take sulfonylurea drugs, you need to follow similar restrictions. You and your doctor must adjust your dosage when your calorie intake falls. Other drugs don't cause hypoglycemia by themselves, but when combined with sulfonylureas they may lower your glucose enough to reach hypoglycemic levels. (Chapter 10 talks more about these other drugs.)

Diet

Your diet plays a major role in helping you avoid hypoglycemia if you take medication. You should try to have a snack in the middle of the morning and in the afternoon — in addition to your usual breakfast, lunch, and dinner — especially if you take insulin. A properly timed snack provides you with a steady source of glucose to balance the insulin that you're taking. Chapter 8 gives much greater detail about proper diet.

You can use your blood glucose level to determine whether to have a snack at bedtime. If your glucose is greater than 180 mg/dL (10 mmol/L), you probably don't need a snack. If your glucose is between 126 and 180 mg/dL (7 to 10 mmol/L), a couple slices of bread and an ounce of cheese will prevent hypoglycemia. If your glucose is less than 126 mg/dL (7 mmol/L), a couple ounces of meat plus a slice of bread will do the trick.

Exercise

Exercise burns your body's fuel, which is glucose, so it generally lowers your blood glucose level. Some people with diabetes use exercise in place of extra insulin to get their high blood glucose down to a normal level. But if you don't adjust your insulin dose or food intake to match your exercise level, exercise can result in hypoglycemia.

One of my patients is dedicated to exercise. He has taken insulin shots for years but requires very little insulin to control his glucose because he burns so much glucose through exercise. He avoids hypoglycemia by measuring his blood glucose level many times a day — especially before vigorous exercise. If his level is low at the beginning of exercise, he eats extra carbohydrates before he starts. Chapter 8 tells you which foods to eat (and when) in order to have the intended effect on your glucose levels.

People who exercise regularly require much less medication and generally can manage their diabetes more easily than nonexercisers can. Chapter 9 covers much more about the benefits of exercise.

Non-diabetes medications

Several drugs that you may take unrelated to your diabetes can lower your blood glucose. One of the most widely used, which you may not even think of as a drug, is alcohol — wine, beer, and other spirits. Alcohol can block your liver's ability to release glucose. It also blocks hormones that raise blood glucose and increases the glucose-lowering effect of insulin. If you're malnourished for some reason or you simply haven't eaten in a while and you drink alcohol before going to bed, you may experience severe fasting hypoglycemia the next morning.

Watch out for these drugs that can lower your blood glucose:

- ✔ **Alcohol:** If you take insulin or sulfonylurea drugs, don't drink alcohol without eating some food at the same time. Food counteracts some of the glucose-lowering effects of alcohol.

- ✔ **Aspirin:** Also, be aware that aspirin (and all of the drugs related to aspirin, called *salicylates*) can lead to hypoglycemia. In adults who have diabetes, aspirin can increase the effects of other drugs that you're taking to lower your blood glucose. In children with diabetes, aspirin has an especially profound effect on lowering blood glucose to hypoglycemia levels. However, the low dose of aspirin taken daily to reduce the risk of heart attacks does not cause hypoglycemia.

Hormonal changes

As type 1 diabetes progresses, your body produces fewer and fewer hormones that counteract insulin when hypoglycemia is present. This situation leads to more severe hypoglycemia later in type 1 diabetes, especially if you and your doctor don't adjust your insulin injections in response to your lower glucose levels. People with type 2 diabetes who take insulin also develop this loss of protective hormones.

These same hormones also play the role of giving you warning signs when your blood glucose drops, such as sweating, a rapid heart beat, and anxiety, so you are prompted to eat. When the hormone levels drop, these warning signs don't occur, so you aren't signaled that it's time to eat. This situation is called *hypoglycemia unawareness*.

Prevention of hypoglycemia

People with diabetes can use a number of simple techniques to prevent hypo-glycemia, including the following:

- ✔ Frequently measuring your blood glucose with a glucose meter (see Chapter 7).

- ✔ Maintaining a realistic goal for your blood glucose level. This subject is one you need to discuss with your doctor.

- ✔ Altering the timing of food and exercise (see Chapters 8 and 9).

- ✔ Altering your insulin and oral drug regimens (see Chapter 10).

- ✔ Becoming totally aware of your own symptoms for low blood glucose. (See the section "Symptoms of hypoglycemia," earlier in this chapter.)

Levels of hypoglycemia

There are three levels of severity of hypoglycemia, defined by the level of the blood glucose:

- ✔ **Mild hypoglycemia:** This level, corresponding to a blood glucose of around 75 mg/dl, is easily treated by the patient himself. It does not cause the patient to change his routine and, in fact, is discovered not so much by symptoms as by the finding of a low blood glucose during routine testing of the blood.

- ✔ **Moderate hypoglycemia:** This level is achieved when the blood glucose is found to be around 65 mg/dl. The patient begins to feel the adrenergic symptoms described above, especially anxiety and a rapid heartbeat. Patients who have moderate hypoglycemia may not recognize they need glucose and have to be helped by someone else.

- ✔ **Severe hypoglycemia:** This level occurs when the blood glucose is less than 55 mg/dl leaving the patient severely impaired and thus requiring outside assistance to restore his or her glucose. An emergency injection of glucagon or intravenous glucose solution is necessary.

Treatment of hypoglycemia

The vast majority of hypoglycemia cases are mild. You can treat hypo-glycemia with a small quantity of glucose in the form of:

✔ Two sugar cubes.

✔ Two or three glucose tablets (Glucose tablets are available in any drugstore, and any person with diabetes who may develop hypoglycemia should carry them.)

✔ A small amount (six ounces) of a sugary soft drink.

✔ Eight ounces of milk or four ounces of orange juice. (These drinks work very well.)

✔ Anything that has about 15 grams of glucose in it.

Sometimes you need a second treatment. Approximately 20 minutes after you try one of these solutions, measure your blood glucose to find out whether your level has risen sufficiently. If it is still low, give a second treatment.

Keep the following tips in mind to aid in your treatment of hypoglycemia:

✔ **You can easily overtreat hypoglycemia,** causing your blood glucose to rise higher than you'd like. However, the high blood glucose resulting from overtreatment of hypoglycemia usually does not last long. You're better off not using a drug or insulin to bring it down, because doing so can result in alternate highs and lows.

✔ **Make sure that your friends or relatives know in advance what hypoglycemia is and what to do about it** because your mental state may be mildly confused when you have it. Inform people about your diabetes and about how to recognize hypoglycemia. Don't keep your diabetes a secret. The people close to you will be glad to know how to help you.

✔ **Try to eat a snack of carbohydrates and protein every hour if you are doing prolonged exercise,** such as playing a baseball or soccer game that lasts several hours. (For example, half a turkey sandwich would work well.) And carry jelly beans at all times, just in case — six or seven are all you need to combat mild symptoms of hypoglycemia.

If you are losing consciousness so that you can't sit up and swallow properly when you have hypoglycemia, no one should try to feed you. One of the following options should be used:

✔ **Someone helping you can use an emergency kit, such as the kit called "Glucagon for Emergencies."** This kit includes a syringe with 1 mg of *glucagon,* one of the major hormones that raises glucose, which your helper should inject into your muscle. The injection of glucagon raises your blood glucose so that you regain consciousness within 20 minutes. Glucagon corrects your hypoglycemic condition for about an hour after you receive an injection.

You need to get a prescription from your doctor for this type of glucagon kit. Make sure the kit doesn't become outdated if you don't use it for a long time.

✔ **If your hypoglycemia recurs shortly after you receive glucagon or doesn't respond to the glucagon, the person helping you should call 911.** (Sulfonylurea drugs are most often the cause of such a severe case of hypoglycemia.) The emergency crew checks your blood glucose and gives you an intravenous (IV) dose of high-concentration glucose. Most likely, you will continue the IV in the emergency room until you show stable and normal blood glucose levels.

Combating Ketoacidosis

In Chapter 3, I talk about the tendency of people with type 1 diabetes to suffer from a severe diabetic complication called *ketoacidosis,* or very high blood glucose with large amounts of acid in the blood. The following sections explain the symptoms, causes, and treatments of ketoacidosis.

The prefix *keto* refers to *ketones* — substances that your body makes as fat breaks down during ketoacidosis. *Acid* is part of the name because your blood becomes acidic from the presence of ketones.

Can ketoacidosis affect you?

Occasionally, ketoacidosis is the symptom that alerts doctors that you have type 1 diabetes, but more frequently it occurs after you already know that you have the disease. Although ketoacidosis occurs mostly in people with type 1 diabetes (who develop diabetes at an early age), the person is usually 40 or more years old when ketoacidosis actually begins.

Ketoacidosis occurs mostly in people with type 1 diabetes because they have no insulin in their bodies except what they inject as medication. Those with type 2 diabetes (or with other forms of the disease) rarely get ketoacidosis because they have some insulin in their bodies, even though the insulin usually isn't fully active due to insulin resistance. People with type 2 diabetes get ketoacidosis mainly when they have severe infections or traumas that put their bodies under great physical stress.

Symptoms of ketoacidosis

The symptoms of ketoacidosis regularly alert doctors to type 1 diabetes in children. But ketoacidosis more often occurs in adults with type 1 diabetes, so they should also keep an eye out for the following symptoms:

- **Nausea and vomiting:** You experience these symptoms because of the buildup of acids and the loss of important body substances.

- **Rapid breathing:** This condition is also known as *Kussmaul breathing*, after the man who first described it. You experience rapid breathing when your blood is so acidic that your body attempts to blow off some of the acid through the lungs. Your breath has a fruity smell due to acetone.

- **Extreme tiredness and drowsiness:** You're tired because your brain is bathed in very thick blood, like syrup, and is missing the essential substances you've lost in the urine.

- **Weakness:** You become weak because your muscle tissue is unable to get its fuel, namely glucose.

In this age of self-monitoring for blood glucose levels, ketoacidosis is becoming more rare, but it still occurs. (See Chapter 7 for more on self-monitoring.) If you use a source of insulin that can be interrupted, you could unexpectedly develop ketoacidosis. For example, if you rely on an insulin pump, which pushes insulin under your skin automatically (as I describe in Chapter 10), the pump could stop for some reason; then your insulin delivery would cease, your glucose level would rise, and ketoacidosis would develop if you don't notice the interruption soon enough.

You may notice that you have some symptoms of ketoacidosis and begin to suspect that you have this complication. But that diagnosis is best made by a doctor — preferably in the hospital, where you can begin treatment at once. Doctors make a diagnosis of ketoacidosis when they see the following abnormalities:

- High blood glucose, usually more than 300 mg/dl (16.6 mmol/L)

- Acid condition of your blood

- Excessive levels of ketones in your blood and urine

- Dry skin and tongue, indicating dehydration

- Deficiency of potassium in your body

- An acetone smell on your breath

When your doctor finds these abnormalities, he or she will want to begin treatment immediately.

Causes of ketoacidosis

The two most common causes of ketoacidosis are the interruption of your insulin treatment and an infection. Your body can't go for many hours without insulin activity before it begins to burn fat for energy and begins to make extra glucose that it can't use. The process of burning fat creates ketones in your blood, which are responsible for your ketoacidosis. (Refer to the earlier section "Combating Ketoacidosis.")

Whether you're person with diabetes or not, if you go on a strict diet to lose weight, your body burns some of its fat stores and produces ketones, similar to how it burns fat when you lack insulin. But in this case, your glucose remains low and (unless you have type 1 diabetes) you have sufficient insulin to prevent the excessive production of new glucose or the release of large amounts of glucose from your liver. So a strict diet doesn't generally lead to ketoacidosis but rather a benign condition called ketosis.

Treatment of ketoacidosis

Ketoacidosis is a serious condition that requires professional treatment. But even though you leave the treatment to a professional rather than trying to manage it yourself, you should know the treatment processes so that you understand what's happening to you or to your loved one.

The basis of ketoacidosis treatment is to restore the proper amount of water to your body, reduce the acid condition of your blood by getting rid of the ketones, restore substances such as potassium that you've lost, and return your blood glucose to its normal level of around 80 to 120. All of these improvements should happen simultaneously after you begin treatment.

The following list gives you a basic understanding of how the treatment process goes:

- ✔ **Your doctor sets up a flowchart to keep track of your levels of glucose, acid, potassium, and ketones, along with other parameters.** Although you've lost a lot of potassium, for example, the initial blood reading of potassium on your flowchart may look normal. As your treatment progresses, more potassium goes into your cells to replenish losses there, so your blood potassium may fall. If that happens, the doctor administers more potassium to fix the problem.

- ✔ **Your doctor gives you insulin intravenously to restore your insulin levels and reverse the abnormalities in your body.** Your lack of insulin got you into this ketoacidosis situation in the first place. At some point, your blood glucose may fall toward hypoglycemia. If it does, your doctor gives you another IV made up of glucose and a solution of salt, potassium, and water.

After you receive insulin, your body stops breaking down fat for energy because your cells can use glucose for energy as they're supposed to. Soon, your body rids itself of the ketones in your bloodstream that caused your complication, and your body takes on a more normal condition.

✔ **Your doctor gives you large volumes of a saltwater solution intravenously to replace the six or more liters of fluids that you lose during ketoacidosis.** Replenishing your body's fluids relieves the nausea and vomiting that you've endured, and you're now able to keep down liquid and solid foods again.

Hopefully, you notice your normal mental functioning returning, which means that you'll soon be ready to resume self-administering your insulin and controlling your own diet. By this time, the doctor has probably found and corrected a malfunctioning insulin pump or an infection that was a factor in causing your ketoacidosis.

Most of the time, your doctor can control ketoacidosis with little or no risk to you. But be aware that ketoacidosis is fatal for 10 percent of people with diabetes who get it — mostly elderly people with diabetes and those with other illnesses that complicate treatment. Recognizing the symptoms early and seeking treatment quickly greatly enhance your chances of an uneventful recovery from ketoacidosis.

Managing the Hyperosmolar Syndrome

The highest blood glucose condition that you may find yourself in is called the *hyperosmolar syndrome*. Like ketoacidosis, the hyperosmolar syndrome, referring to the excessive levels of glucose in the blood, is a medical emergency that needs to be treated in a hospital.

The hyperosmolar syndrome is also like ketoacidosis in its effects on your body. The hyperosmolar syndrome creates ketones in your blood, but it doesn't make your blood as acidic as ketoacidosis does. It also raises your blood glucose levels considerably higher than ketoacidosis does. (See the "Combating Ketoacidosis" section earlier in this chapter for more information.)

Hyper means "larger than normal," and *osmolar* has to do with concentrations of substances in the blood. So hyperosmolar, in this situation, means that the blood is simply too concentrated with glucose. Other hyperosmolar syndromes occur when other substances are at fault.

The following sections explain hyperosmolar syndrome's symptoms, causes, and treatments.

Symptoms of the hyperosmolar syndrome

Because the hyperosmolar syndrome complication is so similar to ketoacidosis, it has many of the same symptoms as ketoacidosis. The main difference is that with hyperosmolar syndrome, you don't experience the rapid Kussmaul breathing, because your blood isn't overly acidic as a part of this complication. Also, the symptoms of the hyperosmolar syndrome develop over many days or weeks, unlike the quick and acute development of ketoacidosis in your body.

If you measure your blood glucose on a daily basis, you should never develop the hyperosmolar syndrome because you'll notice that your blood glucose is getting high before it reaches the critical complication level.

The most important signs and symptoms of the hyperosmolar syndrome are

- ✔ Frequent urination
- ✔ Thirst
- ✔ Weakness
- ✔ Leg cramps
- ✔ Sunken eyeballs and rapid pulse, due to dehydration
- ✔ Decreased mental awareness or (if you delay treatment) coma
- ✔ Blood glucose of 600 or even higher if you delay seeing a doctor

You may also develop more threatening symptoms with this complication. Your blood pressure may be low. Your nervous system may be affected with paralysis of the arms and legs, but these respond to treatment. You may have high counts of potassium, sodium, and other blood constituents (such as white blood cells and red blood cells), but these counts usually fall rapidly and your doctor will replace these elements in your blood as water is restored to your body.

Causes of the hyperosmolar syndrome

The hyperosmolar syndrome afflicts mostly the elderly with diabetes who live alone or in nursing homes where they're not carefully monitored. Age and usually some neglect combine to increase the likelihood that a person with diabetes will lose large quantities of fluids through vomiting or diarrhea and then not replace those fluids. These people tend to have mild type 2 diabetes, and sometimes their diabetes is undiagnosed and untreated.

Another reason age is a contributing cause of the hyperosmolar syndrome is that your kidneys gradually become less efficient as you age. When your kidneys are in their prime, your blood glucose level needs to reach only 180 mg/dl before your kidneys begin to remove some excess glucose through your urine. But as your kidneys grow older and slower, they require a gradually higher blood glucose level before they start to send excess glucose to your urine. If you're at an age (usually 70 or older for people in average health) when your kidneys are really laboring to remove the excess glucose from your body and you happen to lose a large amount of fluids from sickness or neglect, your blood volume decreases, which makes it even harder for your kidneys to remove glucose. At this point, your blood glucose level begins to skyrocket. If you don't replace some of the lost fluids quickly, your glucose rises even higher.

If you allow your blood glucose to rise and don't get the fluids that you need, your blood pressure starts to fall and you get weaker and weaker. As the concentration of glucose in your blood continues to rise, you become increasingly confused, and your mental state diminishes until you eventually fall into a coma.

Other factors — such as infection, failure to take your insulin, and taking certain medications — can raise your blood glucose to the hyperosmolar syndrome levels, but not replacing lost body fluids is the most frequent cause.

Treatment of the hyperosmolar syndrome

Even more so than ketoacidosis (see the section "Treatment of ketoacidosis" earlier in this chapter), the hyperosmolar syndrome requires immediate and skilled treatment from a doctor. By no means should you try to treat the hyperosmolar syndrome yourself. In fact, you should avoid doctors who are not experienced in treatment of this condition. You need the proper treatment from an experienced doctor — and you need it fast. The death rate for the hyperosmolar syndrome is high because most people who suffer from it are elderly and often have other serious illnesses that complicate treatment.

When you arrive at your doctor's office or emergency room with the hyperosmolar syndrome, your doctor must accomplish the following tasks fairly rapidly:

- ✔ Restore large volumes of water to your body
- ✔ Lower your blood glucose level
- ✔ Restore other substances that your body has lost, such as potassium, sodium, chloride, and so on

Your doctor creates a chart to monitor your levels of glucose, blood concentration (osmolarity), potassium, sodium, and other substances, which are measured hourly in some cases. You may think that you need to receive large amounts of insulin to lower your high glucose level, but the large doses of fluids that your doctor gives you do so much to lower your glucose that you need only smaller doses of insulin. As your body fluids return to normal, your kidneys begin to receive much more of the blood that they need in order to rid your body of the excess glucose, and your kidney function improves.

Chapter 5

Preventing Long-Term Complications

*I*f you're preventing short-term complications (see Chapter 4), you're also preventing long-term complications, which I describe in this chapter. So, you're preventing two sets of complications with just one treatment. The difference you need to remember between short-term and long-term complications is that short-term complications result from the immediate effects of very high and very low blood glucose levels, and short-term complications are reversible. On the other hand, long-term complications result from damage done by high blood glucose levels as well as abnormal fat levels and abnormal blood pressure. But, unlike short-term complications, after a while, long-term complications aren't reversible.

The complications detailed in this chapter are the problems that occur if you permit your blood glucose to rise and remain high over many years. The point that I stress throughout this book is that you have a choice. Working with your doctor and other helpers, you can keep your blood glucose near normal so that you never have to deal with these long-term complications.

The struggle to live an uncomplicated life with diabetes reminds me of a commercial airplane pilot who took the airplane down for a rough landing. As was his custom, after the plane landed the pilot stood at the exit; he waited for passengers to make nasty comments about the landing, but no one mentioned it. Finally, a little old lady walked to the exit with her cane and said to the pilot, "Tell me, did we land, or were we shot down?"

The choice is yours: You can have a smooth landing, free of complications, that goes relatively unnoticed by you and those around you. Or you can have the feeling that you have been shot down.

How Long-Term Complications Develop

Doctors aren't sure of the precise reason that long-term complications of diabetes develop. They have lots of theories, many of them strongly based on findings in animals and human beings. For most long-term complications except heart disease — such as kidney disease, eye disease, and nerve disease — doctors believe that years of high blood glucose levels initiate the complications. (In the case of heart disease, high blood glucose levels may make the disease worse or more complicated but not actually cause it.) Most long-term complications require ten or more years to develop, which seems like a long time until you consider that many people with type 2 diabetes have it for five or more years before a doctor diagnoses it.

Often the long-term complication itself (rather than a high blood glucose level) is the clue that leads a doctor to diagnose diabetes in a patient. Therefore, doctors need to look for long-term complications immediately after diagnosing diabetes, because the diabetes and any long-term complications may have been with the patient for quite some time already. Because of the possibility of long-term complications being present at the diagnosis of diabetes, your doctor also must immediately take steps to control your glucose levels.

Kidney Disease

Your kidneys rid your body of many harmful chemicals and other compounds produced during the process of normal metabolism. Your kidneys act like a filter through which your blood pours, trapping the waste and sending it out in your urine, while the normal contents of the blood go back into your bloodstream. They also regulate the salt and water content of your body. When kidney disease (also known as *nephropathy*) causes your kidneys to fail, you must either use artificial means, called *dialysis,* to cleanse your blood and control the salt and water or receive a new working donor kidney, called a *transplant.*

How high glucose leads to complications

Although doctors aren't certain about the causes of most long-term complications of diabetes, I mention the current theories about the causes of the complications as I explain each complication in this chapter. All long-term complications share some common characteristics:

✔ *Advanced glycated end products* (AGEs) are one of the substances that damage tissues. AGEs can damage the eyes, the kidneys, the nervous system, and other organs in your body. You always have glucose in your blood, and some of that glucose attaches to other substances in your bloodstream to form *glycated* (glucose-attached) products. In this way, hemoglobin, which carries oxygen through your blood to cells and tissues throughout your body, attaches to glucose to form hemoglobin A1c. Albumin, a protein in blood, forms glycated albumin. Glucose can attach to red blood cells and white blood cells, as well as to other cells and molecules in the bloodstream. When these normal body substances attach to glucose, they no longer work normally.

When glucose attaches to other substances and cells, it alters their functions, usually in a negative fashion. For example, hemoglobin A1c holds on to oxygen more strongly than hemoglobin, so the cells that need oxygen don't get it as easily. Red blood cells that are glycated do not last as long in your blood circulation. Glycated white blood cells can't fight infection as well as unglycated white cells can.

Your body handles a certain level of glycated substances. But when your blood glucose is elevated for prolonged periods of time, the level of glycated cells and substances becomes excessive, and the complications I describe in this chapter result.

An interesting study in *Diabetes Care* in August 2005 showed that AGEs are present in higher amounts in patients with T2DM who develop peripheral arterial disease (see below) compared to those who don't develop it. It suggests that AGEs play a role in large blood vessel disease as well as small blood vessel disease.

✔ The Polyol Pathway is another major source of damage to the body in diabetes. *Polyol Pathway* refers to one direction, or pathway, that glucose can take as it is *metabolized* (broken down). For example, the common pathway is to form carbon dioxide and water as energy is produced. When you have a lot of glucose in your blood, an abnormal amount is metabolized to become a product called *sorbitol.* Sorbitol is a member of a class of substances called *polyols.* Sorbitol accumulates in many tissues where it can damage them in various ways:

Damage from swelling: Body water enters the cells to make the concentration of substances equal outside and inside, because sorbitol does not pass out of the cell. This causes damage and destruction of cells.

Damage from chemical reactions: During the production of sorbitol, other compounds are produced that chemically damage the cells and tissues.

Damage from autoantibodies: An article in August 2005 in *Diabetes Care* showed that autoantibodies to autonomic nerves (see below) are present in patients with diabetes long before they suffer from autonomic neuropathy involving the heart and the peripheral autonomic nervous system. Autoimmunity may be yet another mechanism by which diabetes causes long-term complications.

In the United States today, half the patients who require long-term dialysis require it because of diabetes. Fortunately, this number is on the decline because of the increasing awareness among people that they need to control their blood glucose. The incidence of kidney disease is only about 5 percent among people with type 2 diabetes, compared to 30 percent among people with type 1 diabetes; however, the absolute number of patients with kidney disease is about the same for the two groups because type 2 diabetes is so much more common than type 1. The following sections on kidney complications tell you how diabetes affects your kidneys, the changes that are occurring in your body and how you can both check for them while they are still reversible and prevent them from getting any worse.

The impact of diabetes on your kidneys

Chronic kidney disease is more prevalent now than it has been in the past. The major source of all these new cases is diabetes. This section tells you what you need to know to prevent and manage diabetic kidney disease.

Your kidneys consist of about a million units called nephrons. Each nephron contains a structure called the *glomerulous* (the plural is *glomeruli*) (see Figure 5-1). Glomeruli cleanse your blood through the following process:

1. **Your blood passes through tiny glomerular capillaries.**

2. **Your filtered blood travels through tubules connected to the glomerular capillaries.**

3. **As your filtered blood passes through the tubules:**

   - Your body reabsorbs most of the water and the normal contents of the blood.

   - A small amount of water and waste passes from the kidney into the ureter and then into the bladder and out through the urethra.

When you first get diabetes, your kidneys are enlarged and seem to function abnormally well, judging by how fast they clear wastes from your body. Your kidneys seem to function so well because you have a large amount of glucose entering your kidneys, which draws a lot of water with it and causes an increase in the pressure inside each glomerulous. This more rapid transit of blood through the kidneys is known as an increased *glomerular filtration rate* (GFR). Early in the development of your diabetes, the membrane surrounding your glomeruli, called the *glomerular basement membrane,* thickens, as do other adjacent structures. These expanding membranes and structures begin to take up the space occupied by the capillaries inside the glomeruli so that the capillaries are unable to filter as much blood.

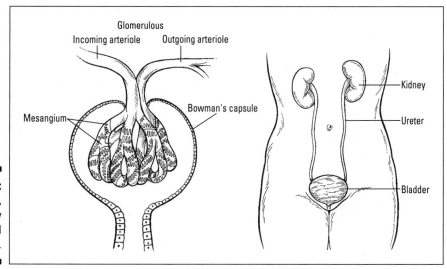

Figure 5-1:
The kidney,
internally
and
externally.

Fortunately, you have many more glomeruli than you really need. In fact, you can lose a whole kidney and still have plenty of reserve to clean your blood. If your kidney disease goes undetected for about 15 years, damage may become so severe that your blood shows measurable signs of the beginning of kidney failure, called *azotemia.* If the neglect of the disease reaches 20 years, your kidneys may fail entirely.

Not every person with diabetes is at equal risk for kidney disease and kidney failure. This complication seems to be more common in certain families and among certain racial groups, especially African Americans, Mexican Americans, and Native Americans. It is certainly more common when high blood pressure is present. Although we believe that high blood glucose is the major factor leading to nephropathy, only half of the people whose blood glucose has been poorly controlled go on to develop nephropathy.

Early indications of kidney disease

If your kidneys are on their way to being damaged by *diabetic nephropathy* (kidney disease caused by diabetes), doctors can detect *microalbuminuria* in your urine. A healthy kidney permits only a tiny amount of *albumin,* a protein in the blood, to enter the urine. However, a kidney being damaged by nephropathy is unable to hold back as much albumin, and the level in the urine increases, causing *microalbuminuria.*

Recent evidence suggests, however, that an abnormal amount of albumin in the urine is not always present when diabetic neuropathy is developing. A study in *Diabetes Care* in January 2004 showed that as many as 25 percent of people with diabetes have kidney disease even though there is no increase in the albumin in their urine. Blood tests for kidney function show some loss of function, yet the test for increased albumin is negative. In other words, the absence of microalbuminuria does not always indicate that no kidney damage is taking place. Rather, this finding suggests that treatment with drugs that protect the kidneys should be done for all patients with diabetes, not just those with microalbuminuria.

For three-quarters of the patients in the early stages of kidney disease, however, the amount of albumin in your urine is so small that it won't trigger a positive result when the traditional urine dipstick test is used. Therefore, your doctor should perform a more sophisticated test for *microalbuminuria* (the presence of tiny but abnormally high amounts of albumin in your urine). This test can be done by collecting a 24-hour urine specimen (meaning you save all the urine you produce in 24 hours and have it tested), by taking a random urine sample, or by collecting a specimen over a certain time period, usually four hours. If the level of albumin is abnormally high, it needs to be checked once again to be certain, because some factors (such as exercise) can trigger a false positive test. A second positive test should lead to action to protect your kidneys.

Because microalbuminuria can be detected about five years before a urine dipstick would test positive for albumin, you have time to treat the onset. Furthermore, treatment during the stage of microalbuminuria can reverse the kidney disease. After *macroalbuminuria* is found using the dipstick method, the disease can be slowed but not stopped.

If you have had type 1 diabetes for five years or more, or if you've recently been diagnosed with type 2 diabetes, *your doctor must check for microalbuminuria* unless you've already tested positive for albumin with a urine dipstick. If your test comes back negative, you should have it rechecked annually.

In June 2003 in the *New England Journal of Medicine,* researchers showed that microalbuminuria does not always lead to kidney failure. Patients with type 1 diabetes who improved their blood glucose levels, blood pressure, and abnormal blood fats (which I discuss in the next section) experienced a decline in microalbuminuria and, therefore, a decline in kidney damage. The levels of improvement indicated by this study are as follows:

- ✔ Lowered blood glucose as indicated by a hemoglobin A1c of less than 8 percent (see Chapter 7)
- ✔ Lowered blood pressure, with the upper number (the *systolic blood pressure*) kept under 115 mg mercury
- ✔ Cholesterol kept under 198 mg/dl (5.12 mmol/L)
- ✔ Triglycerides kept below 145 mg/dl (1.64 mmol/L)

Progressive changes

If diabetes is poorly controlled for five years or more, your kidney experiences a significant expansion of the *mesangial tissue,* the cells between the capillaries in the kidneys. The amount of microalbuminuria correlates to the amount of mesangial expansion. Thickening of the glomerular basement membrane is taking place at the same time but does not correlate as well with the amount of microalbuminuria.

Over the next 15 to 20 years, the open capillaries and tubules are squeezed shut by the encroaching tissues; they appear like round nodules (known as *Kimmelstiel-Wilson nodules,* after the names of their discoverers), and they are diagnostic of diabetic nephropathy. As the glomeruli are replaced by nodules, less and less filtration of the blood can take place. The *blood urea nitrogen* (a handy blood test that indicates how well the kidneys are working) begins to rise, ultimately ending in *uremia,* a condition in which the kidneys are not doing any cleansing.

Other factors besides high blood glucose contribute to the continuing destruction of the kidneys. They include the following:

✔ **High blood pressure (hypertension):** This factor may be almost as important as the glucose level. If your blood pressure is controlled by drugs, the damage to your kidneys slows very significantly. We know this fact is true because occasionally someone with diabetes suffers both from high blood pressure and from disease of one of the arteries to his kidney. The kidney whose artery is diseased doesn't feel the force of the high blood pressure. While the other kidney goes on to develop nephropathy, this kidney is protected and does not develop it.

✔ **Factors of inheritance:** Certain families and ethnic groups have a higher incidence of diabetic nephropathy, as I discuss in the section "The impact of diabetes on your kidneys," earlier in this chapter.

✔ **Abnormal blood fats:** Research shows that elevated levels of certain cholesterol-containing fats promote enlargement of the mesangium.

Diabetic nephropathy does not occur alone. If you experience kidney disease, you need to be aware that the following complications are associated with it:

✔ **Diabetic eye disease:** When someone experiences complete failure of the kidneys, called *end stage renal disease,* diabetic retinopathy (eye disease) is always present (see the section "Eye Disease," later in this chapter). As kidney disease gets worse, retinopathy accelerates. But only half the people with retinopathy also have nephropathy.

If you test positive for microalbuminuria, you will also have some retinopathy if diabetes is the cause of your kidney problems. If you have diabetes and have microalbuminuria but retinopathy is not present, your doctor should look for another cause of kidney disease besides diabetes.

✔ **Diabetic nerve disease (neuropathy):** There is not as great an association between nephropathy and neuropathy. Fewer than 50 percent of patients with nephropathy also experience neuropathy. Neuropathy gets worse as kidney disease gets worse, but after dialysis has begun, some of the neuropathy disappears. This situation indicates that part of the neuropathy may be due to wastes that are retained because of the failing kidney rather than true damage to the nervous system. (For more on this condition, see the section "Nerve Disease, or Neuropathy" later in this chapter.)

✔ **High blood pressure (hypertension):** Hypertension plays an important role in accelerating kidney damage. One-third of patients who have urine dipstick tests that are positive for albumin also have high blood pressure. As the blood tests for kidney failure begin to rise, two-thirds of patients are hypertensive. With end stage renal disease, almost all have high blood pressure.

✔ **Edema:** *Edema,* or water accumulation, in the feet and legs occurs as the amount of protein in the urine exceeds one or two grams a day.

Treatment for diabetic nephropathy

If the information in the previous section is making your blood pressure rise, take a deep breath. I'm happy to report that all the inconvenience and discomfort associated with diabetic nephropathy can be avoided. Following are a few key treatments that you can do to prevent the disease or significantly slow it down after it begins:

✔ **Control your blood glucose:** This crucial step has been shown to avoid the onset of nephropathy and to slow it down once it starts. Both the Diabetes Control and Complications Trial (DCCT) in the United States, which studied glucose control in type 1 diabetes, and the United Kingdom Prospective Diabetes Study Groups in type 2 diabetes have proved this point. If you keep your blood glucose close to normal, you will not develop diabetic nephropathy. (For information on controlling your blood glucose, see Part III.)

One of the best findings from the DCCT is that even eight years after the trial ended, participants experienced persistent benefits of reduced blood pressure and reduced albumin excretion (a marker for kidney damage). Controlling your blood glucose now will pay off years in the future.

✔ **Control your blood pressure:** This step protects the kidneys from rapid deterioration. Treatment begins with a low-salt diet, but drugs are usually needed. High blood pressure can be controlled by a variety of drugs, but one class of drugs seems particularly valuable in nephropathy. This class is called the *angiotensin converting enzyme inhibitors,* or ACE inhibitors. (For more on ACE inhibitors, see the sidebar "ACE inhibitors to the rescue.") If ACE inhibitors can't be used for any reason, a similar class of drugs called angiotensin II receptor blockers are equally or more effective.

✔ **Control the blood fats:** Because abnormalities of blood fats seem to make kidney disease worse, you must lower your bad, or LDL, cholesterol and raise your good, or HDL, cholesterol while lowering the other fat that is damaging — the triglycerides. A number of excellent drugs, in a class called *statins,* can accomplish this task. The ACE inhibitors also seem to help the levels of fats. (See the sidebar on ACE inhibitors for more information.)

✔ **Avoid other damage to the kidneys:** People with diabetes tend to have more urinary tract infections, which damage the kidneys. Urinary tract infections must be looked for and treated. People with diabetes also have damage to the nerves that control the bladder, producing a neurogenic bladder. (See the section "Disorders of automatic (autonomic) nerves," later in this chapter.) When the nerves that detect a full bladder fail, proper emptying of the bladder is inhibited, which can lead to infections.

If you have disease in the urinary system, your doctor may want to do an *intravenous pyelogram* (IVP), a study to observe the appearance and function of your kidneys and the rest of your urinary tract. But people with diabetes with some kidney failure are at high risk for complete failure of the kidneys as a result of an IVP. Your doctor should use another type of study that does not put your kidneys at risk.

If these preventative treatments fail, the patient undergoes dialysis or a kidney transplant.

When the kidneys fail, a main source for the breakdown of insulin is gone, and the patient requires much less or no insulin, so control of the blood glucose may actually get easier.

✔ **Dialysis:** Two dialysis techniques are currently in use.

• **Hemodialysis:** The patient's artery is hooked into a tube that runs through a filtering machine that cleanses the blood and then sends it back into the patient's bloodstream. When the patient is moderately well, hemodialysis is done three times a week in a hospital-like setting. The potential exists for many complications, including infection and low blood pressure.

• **Peritoneal dialysis:** A tube is inserted into the body cavity that contains the stomach, liver, and intestines, called the *peritoneal cavity.* A large quantity of fluid is dripped into the cavity, and it draws out the wastes, which are then removed as the fluid drains out of the cavity. Peritoneal dialysis is done at home, often on a daily basis. Peritoneal dialysis requires the use of sugar in the fluid so that people with diabetes will have very high blood glucose levels, which is undesireable, unless insulin is added to the bags of dialysis fluid. Peritoneal dialysis is also associated with a high rate of infection where the tube enters the peritoneal cavity.

Little difference exists in the long-term survival of patients treated with hemodialysis compared with peritoneal dialysis, so the choice becomes one of convenience and whether one is covered by insurance more than the other. People with diabetes do not tolerate kidney failure well, so dialysis tends to be started earlier in them than in people without diabetes.

✔ **Kidney transplant:** Patients who receive a kidney transplant seem to do better than dialysis patients, but in the United States, because of a lack of kidneys, 80 percent of patients have dialysis and 20 percent have a transplant. Obviously, a transplanted kidney is foreign to the person who receives it, and the body tries to reject it. To avoid this result, the patient is given antirejection drugs, some of which make diabetic control more complicated. The kidney that is least rejected is the one from a donor who is most closely related to the patient.

When a healthy kidney enters the body of a person with diabetes, it is subject to the damage done by elevated glucose levels. After a transplant, controlling your blood glucose is crucial.

ACE inhibitors to the rescue

The class of drugs called *angiotensin converting enzyme inhibitors,* or ACE inhibitors, has long been known to lower blood pressure. Recent studies show that these drugs also lower the pressure inside the *glomeruli* (the structures inside your kidneys that cleanse your blood). The result is a 50 percent reduction in death due to diabetic nephropathy and an equal reduction in the need for dialysis or a kidney transplant.

Your doctor should prescribe one of these medications if your blood pressure is 140/90 or higher. The target blood pressure is 120/80 and even lower in younger people. ACE inhibitors can even be used if you have microalbuminuria without hypertension, because the microalbuminuria suggests that there is increased pressure within the kidney. When ACE inhibitors are used, the excretion of albumin begins to fall; if you are leaking albumin into the urine, your urine albumin level can be used to monitor the drugs' effectiveness if your blood pressure is normal.

ACE inhibitors are not perfect: They do cause a cough in some patients, which some people find hard to tolerate, but the choice of a particular ACE inhibitor may solve this problem. In addition, ACE inhibitors tend to raise the potassium level in the blood. The potassium level is already an issue with failing kidneys, so a higher potassium level may add to the problem. A very high potassium level can cause abnormalities in the heart. Angiotensin II receptor blockers can replace ACE inhibitors when necessary. They're not associated with the cough but do raise potassium.

Other drugs used for high blood pressure include the calcium channel blockers, which may be as useful as ACE inhibitors. Other antihypertensives that have been standards in the past for hypertension may cause unacceptable side effects. Water pills (diuretics such as hydrochlorothiazide) raise the blood glucose. Beta blockers like propranolol make the abnormal fats worse. They also cause a difficulty in recognizing when the blood glucose has gone down to very low levels.

Eye Disease

The eyes are the second major organ of the body affected by diabetes over the long term. Some eye diseases, such as glaucoma and cataracts, also occur in the nondiabetic population, though they appear at a higher rate and earlier in people with diabetes. Glaucoma and cataracts respond to treatment very well. Diabetic retinopathy, however — which I explain in the next section — is limited to the diabetic population and may lead to blindness. In the past, blindness was inevitable, but that is not the case today. In the next sections you will learn about the normal function of the eye and how diabetes can damage or even eliminate that function. You will also discover the importance of early diagnosis by regular eye exams and how you can stop the progress of eye disease should it occur.

Understanding how the eye works

In order to understand how diabetes affects the eyes, Figure 5-2 shows you the different parts of the eye.

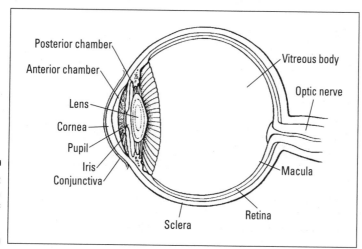

Figure 5-2:
The structure of the eye.

Light enters the eye through the lens where it is bent and focused upon the retina. The place in the retina where the lens focuses is called the *macula*. The retina collects an image and transfers it to the optic nerve, which carries it to the brain where the image is interpreted. Between the lens and the retina is a transparent material called the *vitreous body*. Many more structures exist within the eye, but they're not important for my purposes in this chapter.

The eye muscles surround the eye on all sides and are attached to it. These muscles permit you to look up, down, and sideways without moving your head. These eye muscles are important in the discussion of diabetic nerve damage, called *neuropathy*. (For more on this condition, see the section "Nerve Disease, or Neuropathy," later in this chapter.)

Following is a list of common eye diseases found in people with diabetes:

- **Cataracts:** These opaque areas of the lens can block vision if they're large enough. Cataracts tend to be more common in people with diabetes, even at a young age, both as a result of advanced glycated end products (AGEs) that form within the lens, and as a result of the increased concentration of sorbitol in the lens. (I discuss AGEs and sorbitol in the sidebar "How high glucose leads to complications," earlier in this chapter.) Cataracts can be surgically removed by a fairly routine operation. The entire lens is removed, and an artificial lens is put in its place. With removal, you have an excellent chance for the restoration of your vision.

- **Glaucoma:** This high pressure inside the eye is enough to do damage to the optic nerve. Glaucoma is found more often in people with diabetes than in the nondiabetic population. If left unchecked, the high pressure can destroy the optic nerve and destroy your vision. Fortunately, medical treatment can lower the eye pressure and save the eye. Eye doctors check for glaucoma on a routine basis.

- **Retinopathy:** *Diabetic retinopathy* refers to a number of changes that are seen on the retina of the eye. These changes indicate that the patient has been exposed to high levels of blood glucose over time. If untreated at the appropriate time, retinopathy can lead to blindness. The first changes are seen after ten years of diabetes in both type 1 and 2. Because retinopathy is much more complicated and less treatable than the other two conditions, I discuss it in detail in the next section.

If you have diabetes, you must get an annual eye examination by an ophthalmologist or optometrist to preserve your vision. This situation is one where an expert is definitely needed. Doctors who are not ophthalmologists or optometrists diagnose retinopathy correctly only 50 percent of the time, while ophthalmologists and optometrists are correct more than 90 percent of the time. You need to get an eye examination as soon as you are diagnosed with type 2 diabetes or five years after the diagnosis of type 1 diabetes, and you need to be rechecked every year after that.

Retinopathy

Ophthalmologists break down retinopathy into two major types, according to their potential to cause visual loss:

✔ **Background retinopathy:** This type is usually benign but can be a predictor of worse problems. The first changes noted by the ophthalmologist are *retinal aneurysms,* which are the result of weakening of the capillaries of the eye; they produce outpocketing of the capillaries, which look like tiny balloons. These aneurysms appear as small red dots on the back of the eye. They are benign and disappear over time. The weakened capillaries also rupture sometimes and release blood to form *retinal hemorrhages* and *hard exudates.* The hard exudates, which are yellowish and appear round and sharp, are scars from the hemorrhage. If they extend into the macular area, they reduce vision. If the capillaries in the retina allow fluid to flow into the macula, you get *macular edema,* which also causes loss of vision. These exudates and hemorrhages can last for years. As the capillaries close, you have a decreased blood supply to the retina, and *cotton wool spots* or *soft exudates* appear. These spots represent destruction of the nerve fiber layer because of the lack of blood.

These changes usually do not cause complete loss of vision, but in about 50 percent of cases, they go on to the more serious proliferative retinopathy.

✔ **Proliferative retinopathy:** This condition results in vision loss if untreated. Just as in many other parts of the body, when the blood supply in the eye is reduced, new blood vessels form to carry more blood to the retina. This is the stage of proliferative retinopathy. This condition is when some visual loss becomes more certain. The growth of blood vessels takes place into the vitreous body. Hemorrhage into the vitreous body blocks vision. As the hemorrhage forms a clot and contracts, it may pull up the retina to produce *retinal detachment.* Because the lens can no longer focus the light onto the macula, you have a complete loss of vision.

Like diabetic nephropathy, retinopathy has a number of important associations:

✔ Certain ethnic groups are at very high risk for retinopathy. These include certain American Indian groups, like the Pima Indians, as well as Mexican Americans. Researchers aren't yet certain if African Americans are at higher risk.

✔ Specific genetic material, if found in a person with diabetes, increases the incidence of retinopathy. This material can be found by doing a chemical analysis of a person's *chromosomes,* the material in each cell that holds the genes. If the genetic material is found, that person has a higher likelihood of developing retinopathy.

✔ Males and females get retinopathy equally.

✔ Greater duration of diabetes results in more eye disease.

✔ High blood pressure worsens the eye disease.

✔ Nephropathy occurs along with the eye disease. (See the "Progressive changes" section, earlier in this chapter.)

✔ Smoking and alcohol use probably worsen retinopathy (but the final word on their influence is not in).

✔ Patients with severe diabetic retinopathy are at increased risk for heart attacks. A recent article in *Diabetes Care* in July 2007 strongly confirmed this relationship. People with diabetic retinopathy are twice as likely to have a heart attack as people with diabetes who don't have retinopathy. If they have a heart attack they are three times as likely to have a fatal heart attack.

No drugs are currently available to treat retinopathy, but laser surgery is an excellent treatment option. And the use of laser surgery to create many burns in the retina has been shown to save many eyes. Only 5 percent of diabetics with proliferative retinopathy who undergo laser treatment develop severe visual loss. Because the retina is being burned, you have some minor loss of vision. You also have a mild decrease in night vision and a minor decrease in the size of the field that your eye can take in at one time. The procedure is done outside the hospital. It is used for treating macular edema with success as well.

Tight control of the blood glucose (maintaining a hemoglobin A1c under 7 percent) is associated with a much better response to laser surgery than loose control.

Laser surgery cannot treat a retinal detachment that has already occurred. To do so, a surgical procedure called *vitrectomy* is used. This operation, done under general anesthesia, involves removing the vitreous body and replacing it with a sterile solution. Attachments to the retina are cut, and the retina returns to its place. Any hemorrhages in the vitreous body are removed at the same time. Vitrectomy is successful in restoring some vision about 80 to 90 percent of the time. If a retinal detachment is present in addition to hemorrhage, the amount of improvement depends upon the extent and duration of the retinal detachment, with restoration of vision occurring about 50 to 60 percent of the time.

Resources for the blind and visually impaired

A search for resources for the blind and visually impaired must begin with the World Wide Web. Using a search engine, you can come up with more than 8,000 sites that have something to do with loss of vision and blindness. One of the first sites is the Blindness Resource Center, sponsored by the New York Institute for Special Education. You can find this site, which contains a huge list of other sources of information, at www.nyise.org/text/blindness.htm. The site itself uses large print, so a person with impaired vision can easily read it.

The Blindness Resource Center is filled with useful information. Just to give you the flavor of what is available, here are some of the other sites described to which you can link from this site:

- A Blind Net (`www.blind.net/blindind.htm`), which contains useful information about blindness

- New York Institute For Special Education's Blindness Resource Center (`www.nyise.org/blind.htm`), which provides programs for children who are blind or visually disabled

- *Dialogue* magazine (`www.blindskills.com`), written specifically for the blind

- Guidedogs for the Blind (`www.guidedogs.com`), which explains everything you want to know about these amazing animals

Undoubtedly, one of its best links is to the American Foundation for the Blind (AFB) at `www.afb.org/`. It would take a good part of a lifetime to read all of the resource materials that the AFB provides on thousands of pages. The AFB is the organization that Helen Keller devoted her life to, and it has every imaginable resource — and some that are unimaginable. Just a few of the AFB's reports and fact sheets include

- A profile of the blind and visually impaired audience for television and video

- A fact sheet on Braille

- Information on synthetic speech systems

- A list of catalog houses that sell specialty products

- Information on accommodating applicants or employees who are blind or visually impaired

- A bibliography of art for and by the blind

The Web is a tremendous resource for the visually handicapped and should be utilized by friends, relatives, or the impaired person if that is possible. You have no reason to feel alone with your visual problem.

Nerve Disease, or Neuropathy

The third major organ system of the body that is attacked by poorly controlled diabetes is the nervous system. Sixty percent of people with diabetes have some abnormality of the nervous system. These patients usually don't realize it because the disease does not have any early symptoms. These patients usually have poor glucose control, smoke, and are over age 40. Nerve disease is found most often in the people who have diabetes the longest. Diabetic neuropathy often leads to foot infections, foot ulcerations, and amputation — complications that are all entirely preventable. (See the section "Diabetic Foot Disease," later in this chapter.) The sections that follow describe the basics of nerve disease, as well as disorders associated with nerve disease.

Basics of neuropathy

How high glucose levels damage nerves remains uncertain. Doctors do know that the part of the nerve, called the *axon,* that connects to other nerves or to muscle becomes degenerated. The damage may be *vascular* in some cases, resulting from a cut-off of blood to the nerve, and *metabolic* in others, resulting from chemical toxins produced by the metabolism of too much glucose.

Diabetic neuropathy occurs in any situation where the blood glucose is abnormally elevated for ten years or more. It is therefore not limited to type 1 or type 2 diabetes, although these are the most common diseases where it is found. When the elevated blood glucose is brought down to normal, the signs and symptoms improve. In some cases, the neuropathy disappears.

The fact that intensive control of the blood glucose improves the neuropathy suggests that the disease is a consequence of abnormal metabolism that damages the nerves.

The speed with which a nervous impulse travels down a nerve fiber is called the *nerve conduction velocity.* In diabetic neuropathy, the nerve conduction velocity (NCV) is slowed. This slowing may not be accompanied by any symptoms at first; testing the NCV provides a way of diagnosing neuropathy in people without symptoms. If a patient who has very mild symptoms takes medication to control neuropathy, the improvement that follows may be hard to detect except by doing a nerve conduction velocity study. A medication that helps the neuropathy would be expected to speed up the NCV.

In addition to a persistently high blood glucose level, neuropathy is made worse by the following conditions:

- ✔ **Age:** Neuropathy is most common in people over 40.
- ✔ **Height:** Neuropathy is more common in taller individuals, who have longer nerve fibers to damage.
- ✔ **Alcohol consumption:** Even small quantities of alcohol can make neuropathy worse.

Doctors can test nerve function in a variety of ways because different nerve fibers seem to be responsible for different kinds of sensation, such as light touch, vibration, and temperature. The connection between the kind of test and the fiber it tests for is as follows:

✔ **Vibration testing:** Using a tuning fork, for example, can bring out abnormalities of large nerve fibers.

✔ **Temperature testing:** Using a warm or cold item, tests for damage to small fibers, which are very important in diabetes. When small fibers are damaged, the patient can lose the ability to feel that he is entering a burning hot bath for instance.

✔ **Light touch testing:** Perhaps the most important test that is done, reflects the large fibers, which sense anything touching our skin. This test is done using a filament that looks like a hair. The thickness of the filament determines how much force is needed to bend the filament so that it is felt. For example, a filament that bends with 1 gram of force can be felt by normal feet. If a patient can feel a filament that bends with 10 grams of force, it is unlikely that this person will suffer damage to the foot without feeling it. If the patient cannot feel any sensation with a filament that requires 75 grams of force to bend, that area is considered to have lost all sensation.

Either you or your doctor can use the 10-gram filament to discover whether you are at risk for damage to your feet because you cannot feel the pain. This test takes a minute to do and can save your feet from amputation. (See the section about the diabetic foot, later in this chapter.)

Disorders of sensation

Disorders of sensation, the most common and bothersome disorders of nerves in diabetes, occur where the sensory nerves are damaged. Disorders of sensation include a number of different conditions, which break down into two categories:

✔ *Diffuse neuropathies:* involving many nerves.

✔ *Focal neuropathies:* involving one or several nerves.

This section focuses on the diffuse neuropathies affecting sensation.

Distal polyneuropathy

Distal polyneuropathy is the most frequent form of diabetic neuropathy. *Distal* means far away from the center of the body — in other words, the feet and hands. *Poly* means many, and *neuropathy* is disease in nerves. So this disease is one of many nerves, which is noticed in the feet and hands.

Physicians believe that distal polyneuropathy is a metabolic disease (a problem of too much glucose in the blood, specifically) because patients who have other diseases with a general abnormality of metabolism, such as kidney failure or vitamin deficiency, experience a distal polyneuropathy as well.

The signs and symptoms of distal polyneuropathy are

- ✔ Diminished ability to feel light touch (numbness) or feel the position of a foot, whether bent back or forward, resulting from the loss of the large fibers
- ✔ Diminished ability to feel pain and temperature from loss of small fibers
- ✔ Insignificant weakness
- ✔ Tingling and burning
- ✔ Extreme sensitivity to touch
- ✔ Loss of balance or coordination
- ✔ Worsening of symptoms at night

The danger of this kind of neuropathy is that the patient doesn't know, without looking, whether he has trauma to his feet, such as a burn or stepping on a tack. When the small fibers are lost, the symptoms are uncomfortable but not as serious. The patient may feel pain when the bed covers are on his feet or other uncomfortable sensations. The majority of patients with this condition are unaware of the loss of nerve fibers, and the disease is detected by nerve conduction studies.

The complications of this loss of sensation are preventable. If you cannot feel your feet, you must look at them. In the section on feet, later in this chapter, I offer specific techniques to preserve your feet when neuropathy is present.

The most serious complication of loss of sensation in the feet is the neuropathic foot ulcer. A person with normal nerve function feels pains when pressure mounts on an area of the foot. However, a person with diabetic neuropathy doesn't feel this pressure. A callus forms and, with continued pressure, the callus softens and liquifies, finally falling off to leave an ulcer. This ulcer becomes infected. If it isn't promptly treated, it spreads, and amputation may be the only way of saving the patient. In this situation, loss of blood supply to the feet is not an important contributing factor to the ulceration — in fact, the blood supply may be very good.

A less common complication in distal polyneuropathy is *neuroarthropathy,* or Charcot's Joint. In this condition, trauma, which isn't felt, occurs to the joints of the foot or ankle. The bones in the foot get out of line, and many painless fractures may occur. The patient has redness and painless swelling of the foot and ankle. The foot becomes unusable and is described as a bag of bones.

Treatment of distal polyneuropathy starts with the best glucose control possible and extremely good foot care. Your doctor should look at your feet during each visit, particularly if you have any evidence of loss of feeling.

Some drugs, such as the nonsteroidal anti-inflammatory agents ibuprofen and salindac, can reduce the inflammation. Other drugs, such as the antidepressants amitriptylene or imipramine, reduce the pain and other discomfort. A drug called *capsacin,* which is applied to the skin, reduces pain as well. The results of these treatments are variable and seem to work about 60 percent of the time. However, the longer the pain has been present and the worse the pain, the less likely that these drugs will work.

Another drug, called *gabapentin,* has been found to work more often than many of the older drugs, but it causes dizziness and sleepiness, which may make treatment more complicated.

A promising study in *Diabetes Care* in October 2002 describes the use of a spray of isosorbide dinitrate for the treatment of painful diabetic neuropathy. This spray was effective in half of the patients treated. Another large trial, this time using alpha lipoic acid, which has to be injected into a vein, was very successful in improving pain and other symptoms. The trial results were reported in *Diabetes Care* in March 2003.

An even newer and apparently successful therapy is called Anodyne Therapy. It involves the placement of pads that emit an infrared light that increases circulation under the pad. In a study reported in *Diabetes Care* in January 2004, 18 patients were treated with four pads placed one on top and bottom of the foot and one on each side of the calf above the ankle. One foot received the treatment while the other received "sham" treatment. This therapy was done for 40 minutes three times a week for 2 weeks. The treatment improved sensation in the feet, improved balance and reduced pain in the treated foot compared to the untreated foot. Those patients who had the greatest impairment did not improve, however.

Polyradiculopathy-diabetic amyotrophy

Polyradiculopathy-diabetic amyotrophy is a mixture of pain and loss of muscle strength in the muscles of the upper leg so that the patient cannot straighten the knee. Pain extends down from the hip to the thigh. This nerve condition is second in occurrence after distal polyneuropathy in the diabetic population. Polyradiculopathy-diabetic amyotrophy generally has a short course but may continue for years and doesn't particularly improve with better diabetic control. Patients often improve just after the passage of time.

Radiculopathy-nerve root involvement

Sometimes a severe pain in a particular distribution suggests that the root of the nerve, as it leaves the spinal column, is damaged. The clinical picture is pain distributed in a horizontal line around one side of the chest or abdomen. The pain can be so severe that it is mistaken for an internal abdominal emergency.

Fortunately, the pain goes away after a variable period of time — anywhere from 6 to 24 months. In the meantime, good glucose control and pain management are helpful.

Disorders of movement (mononeuropathy)

Neuropathy can affect nerves to various muscles. Disorders of movement occur when you lose motor nerves that carry the impulses to muscles to make those muscles move. When you lose those nerves, you lose the ability to move or use those muscles. These disorders are believed to originate as a result of the sudden closing of a blood vessel supplying the nerve. The clinical picture depends on which nerve or nerves are affected. If one of the nerves to the eyeball is damaged, the patient cannot turn his eye to the side that nerve is on. If the nerve to the face is affected, the eyelid may droop or the smile on one side of the face may be flat. The patient can have trouble with vision or problems with hearing. Focusing the eye may not be possible. No treatment really exists, but fortunately the disorder goes away on its own after several months.

Disorders of automatic (autonomic) nerves

Even as you're reading this page, many movements of muscles are going on inside your body, but you're unaware of them. Your heart muscle is squeezing down and relaxing. Your diaphragm is rising up to empty the lungs of air and relaxing to draw air in. Your esophagus is carrying food from the mouth to the stomach and, in turn, the stomach pushes it into the small intestine, which pushes it into the large intestine. All these muscle functions are under the control of nerves from the brain, and diabetic neuropathy can affect all of them. These automatic functions are called the *autonomic nerves.* Sensitive tests determine that as many as 40 percent of people with diabetes have some form of autonomic neuropathy.

The clinical presentation of this type of neuropathy depends upon the involved nerve. Some possibilities include

- **Bladder abnormalities, starting with a loss of the sensation of bladder fullness:** The urine is not eliminated, and urinary tract infections result. After a while, loss of bladder contraction occurs, and the patient has to strain to urinate or loses urine by dribbling. The doctor can easily diagnose this abnormality by finding out how much urine is left in the bladder after urinating. The treatment is to remember to urinate every four hours or take a drug that increases the force of bladder contraction.

- **Sexual dysfunction, which occurs in 50 percent of males with diabetes and 30 percent of females with diabetes:** Males cannot sustain an erection, and females have trouble lubricating the vagina for intercourse. (See Chapter 6 for more information on these problems.)

✔ **Intestinal abnormalities of various kinds:** The most common abnormality is constipation. In one quarter of all patients with diabetes, nerves to the stomach are involved, so the stomach does not empty on time. This condition is called gastroparesis. It can lead to what's called *brittle diabetes,* where the insulin is active when there is no food. Fortunately, a drug called *metocloprimide* helps to empty the stomach. A new treatment that has worked well is the implantation of a device that stimulates the stomach electrically. It greatly diminishes the symptoms. This treatment was described in a report in *Diabetes Care* from the University of Kansas Medical Center in May 2004.

✔ **Involvement of the gallbladder, which leads to gallstones:** Normally, the gallbladder empties each time you eat, especially if you eat a fatty meal, because the substances in the bile (within the gallbladder) help to break down fat. If disease of the nerve to the gallbladder prevents it from emptying, these same substances will form stones.

✔ **Involvement of the large intestine that can result in diabetic diarrhea with as many as ten or more bowel movements in a day:** Accidental loss of bowel contents can occur, and bacteria can grow abnormally in the intestine. This problem responds to antibiotic treatment. Diarrhea is treated with one of several drugs that quiet the large intestine.

✔ **Heart abnormalities:** If loss of nerves to the heart occurs, the heart may not respond to exercise by speeding up as it should. The force of the heart may not increase when the patient stands, and the patient then becomes lightheaded. A fast fixed heart rate also may occur, and the rhythm of the heart may not be normal. Such patients are at risk for sudden death.

✔ **Sweating problems, especially in the feet:** The body may try to compensate for the lack of sweating in the feet by sweating excessively on the face or trunk. Heavy sweating can occur when certain foods, such as cheese, are eaten.

✔ **Abnormalities of the pupil of the eye:** The pupil determines the amount of light that is let in. As a result of the neuropathy, the pupil is small and does not open up in a dark room.

Entrapment neuropathies

These neuropathies result from squeezing of individual nerves as they pass through bony or ligamentous areas that do not allow expansion so the nerve is trapped if there is swelling for any reason. The entrapment neuropathies can produce symptoms similar to the mononeuropathies described above but they differ in several ways:

✔ Onset of mononeuropathies is sudden while entrapment neuropathies have a gradual onset.

✔ Mononeuropathies are self-limited, usually resolving over six weeks while entrapment neuropathies persist unless the nerve is released by surgery.

✔ Mononeuropathies are painful from the start while entrapment neuropathies gradually get more and more painful.

Entrapment neuropathies are very common in people with diabetes, occurring in one in every three patients.

The entrapment neuropathies include

✔ **Carpal tunnel syndrome:** produces reduced sensation in the fingers and weakness touching the thumb to the fifth finger. The median nerve is trapped at the wrist.

✔ **Ulnar entrapment:** produces reduced sensation in part of the fourth finger and the entire fifth finger as well as the hand between the fifth finger and the wrist. The ulnar nerve is trapped at the elbow.

✔ **Radial nerve entrapment:** produces loss of sensation in the back of the hand and "wrist drop" from weakness of the muscles that straighten up the wrist. The radial nerve is trapped at the elbow.

✔ **Common peroneal entrapment:** produces loss of sensation in the side of the leg and top of the foot and "drop foot" from weakness of the muscles that pull up the foot. The common peroneal nerve is trapped as it passes the head of the fibula, one of the two bones that begin at the knee joint and end at the ankle.

✔ **Tarsal tunnel syndrome:** produces loss of sensation on both sides of the foot and wasting of the muscles of the foot resulting in decreased toe movement. It is like the carpal tunnel syndrome in the foot and results from trapping of the tibial nerve between two of the small foot bones.

✔ **Lateral femoral cutaneous nerve entrapment:** produces loss of sensation on the outside of the thigh but no muscle weakness. It results from trapping of that nerve at the groin.

The entrapment neuropathies respond to rest, splints, drugs that promote water loss, injections of steroids and surgery if necessary. The important thing is not to confuse them with mononeuropathies.

You can see that you can run into all kinds of problems if you develop diabetic neuropathy. None of them need ever bother you, though, if you follow the recommendations in Part III — the closest you will ever get to a nerve problem will be when you try to get a date with that cute neighbor.

Heart Disease

In the last three decades, the number of deaths due to heart disease has fallen dramatically, thanks to all kinds of new treatments as well as improved diets. However, the tremendous increase in the number of type 2 diabetes patients predicted for the next few decades may reverse this trend. In this section, you find out about the special problems that diabetes brings to the heart.

Risks of heart disease to diabetic patients

Coronary artery disease (CAD) is the term for the progressive closure of the arteries, which supply blood to the heart muscle. When one or more of your arteries closes completely, the result is a heart attack (or *myocardial infarction*). In diabetes, the incidence of CAD is increased even in the young type 1 patient. The duration of time with diabetes promotes CAD in type 1 patients. CAD affects males and females with type 1 diabetes in the same way.

Type 2 diabetes is different. CAD is the most common reason for death in type 2 patients. Women with type 2 are at increased risk for CAD compared to men. Many risk factors promote CAD in the type 2 patient, including the following:

- ✔ **Increased production of insulin** because of insulin resistance

- ✔ **Obesity**

- ✔ **Central adiposity,** which refers to the distribution of fat particularly in the waist area

- ✔ **Hypertension (high blood pressure)**

- ✔ **Abnormal blood fats,** especially reduced HDL (good cholesterol) and increased triglyceride. The abnormal fats may persist even when the patient's glucose is controlled. People without diabetes but with impaired glucose tolerance may show the same abnormalities.

People with diabetes have more CAD than people without diabetes. When X-ray studies of the heart blood vessels are compared, people with diabetes have more arteries involved than people without diabetes.

If a heart attack occurs, the risk of death is much greater for the person with diabetes. More than half of all people with diabetes die of heart attacks. If people without diabetes have heart attacks, they die 15 percent of the time, but people with diabetes die 40 percent of the time. The death rate is worse for the person with diabetes who was in poor glucose control before the heart attack. That same poorly controlled person has more complications, such as shock and heart failure, from a heart attack than the person without diabetes. After a heart attack occurs, the outlook is much worse for the person with diabetes. A second heart attack occurs in 50 percent of people with diabetes (as opposed to 25 percent of people without diabetes), and the death rate in five years is 80 percent (versus 25 percent for people without diabetes).

The picture is not a pretty one for the person with diabetes who has coronary artery disease. The treatment options are the same for people with and without diabetes. Therapy to dissolve the clot of blood that is obstructing the coronary artery can be used, but people with diabetes do not do as well with *angioplasty,* the technique by which a tube is placed into the artery to clean it out and open it up. New techniques using certain chemicals in the tube are making this better therapy. People with diabetes do as well with surgery to bypass the obstruction (called *bypass surgery*) as people without diabetes, but the long-term prognosis for keeping the graft open is not as good.

Metabolic syndrome

The earliest abnormality in type 2 diabetes is insulin resistance, which is found in people even before diabetes can be diagnosed. People with impaired glucose tolerance, and even 25 percent of the population with normal glucose tolerance, have evidence of insulin resistance. The condition, formerly known as the *insulin resistance syndrome,* is now called the *metabolic syndrome.* It is particularly worrisome because it is being found in obese children and adolescents, resulting in greater danger of diabetes and an early heart attack in these children. The next twenty years will show us how these risks play out.

Several features accompany insulin resistance, which is associated with three times the incidence of coronary artery disease compared to people with normal insulin sensitivity:

- **Hypertension:** High blood pressure may be a consequence of the increased insulin required to keep the glucose normal when a patient is insulin resistant. When people are given insulin to control the glucose, a rise in blood pressure often occurs.

- **Abnormalities of blood fats:** The level of triglycerides is elevated, as is the amount of small, dense LDL (low density lipoprotein), a particle in the blood that carries bad cholesterol. At the same time, you see a decline in the amount of HDL (high density lipoprotein), the good cholesterol particle that helps to clean out the arteries.

- **Microalbuminuria:** The presence of microalbuminuria strongly correlates with the development of coronary artery disease. (See the section "Early indications of kidney disease," earlier in the chapter.)

- **C-reactive protein:** This marker for inflammation in the body (easily obtained by a blood test) rises as the severity of the metabolic syndrome increases. It indicates that inflammation plays an important role in coronary artery disease. The important role of inflammation is confirmed by the presence of inflammatory factors in the blood that come from fat tissue and that increase production of fats while they block glucose metabolism, as well as the presence of inflammatory cells that promote atherosclerosis in the arteries.

✔ **Increased plasminogen activator inhibitor-1:** This chemical, which blocks the activity of plasminogen activator, prevents the breakdown of blood clots that form in the arteries of the heart and other areas.

✔ **Increased abdominal visceral fat:** You can lose a lot of this fat, which is found at the waistline, by dieting and losing 5 to 10 percent of your body weight.

✔ **Obesity:** Many people with the metabolic syndrome are obese, but not all. Likewise, many people who are obese do not have the metabolic syndrome.

✔ **Sedentary lifestyle:** This feature is also often found, but an active lifestyle does not preclude the metabolic syndrome.

The preceding features, plus some others that I do not list, are found in people who have an increased tendency to have coronary artery disease and heart attacks. Keep in mind that the metabolic syndrome may be present even when diabetes is not. The metabolic syndrome is probably a primary abnormality and not a consequence of an elevated blood glucose over time.

When insulin resistance is present in diabetes, lowering the blood glucose may decrease the complications of a heart attack, which are related to high blood glucose. But lowering blood glucose does not impact the increased tendency to have a heart attack in the first place, which is not dependent on a high blood glucose.

A number of treatments are available for the metabolic syndrome. If you are obese and have a sedentary lifestyle, you should correct these problems. Even a small amount of weight loss or exercise can make a major contribution toward decreasing the risk of a heart attack.

You can treat elevated triglyceride and reduced HDL with drugs such as the class called *statins*. The *thiazolidendione drugs* (glitazones) — a new class of drugs of which rosiglitazone and pioglitazone are the only ones currently available (see Chapter 10) — directly attack the insulin resistance. However, I no longer recommend rosiglitazone (see Chapter 10) People with diabetes, as well as people without diabetes but with the features of the metabolic syndrome, may find these drugs useful.

There are some new and interesting features of the metabolic syndrome that remain to be clarified:

✔ Men with elevated levels of parathyroid hormone, a chemical that controls the calcium in the blood are at higher risk of developing metabolic syndrome.

✔ Women with reduced intake of magnesium have a higher incidence of metabolic syndrome.

✔ Abdominal obesity, the presence of visceral fat (see above) is a stronger predictor of insulin resistance than physical fitness in older men and women.

✔ Bariatric surgery to produce a small stomach and divert food lower down the small intestine reverses all the major components of metabolic syndrome.

✔ Low blood levels of the male hormone testosterone predict the occurrence of metabolic syndrome and diabetes in middle-aged men.

✔ The DASH diet, the dietary approach to stop hypertension, improves the metabolic abnormalities of the metabolic syndrome in both men and women. See my book, High Blood Pressure For Dummies (Wiley).

Cardiac autonomic neuropathy

I discuss cardiac autonomic neuropathy briefly in the section on neuropathy, earlier in this chapter. Basically, the heart is under the control of nerves, and high glucose levels can damage these nerves. Your doctor can test for this condition in a number of ways:

✔ **Measure the resting heart rate:** It may be abnormally high (greater than 100).

✔ **Measure the standing blood pressure:** It may fall abnormally low (a decrease of 20 mm sustained for 3 minutes) compared to the sitting blood pressure.

✔ **Measure the variation in heart rate** when the patient breathes in compared to breathing out: The variation may be abnormally low (under 10).

The presence of cardiac autonomic neuropathy results in a diminished survival even among patients who don't have coronary artery disease.

Cardiomyopathy

Cardiomyopathy refers to an enlarged heart and scarring of the heart muscle in the absence of coronary artery disease. As a result, the heart does not pump enough blood with each stroke. The patient may be able to compensate by a more rapid heart rate, but if hypertension is present, a stable condition can deteriorate.

The key treatment in this condition is control of the blood pressure as well as control of the blood glucose. Studies in animals in which diabetic cardiomyopathy has been induced have shown healing by controlling the blood glucose.

Diabetic Blood Vessel Disease Away from the Heart

The same processes that affect the coronary arteries can affect the arteries to the brain, producing cerebrovascular disease, and the arteries to the rest of the body, producing peripheral vascular disease. I explain each condition in the following sections.

Peripheral vascular disease

Peripheral vascular disease (PVD) occurs much earlier in the person with diabetes than in the person without diabetes and proceeds more rapidly. This clogging of the arteries to parts of your body other than the heart and brain results in the loss of pulses in the feet; after ten years of diabetes, a third of men and women no longer feel a pulse in their feet. The most common symptom of PVD is intermittent pain in the calves, thighs, or buttocks that begins after some walking and subsides with rest. People with PVD have a reduction in life expectancy. When PVD occurs, just as when CAD occurs, it is much worse in people with diabetes because more of their arteries are involved.

The major screening test for peripheral vascular disease is the anklebrachial index (ABI). The systolic blood pressure in the ankle is divided by the systolic blood pressure in the arm. A result of .95 or greater is normal. A result of less than .75 suggests serious peripheral vascular disease. Some people with diabetes have a lot of calcium in their arteries and get a higher blood pressure in the ankle than the arm. If the ABI is more than 1 and the systolic blood pressure in the ankle is more than 300 mm mercury or 75 greater than the arm, this condition also suggests PVD.

An ABI in a person with diabetes that is less than .9 is associated with a much higher risk of death from a heart attack according to a study published in *Diabetes Care* in March 2006.

In addition to diabetes, certain risk factors increase the severity of PVD. The following risk factors are unavoidable:

- ✔ **Genetic factors:** PVD is more common in some families and certain ethnic groups, especially African Americans.
- ✔ **Age:** The risk of PVD increases as you age.

The following risk factors are within your control:

- ✔ Smoking, which clearly promotes early foot amputation
- ✔ Hypercholesterolemia (high cholesterol)

✔ High glucose

✔ Hypertension

✔ Obesity

In addition to controlling the preceding factors as much as possible, you may need to take drugs that help prevent closure of the arteries and loss of blood supply. Aspirin, which inhibits clotting, is among the most useful. Trental improves the circulation of cells in the blood. In addition, exercise improves blood flow and promotes the development of blood vessels around an obstruction. If none of these measures reverses the symptoms, some form of surgery that opens or bypasses the blocked arteries may be necessary.

Cerebrovascular disease

Cerebrovascular disease (CVD) is a disease of the arteries that supply the brain with oxygen and nutrients. What I say about peripheral vascular disease in the preceding section also covers cerebrovascular disease, with some exceptions. The risk factors and the approach to treatment are similar. However, the symptoms are very different because the clogged arteries in CVD supply the brain.

If a temporary reduction in blood supply to the brain occurs, the person suffers from a *transient ischemic attack,* or TIA. This temporary loss of brain function may present itself as slurring of speech, weakness on one side of the body, or numbness. TIA may disappear after a few minutes, but it comes back again some hours to days later. If a major artery to the brain completely closes, the person suffers a stroke. Fortunately, stroke victims who are seen soon enough after the stroke can take advantage of clot-dissolving materials.

Smoking and diabetes

As we all know, smoking has a number of ill effects on people without diabetes, but the effects are even worse in people with diabetes. Among other things, smoking:

✔ Reduces blood flow in arteries and blocks increased flow when it is needed

✔ Increases pain in the legs in people with peripheral vascular disease and in the heart in people with coronary artery disease

✔ Increases *atheromatous plaques,* the changes in arteries in the heart and other

areas (like the brain and the legs) that precede closing of the blood vessels

✔ Increases clustering of *platelets,* the blood elements that form a plug or clot that blocks the artery

✔ Increases blood pressure, which also worsens atheromatous plaques

These problems don't even take into account the effects of smoking on the lungs, the bladder, and the rest of the body.

People with diabetes are at increased risk for CVD just as they are for PVD. Their disease tends to be worse than the disease in a person without diabetes, and they can have blockage in many small blood vessels in the brain that leads to the loss of intellectual function, a symptom similar to Alzheimer's disease.

The treatable risk factors for CVD are the same as those for PVD (see the preceding section). You should make attempts to improve them, particularly the high blood pressure.

Diabetic Foot Disease

If I ever have an opportunity to save people from the consequences of diabetes, it's in this section of the book. About 70,000 amputations occur in the United States each year, and more than half of them are done on people with diabetes. Despite the wonderful surgery to bring more blood into the feet, the number of amputations is actually rising.

Good medical care can prevent amputations. Your doctor should look at your feet as routinely as he or she measures your weight.

In the section on neuropathy, earlier in this chapter, I point out that a filament that requires a pressure of 10 grams to be felt can differentiate the patient who will not suffer damage to the feet under normal walking conditions from the patient who will. All doctors who have patients with diabetes should have this filament to test the feet at least annually. Even better, you should have your own filament and test yourself any time you feel like it. If you can't feel the filament, you had better start looking at your feet every day. See Chapter 7 for where to obtain a filament.

If your feet are dry, you may have loss of sweating. Loss of sweating is usually accompanied by the loss of touch sensation and the development of ulcers. You need to moisturize your feet, first by soaking them in water (which you test with your hand for its temperature), and then by drying them with a towel and applying a moisturizer.

Ulcers of the foot can develop in a number of ways:

- ✔ Constant pressure
- ✔ Sudden higher pressure
- ✔ Constantly repeated moderate pressure

It takes very little pressure, if constantly applied, to damage the skin. If you have diminished sensation, some of the following tips may save your feet:

- ✔ Change your shoes about every five hours.

- ✔ If you have new shoes, change them every two hours at first. Your shoes should not be too tight or too loose.

- ✔ Never walk barefoot.

- ✔ Shake out your shoes before you put them on.

- ✔ Inspect your feet daily, with a mirror if necessary.

- ✔ Do not use a heating pad on your feet.

- ✔ Stop smoking. If you smoke, you are asking for an amputation.

If you do develop an ulcer, the treatment is to take pressure off the site by resting the foot and elevating it. When the infection is localized in a foot with adequate blood supply, a plaster cast is applied to overcome the natural tendency to want to stand or walk. The cast protects the ulcer from slight trauma that could prevent healing.

There is a product that has been shown to speed the healing of deep diabetic foot ulcers when it is combined with good wound care. (Good wound care means carefully removing dead tissue and keeping your weight off the ulcer, along with treating any infection and controlling your blood glucose.) The product, called Regranex Gel, is distributed by Ortho-McNeil and is applied to a clean wound bed once daily. You should see significant reduction in the size of the ulcer within 10 weeks and complete healing by 20 weeks. The long duration for healing is a problem, because Regranex Gel is very expensive. However, a typical deep diabetic ulcer is very expensive to treat in any case, and if this product can speed up your healing, it may be worthwhile.

I must reiterate that ulcers of the foot, which can lead to amputation in people with diabetes, are entirely preventable. If your feet lack sensation, your doctor must examine them at every visit, and you must examine them daily. At the first sign of a problem, take appropriate action.

Skin Disease in Diabetes

Many conditions involving the skin are unique to the person with diabetes because of the treatment and complications of the disease. The most common and important complications include the following:

- ✔ Bruises occur due to the cutting of blood vessels by the insulin needle.

- ✔ *Vitiligo* (loss of skin pigmentation) is part of the autoimmune aspect of type 1 diabetes and cannot be prevented.

✔ *Necrobiosis lipoidica,* which also affects people without diabetes, creates patches of reddish-brown skin on the shins or ankles, and the skin becomes thin and can ulcerate. Females tend to have this condition more often than males. Steroid injections are used to treat this condition, and the areas eventually become depressed and brown.

✔ *Xanthelasma,* which are small yellow flat areas called *plaques* on the eyelids, occur even when cholesterol is not elevated.

✔ *Alopecia,* or loss of hair, occurs in type 1 diabetes, but the cause is unknown.

✔ *Insulin hypertrophy* is the accumulation of fatty tissue where insulin is injected. This condition is prevented by moving the injection site around.

✔ *Insulin lipoatrophy* is the loss of fat where the insulin is injected. Although the cause is unknown, this condition is rarely seen now that human insulin has replaced beef and pork insulin (see Chapter 10).

✔ Dry skin is a consequence of diabetic neuropathy, which leads to a lack of sweating.

✔ Fungal infections occur under the nails or between the toes. Fungus likes moisture and elevated glucose. Lowering your glucose and keeping your toes dry prevents these infections. Medications may cure this problem, but it recurs if glucose and moisture are not managed.

✔ *Acanthosis nigricans,* a velvety-feeling increase in pigmentation on the back of the neck and the armpits, causes no problems and needs no treatment. This condition is usually found when insulin resistance exists. It is seen in children with type 2 diabetes.

✔ Diabetic thick skin, which is thicker than normal skin, occurs in people who have had diabetes for more than ten years.

Gum Disease in Diabetes

The major problem that people with diabetes may have in their mouths is gum disease. This problem develops because the higher concentration of glucose in the mouth promotes the growth of germs, which mix with food and saliva to form plaque on your gums. If you do not brush your teeth twice a day and floss your teeth once a day, the plaque may harden into tarter, which is very hard for you to remove. The gums may become brittle and bleed easily, and then you have gingivitis. You may experience pain and bad breath, and eventually the gums may become so weakened that they cannot support your teeth.

Controlling your blood glucose is a key step in preventing gum disease. Visiting your dentist for routine cleanings of your teeth twice a year is another important way to keep your gums healthy. Interestingly, people with diabetes do not seem to develop cavities more often than people who do not have the disease.

Chapter 6

Diabetes, Sexual Function, and Pregnancy

*N*othing is quite so pleasant as walking into the hospital room of a mother with diabetes holding her healthy newborn. Pregnancy associated with diabetes used to be a disaster for both the baby and the mother. No longer. With the proper precautions, the diabetic pregnancy can proceed like a pregnancy without diabetes. This chapter describes everything you need to know from start to finish, including overcoming obstacles to intercourse, enjoying a healthy pregnancy, and delivering a healthy baby.

Examining Erection Problems

If carefully questioned, up to 50 percent of all males with diabetes admit to having difficulty with sexual function. This difficulty usually takes the form of *erectile dysfunction (ED)*, the inability to have or sustain an erection sufficient for intercourse. It develops 10 to 15 years earlier in men with diabetes than in men without diabetes. After the age of 70 more than 95 percent of men with diabetes have erectile dysfunction. Many factors besides diabetes can cause the same problem, and you should rule them out before blaming diabetes. After you eliminate the following possibilities for erectile dysfunction, you can feel confident that diabetes is the source of the problem:

✔ Trauma to the penis

✔ Medications, such as certain antihypertensives and antidepressants

✔ Hormonal abnormalities, such as insufficient production of the male hormone testosterone or overproduction of a hormone from the brain called *prolactin.* Although prolactin is the hormone in women that causes breast enlargement in pregnancy and later production of milk, its role in men is not clear.

✔ Poor blood supply to the penis due to blockage of the artery by peripheral vascular disease (see Chapter 5), which can be treated very effectively by microvascular surgery.

✔ *Psychogenic impotence,* an inability to have an erection for psychological rather than physical reasons. This would be managed by a therapist, especially a sex therapist rather than drugs.

In order to understand how diabetes affects an erection, you need to first understand how an erection is normally produced.

The erection process

As a result of some form of stimulation — such as touch, sight, or sound — the brain activates nerves in the *parasympathetic nervous system,* which is part of the autonomic nervous system. These nerves cause muscles to relax so that blood flow into the penis greatly increases. As blood flow increases, the veins through which blood leaves the penis compress, and the penis becomes erect. An erect penis contains about 11 times as much blood as a flaccid penis. With sufficient stimulation, muscles contract, propelling semen through the *urethra* (the tube in the penis that normally carries urine from the bladder) to the outside of the body. The pleasant sensation that occurs along with the muscle contractions (*ejaculation*) is called *orgasm.*

Orgasm and ejaculation are the result of stimulation by the other side of the autonomic nervous system, the sympathetic nervous system. As the stimulation causes contraction of the muscles, it closes the muscle over the bladder so that urine does not normally accompany expulsion of semen and the semen does not go back into the bladder.

Diabetes can damage the parasympathetic nervous system so that the male cannot get an erection sufficient for sexual intercourse. The sympathetic nervous system is spared, so that ejaculation and orgasm can occur, but intercourse may be unpleasant for both partners because of the psychological consequence of not being able to sustain a firm erection.

The onset of failure of erection is determined by the following factors:

✔ **Degree of control of the blood glucose:** Better control is associated with fewer problems.

✔ **Duration of the diabetes:** The longer you have diabetes, the more likely you will be unable to have an erection.

> ✔ **Interaction with your partner:** A positive relationship is important.
>
> ✔ **Use of drugs, tobacco, or alcohol:** Both may prevent erection.
>
> ✔ **State of mind:** A positive frame of mind is associated with more success-ful erections.

Discussing ED with your doctor

Although sexual intercourse tends to be an embarrassing topic for many men and women, if you have diabetes and have a problem in this key area of life, you need to discuss it with your doctor. Some doctors find this topic just as embarrassing as some patients. Any doctor who treats patients with diabetes should bring the topic up in the first meeting and annually thereafter. If he or she does not, it is up to you to broach the subject. If you read the explanation of the normal development of an erection and your experience differs from that, discuss it with your physician. There are so many ways to treat it, and the lack of an erection can have such a profound effect upon your self-esteem and your relationship with another person that it is sad to discover how often a new patient has been suffering in silence for years.

Treatment for erectile dysfunction

Fortunately for the male with diabetes with erectile dysfunction, numerous approaches to treatment exist, beginning with drugs, continuing with exter-nal devices to create an erection, and ending with implantable devices that provide a very satisfactory erection. Treatment is successful in 90 percent or more of men, but only 5 percent ever discuss the problem with their doctors. The following sections discuss these treatment options:

Viagra and similar medications

Viagra, also called *sildenafil,* has been specifically studied in males with dia-betes and is successful in 70 percent of patients.

Viagra does not seem to affect diabetic control, but it is not free of side effects. Some men experience headaches, facial flushing, or indigestion, which gener-ally decline with continued use of the drug. Viagra has also been found to cause a temporary color tinge to a man's vision, as well as increased sensitiv-ity to light and blurred vision. These side effects also decline with continued use of the drug.

Viagra is taken no more than once a day, about an hour before sexual activity. While the starting dose is 50 milligrams for men, when diabetes is present, 100 mg is often required. The drug itself doesn't cause erections; an erection occurs only as a result of some kind of sexual stimulation. But Viagra does prevent an erection from subsiding so that it lasts longer. The effects of Viagra can last for four to six hours after taking it.

Pfizer, which makes Viagra, could not expect to have the playing field to itself for very long, given that the game is something most men want to play. Bayer Pharmaceuticals and GlaxoSmithKline have now brought vardenafil, which they call *Levitra,* to the marketplace. Its characteristics are very similar to Viagra but the dosage is 10 mg, which probably means 20 mg for men with diabetes.

Eli Lilly and ICOS Corporation have brought out tadalafil, which they call *Cialis.* It works like Viagra and Levitra but stays active for 36 hours. In addition, its onset of action is 20 minutes, half the time of Viagra or Levitra. Cialis has been nicknamed the "weekender pill" because it permits spontaneous sexual activity from Friday to Sunday. The starting dose for Cialis is 20 mg, but, again, the male with diabetes may need to start at twice that amount.

Some men must not take Viagra or the other two drugs. Men who have chest pain often take nitrate drugs, the most common of which is nitroglycerine. The combination of Viagra and nitrates may cause a significant and possibly fatal drop in blood pressure.

In October 2007, the U.S. Food and Drug Administration began to receive reports of sudden loss of hearing in men taking the drugs described above. Some of the men also reported dizziness and ringing in the ear. The hearing loss was temporary in one third of cases and too recent in the others. It begins within hours to a day or two of starting these drugs. It involves only one ear. There have been only 29 cases among the millions who have taken the drugs beginning in 1996. If you experience hearing loss, take no more of the drug and report it to your doctor. Since the side effect is so rare, it should not prevent you from using the drugs, but you should be aware of it.

Injection into the penis

The patient himself can use two different kinds of injections to create an erection. The first one, a mixture of the drugs papaverine and phentolamine, has for the most part been replaced by alprostadil (Caverject or Edex), a chemical that relaxes the blood vessels in the penis to allow more flow. Alprostadil does not require sexual stimulation in order to work.

The drug is injected about 30 minutes before intercourse and no more than once in 24 hours and three times per week. An injection of either preparation gives a full erection lasting about an hour in 85 to 95 percent of men, except for those who have the most severe loss of blood flow to the penis.

Complications of injections are rare but include bruising, pain, and the formation of nodules at the injection site. A very rare complication is *priapism,* where the penis maintains its erection for many hours. If the erection lasts more than four hours, the patient must see his doctor to get an injection of a *vasoconstrictor,* a drug that squeezes down the arteries into the penis so that blood flow is interrupted.

Suppository in the penis

Alprostadil — the chemical that can be injected into the penis — also comes in a suppository form. The patient inserts a tube containing this small pill into the opening of the penis after urination. When the tube is fully in the opening, the man squeezes the top so that the pill exits the tube. This preparation, called *MUSE,* comes in several different strengths so that patients can use a higher dose if the lower dose does not result in a satisfactory erection. It may safely be used twice in 24 hours. A few men experience pain with this procedure. Sexual stimulation is unnecessary to achieve an erection.

Vacuum constriction devices

These tubes, which fit over the penis, create a closed space when pressed against the patient's body. A pump draws out the air in the tube, and blood rushes into the penis to replace the air. When the penis is erect, a rubber band is placed around the base of the penis to keep the blood inside it. Sometimes pain and numbness of the penis occur. Because a rubber band is constricting the penis, semen does not get through, so conception does not take place. The rubber band may be kept on for up to 30 minutes.

Implanted penile prostheses

If the patient doesn't like the idea of injecting himself in his penis or using a vacuum device, and if Viagra does not work for him, a *prosthesis* (an artificial substitute) can be implanted in the penis to give a very satisfactory erection. Prostheses come in several varieties. A semi-rigid type produces a permanent erection, but some men do not like the inconvenience of a permanent erection. An inflatable prosthesis involves a pump in the scrotal sac that contains fluid. The pump can be squeezed to transfer the fluid into balloons in the penis to stiffen it. When not pumped up, the penis appears normally soft. In the past few years, the surgery to insert these prostheses has become very satisfactory.

Facing Female Sexual Problems

Because women don't have penises that must enlarge during sex, sexual dysfunction is not as visually obvious as it is in men. But as many as half of the women with diabetes have problems with sexual function, and, the problems can be just as difficult to handle as they are for men. The following problems are associated with diabetes:

- ✔ You may have a dry mouth and dry vagina because of the high blood glucose.
- ✔ Your menstrual function may be irregular when your diabetes is out of control.
- ✔ You may develop yeast infections of the vagina that make intercourse unpleasant.

- Because type 2 diabetes is usually associated with obesity, you may feel fat and unattractive.

- You may feel uncomfortable discussing the problem with your partner or your physician.

- You may have loss of bladder control due to a neurogenic bladder (see Chapter 5).

- Your increasing age may cause a reduction in estrogen secretion and the vaginal thinning and dryness associated with that change.

Menopause can cause several of the same difficulties as diabetes-related sexual dysfunction, particularly the dry vagina and irregular menstrual function. You must rule out menopause before assuming that diabetes is the source of the problem. Unlike the case with men with diabetes, this is the only important abnormality that is known to cause sexual problems in women that may simulate the problems of diabetes.

The female with long-standing diabetes may have several other problems that are specific to her sexual organs. These problems include

- **Reduced lubrication because of parasympathetic nerve involvement:** Lubrication serves to permit easier entry of the penis, but it also increases the sensitivity of the vagina to touch, thus increasing pleasant sensations.

- **Reduced blood flow because of diabetic blood vessel disease:** Some of the lubrication comes from fluid within the blood vessels.

- **Loss of skin sensation around the vaginal area:** This loss reduces pleasure.

Most women who have problems with lubrication, whether due to diabetes or menopause, medicate themselves with over-the-counter preparations. These preparations fall into three categories:

- Water-based lubricants, like K-Y jelly and In Pursuit of Passion, which are probably the easiest to use and clean up

- Oil-based lubricants, like vegetable oils

- Petroleum-based lubricants, which are not recommended because of the possibility of bacterial infection

Estrogen, which can be taken by mouth or placed in the dry vagina in suppository form, also may be useful for the menopausal woman.

When psychological or interpersonal issues exist, a discussion with a therapist, the use of antidepressant medications (some of which can dry the vagina, by the way), and sex therapy with your partner are important steps to take to improve sexual pleasure.

As with all of the diabetic problems you read about in this book, maximum control of the blood glucose prevents or slows down a lot of these complications.

Striving for a Healthy Pregnancy

Pregnancy in a mother with diabetes is definitely more complicated than in a mother without diabetes. For this reason, diabetes centers around the country employ the latest techniques and equipment and make knowledgeable health care workers available.

About 0.4 percent of pregnancies occur in women with preexisting diabetes, called *pregestational diabetes,* and an additional 2 to 4 percent occur in women who develop diabetes sometime in the second half of the pregnancy, called *gestational diabetes.* Four million births occur in the United States annually, and diabetes affects 100,000 or more pregnancies each year.

If you have diabetes and want to become pregnant, you need to confer with an expert in pregnancy and diabetes before you conceive. In the following sections, I explain potential complications you may experience and some steps you should take to ensure the healthiest pregnancy possible.

Realizing the body's reaction to pregnancy

In a nondiabetic pregnancy, the woman's body makes enough insulin to overcome the effect of pregnancy hormones (which block insulin action), and her blood glucose stays normal. But a woman with type 1 diabetes can't make more insulin, and during pregnancy she needs two or three times her usual dose to counteract the effect of her hormones. This increased need for insulin in a woman with type 1 diabetes usually stabilizes in the last several weeks of the pregnancy; by the last one or two weeks, the mother-to-be may actually begin to have hypoglycemia. After the baby and the placenta are delivered, her insulin needs plummet immediately.

A woman with type 1 diabetes may have some retinopathy (see Chapter 5) before she becomes pregnant. If the condition is severe, her eyes may deteriorate during the pregnancy. Although scientists aren't yet clear on why this tendency to deteriorate increases during pregnancy, the deterioration probably results from rapid improvement of blood glucose control in a woman who has been poorly controlled previously. If glucose control is improved or if laser photocoagulation (see Chapter 5) is carried out before the pregnancy, this deterioration does not take place. After the baby is delivered, her eyes will return to their previous state.

There is much more about pregnancy in the woman with type 1 diabetes in my book *Type 1 Diabetes For Dummies* (Wiley).

If you're thinking about becoming pregnant and you have diabetes-related eye disease, that condition must be stabilized before you try to conceive.

Kidney disease, or *nephropathy* (see Chapter 5), increases the danger of complications of pregnancy for both the mother and baby. Severe, permanent worsening of the nephropathy is unusual as a result of pregnancy, but a temporary decline in kidney function in the mother may occur. The baby may have to be delivered early and may suffer some growth retardation.

Being proactive before and during pregnancy

You must take action in advance to avoid potential problems by controlling your glucose before conception. (See Part III for more on how to manage your diabetes.) In addition, you need to monitor your diet after you become pregnant.

Following are some other key steps you should take to improve your chances or a problem-free pregnancy:

- ✓ **Lose weight:** Obesity, which is prevalent in type 2 patients, puts a mom-to-be at greater risk for hypertension during pregnancy.

- ✓ **Quit smoking:** Children of mothers who smoke during pregnancy are at much greater risk of developing obesity and diabetes later in life.

- ✓ **Use insulin for glucose control:** If you have type 2 diabetes and are taking oral agents to lower your glucose, you need to switch to insulin to control your glucose during pregnancy.

For more detailed information about what to do during pregnancy, see the section "Treating diabetes during pregnancy," later in the chapter.

Most diabetic pregnancies can be allowed to go to term at 39 weeks. However, if the mother-to-be has hypertension or a previous history of delivery problems, her doctor may advocate earlier delivery.

Diagnosing gestational diabetes

Experts disagree as to whether all pregnant women who don't already have diabetes need to be checked for it. Some advocate selective screening, suggesting that a thin pregnant woman with no family history of diabetes who is physically active is an unlikely candidate for diabetes. You are unlikely to develop gestational diabetes if you have the following characteristics:

✔ You are less than 25 years old

✔ Your weight is normal before the pregnancy

✔ You are not a member of an ethnic group with a high incidence of type 2 diabetes (Hispanic Americans, African Americans, Native Americans, Pacific Islanders)

✔ There is no family history of diabetes in mother, father, sisters, brothers, or other children

✔ You have no previous history of abnormal tolerance to glucose

✔ You have no previous history of poor outcome of a birth or have previously given birth to a large baby

However, the current consensus is to screen all women because a small but significant number of patients with gestational diabetes will be missed if all women are not screened.

Everyone agrees that if your glucose tolerance is normal in weeks 27 to 31 of the pregnancy, you don't need to do more screening. If you experienced gestational diabetes during a previous pregnancy, the screening test is done much earlier — as early as the 13th week. Other reasons for earlier screening are

✔ Previous delivery of a large baby

✔ Obesity

✔ Glucose in the urine

✔ Close family members with diabetes

The screening test is done between weeks 24 and 28 of the pregnancy. No preparation is necessary. You consume 50 grams of glucose, and a blood glucose level is obtained from a vein one hour later. If the glucose level is less than 140, it's considered normal. If it's greater than 140, a further test is done before making a diagnosis of gestational diabetes, because many women who have a value greater than 140 do not necessarily have diabetes. The definitive test is done as follows:

✔ The woman prepares by eating at least 150 grams of carbohydrate daily for three days and then fasting for at least eight hours before the test.

✔ The woman drinks 100 grams of glucose to begin the test.

✔ Blood glucose is measured before the glucose meal and at one hour, two hours, and three hours after drinking the glucose.

✔ A diagnosis of gestational diabetes is made if two or more of the samples exceed the levels in Table 6-1.

Table 6-1	Excessive Glucose Levels That Signal Gestational Diabetes		
Before	*1 Hour*	*2 Hours*	*3 Hours*
95 mg/dl (5.3 mmol/L)	180mg/dl (10.0 mmol/L)	155 mg/dl (8.6 mmol/L)	140 mg/dl (7.8 mmol/L)

Realizing risks to mother and baby

Whether you have diabetes before pregnancy or develop gestational diabetes, you face many considerations regarding your own health and the health of your baby.

Persistently high blood glucose left untreated has major consequences for both mother and fetus. If high glucose is present early in the pregnancy, the result may be *congenital malformations* (physical abnormalities that may be life threatening) in the fetus. In the third trimester, the growing fetus may exhibit *macrosomia* (abnormal largeness; see Figure 6-1) that can lead to an early delivery or damage to the baby or mother during delivery.

Figure 6-1: A baby with macrosomia.

Babies develop normally if their fathers have diabetes but their mothers don't. The environment in which the fetus is developing is responsible for the potential abnormalities. Elevated blood glucose, abnormalities of proteins and fats that result from the elevated glucose, and the loss of sensitivity to insulin explain the problems.

Measuring the risks

The hemoglobin A1c (see Chapter 7) is an excellent measurement of overall glucose control and provides a good indicator for the risk of miscarriage. If a pregnant woman's hemoglobin A1c is high, it indicates that she was in poor glucose control at conception, and the likelihood of a miscarriage is greater. If overall glucose control is normal, the baby of the woman with diabetes is no more likely to be miscarried than that of a woman without diabetes.

The situation for congenital malformations is a little more complicated. The occurrence of these malformations rises with increasing glucose, but the level of *ketones* (the breakdown product of fats) also impacts their occurrence. However, measuring the ketones will not tell you if malformations will definitely occur.

Early pregnancy problems

The major concern of a woman with pregestational diabetes is to be under good blood glucose control at the time of conception. Both miscarriages and congenital malformations are a result of poor glucose control at conception and shortly thereafter. Both high blood glucose and low blood glucose can induce malformations. (For more on managing diabetes, see Part III.)

However, a woman in poor control of her diabetes has more trouble conceiving a baby than a woman with good glucose control, which may be the major reason that more babies aren't born with congenital malformations.

The woman who has gestational diabetes mellitus does not have to worry that her baby's likelihood of having congenital malformations is greater than a baby whose mother does not have diabetes. This likelihood is because her blood glucose did not start to rise until halfway through the pregnancy, long after the baby's important body structures were formed.

Late pregnancy problems

A baby is considered large if it weighs more than 4 kilograms or 8.8 pounds at birth. Keep in mind that most large babies are the healthy offspring of mothers without diabetes. Their growth is proportional throughout the pregnancy so that their shoulders are not out of proportion to their heads, and delivery is not complicated.

However, both the woman with pregestational diabetes and the woman with gestational diabetes need to be concerned about having a large baby. This largeness is not proportional. The areas that are most responsive to insulin, where fat is stored in the baby, are the ones that enlarge the most. (See the sidebar "Why macrosomia occurs" for more information.)

Why macrosomia occurs

Macrosomia, or abnormal largeness in a fetus, has to do with the elevated glucose, fat, and amino acid levels in the second half of pregnancy for a mother with diabetes. If these levels aren't lowered, the fetus is exposed to high levels. The high levels, especially of glucose, stimulate the fetal pancreas to begin to make insulin earlier and to store these extra nutrients. The fetus becomes large wherever fat is stored, such as in the shoulders, chest, abdomen, arms, and legs. Because they are large, macrosomic babies are delivered early in order to make the delivery easier and avoid birth trauma. However, though they are large, they are not fully mature.

Treating diabetes during pregnancy

In addition to controlling your glucose levels before conceiving, if you have pregestational diabetes, you need to do the following:

- ✔ Discontinue taking prescription drugs that can harm a fetus.
- ✔ Have your eyes, kidneys, and blood pressure evaluated to establish a baseline for future damage control.
- ✔ Stop tobacco and alcohol use.

You need to achieve a stricter level of glucose control during pregnancy than when you aren't pregnant. Your fetus is removing glucose from you at a rapid rate, so your blood glucose level is lower than usual. In addition, your body turns to fat for fuel much sooner, so you produce ketones earlier. Too many ketones can damage the fetus as well. The fact that you break down fat so early is termed *accelerated starvation.*

Monitoring your glucose and ketones

In order to maintain your blood glucose at the proper level, you must measure it more frequently. You should measure it before meals, at bedtime, and occasionally one hour after eating. Your goal is to achieve the levels of blood glucose listed in Table 6-2.

Table 6-2	Optimum Levels of Blood Glucose	
Fasting and Premeal	*1 Hour After Eating*	*2 Hours After Eating*
Less than 90 mg/dl (5 mmol/L)	Less than 120 mg/dl (6.7 mmol/L)	Less than 120 mg/dl (6.7 mmol/L)

Recent studies have shown that the glucose level one hour after eating may be the most important for the pregnant woman with diabetes to keep under control. Although you can deliver insulin in other ways besides a syringe and needle (see Chapter 10), several studies indicate that the syringe-and-needle method is as effective as any other for the pregnant woman with diabetes.

You also need to check for ketones in the urine before breakfast and before supper. You can do so by placing a test strip in the stream of urine. The strip indicates whether ketones are present. If the test strip is positive, it means that you are not eating enough carbohydrates and your body is going into accelerated starvation. Too much of this condition is not good for the growing fetus.

Eating well

Your appropriate amount of weight gain depends upon your weight at the time you become pregnant. Your BMI determines your weight gain. You need to determine your BMI (see Chapter 3 if you're not sure how to do this calculation). If your BMI is normal, you should gain 20 to 25 pounds during the pregnancy. However, if you're overweight, you need to gain less weight through the pregnancy, 15 to 20 pounds. If you're obese, you should gain no more than 17 or 18 pounds. And if you're underweight, you may gain 25 to 30 pounds.

Chapter 8 tells you what you need to know about diet and diabetes, but as a pregnant woman with diabetes, you have some special requirements:

- ✔ **Your daily food intake should be 35 to 38 kilocalories per kilogram of ideal body weight.** (In this book, I use the term *kilocalories* rather than *calories,* which is an incorrect term.) You can use your height to determine your ideal body weight (IBW). As a woman, you should weigh 100 pounds if you are 5 feet tall, plus 5 pounds for every inch over 5 feet. For example, a 5-foot 4-inch woman should weigh 120 pounds, ideally (and *approximately,* because these numbers represent a range, not a single weight). You can change that figure to kilograms by dividing the pounds by 2.2. Then multiply that number by 35 to get the low end of the daily calorie intake and by 38 to get the high end. So if you weigh 120 pounds, you weigh 54.6 kilograms. Your daily food intake should be between 1,900 and 2,100 kilocalories.

- ✔ **Your protein intake should be 1.5 to 2 grams per kilogram of IBW.** The woman with the IBW of 54.6 should eat about 110 grams of protein daily. Because each gram of protein contains four kilocalories, protein takes up about 440 of the 2,100 daily kilocalories.

- ✔ **Your carbohydrate intake should be 50 to 55 percent of your daily kilocalories.** If you need approximately 2,000 daily kilocalories, about 1,000 kilocalories should be carbohydrate. Because each gram of carbohydrate has 4 kilocalories, just like protein, this amounts to 250 grams of carbohydrate.

✔ **Your fat intake should be less than 30 percent of the total daily kilocalories.** Using 2,000 kilocalories as our target, that amounts to 630 kilocalories of fat. Because fat contains 9 kilocalories per gram, this equals 70 grams of fat a day.

Translating grams of food into amounts of specific foods would require another whole book. Because an excellent one on the subject has already been written, I refer you to *Nutrition For Dummies,* 3rd Edition, by Carol Ann Rinzler (Wiley) to get this information.

✔ **You need to eat three meals a day plus a bedtime snack.** Frequently eating helps prevent the accelerated starvation that results from the prolonged fast between supper and breakfast.

✔ **You must maintain fasting and premeal glucose levels below 90 mg/dl.** Your glucose should be less than 120 mg/dl one hour after meals.

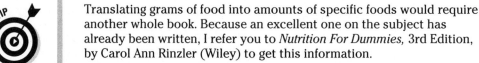

In addition, you can use a good multivitamin and mineral preparation. A moderate amount of exercise is also very helpful in controlling the blood glucose and keeping you in top shape during pregnancy.

Testing for fetal defects

A blood test called a *serum alpha-fetoprotein* can be done 15 weeks into the pregnancy to determine whether neural tube defects exist in the fetus. At 18 weeks, an ultrasound can show any malformations of the growing fetus. An ultrasound, by directing a sound at the fetus and catching it as it bounces back to the machine, produces a picture of the fetus that shows the presence of any abnormalities. This harmless test is not painful for the mother or the fetus.

Another useful study during the diabetic pregnancy is the non-stress test. A device is placed on your abdomen that listens to the fetus's heartbeat. When the fetus moves, its heart rate normally speeds up by 15 to 20 beats per minute. This increase in heart rate should normally occur at least three times in a 20-minute period of listening.

Handling issues of gestational diabetes

If you have gestational diabetes, you need not worry about congenital malformations in your baby, but you need to avoid macrosomia. You need to follow the same dietary prescription as the woman with pregestational diabetes, and you need to use insulin if a careful diet does not keep your fasting blood glucose below 90, your glucose one hour after eating below 120, or your glucose two hours after eating below 120. If you can't bring yourself to use insulin shots, glyburide (see Chapter 10) has been shown not to harm the baby since it does not pass through the placenta, although it is not approved by the FDA for this use. Your insulin regimen will probably be simpler than that of the woman with pregestational diabetes because your pancreas can make its own insulin. If you are taking insulin, you will stop doing so at the time of delivery.

Early ultrasound is not necessary for the woman with gestational diabetes unless your doctor suspects that the diabetes was actually there much earlier. An ultrasound at week 38 can show whether fetal macrosomia exists. If macrosomia is present, your doctor will probably perform a caesarean section, where the baby is removed through an incision made in the abdominal wall and then in the uterus.

Delivering the baby

It's best for a woman with diabetes to deliver her baby at the end of 39 weeks, when it has had a chance to mature completely. If the mother does not go into labor spontaneously, the physician usually induces labor.

If you have been taking insulin during pregnancy, nurses will monitor your blood glucose every four hours after you deliver. You blood glucose will be maintained at 70 to 120 mg/dl with insulin, if necessary. The insulin is given in short-acting form as needed and not in large doses of long-acting insulin, which would be around in the circulation when you no longer need it.

Maintaining your health after pregnancy

If you are breastfeeding, which is always a good idea, you need to consume about 300 kilocalories *above* your usual needs. You cannot take oral agents for diabetes because these pass through the milk into the baby. For more information about breastfeeding, see *Breastfeeding For Dummies* by Sharon Perkins and Carol Vannais (Wiley).

For the woman with gestational diabetes, the disease usually disappears when the pregnancy is over. However, a woman who develops gestational diabetes during pregnancy is at a much higher risk for developing diabetes later in life. If your fasting blood glucose is greater than 130 during pregnancy, the risk of developing diabetes again is as much as 75 to 90 percent in the next 10 to 15 years.

If you had gestational diabetes, you need to have a test for glucose tolerance between 6 and 12 weeks after the pregnancy and annually after that if diabetes is not found.

Several factors predispose the woman with gestational diabetes to develop diabetes later on. Some factors that cannot be changed include the following:

- ✔ **Ethnic origin:** Certain ethnic groups, such as Mexican Americans, Native Americans, Asian Americans, and African Americans, are at a higher risk.

- ✔ **Prepregnancy weight:** Women with a higher prepregnancy weight are at a higher risk.

- ✔ **Number of pregnancies:** The more pregnancies you have, the higher your risk.

✔ **Family history of diabetes:** If a family history is present, you are at a higher risk.

✔ **Severity of blood glucose during pregnancy:** Higher blood glucose levels mean a higher risk.

On the other hand, you can reduce several risk factors:

✔ **Future weight gain:** Gain less weight in future pregnancies.

✔ **Future pregnancies:** Have fewer children.

✔ **Physical activity:** Increase your exercise.

✔ **Dietary fat:** Limit the fat in your diet.

✔ **Smoking and certain drugs:** Stop smoking and using drugs.

Women who have had gestational diabetes can use oral contraceptives with low levels of estrogen and progesterone to prevent conception. These drugs, along with hormonal replacement therapy after menopause, do not increase your risk of later diabetes. They may, in fact, decrease the risk and decrease blood glucose levels in those who have diabetes already. Women with type 1 and type 2 diabetes can use the same preparations.

The story is similar for postmenopausal women. A study in *Diabetes Care* in October 2003 showed that the use of estrogens (with or without progestins) by women with diabetes resulted in a decrease in coronary artery disease. Because women with diabetes are at very high risk for coronary artery disease, this finding is an important one.

Another large study reported that women on hormone replacement therapy have better control of their blood glucose than those not on such treatment. This information was reported in *Diabetes Care* in July 2001.

Focusing on your baby's health

Increased understanding of diabetes's impact during pregnancy has resulted in a great reduction in malformations in these babies as well as the macrosomia that leads to complications at delivery. Unfortunately, many women with diabetes do not have tight glucose control at conception, so some malformations still occur. If an obvious malformation is present at birth, it is important to search for other malformations.

Also, keep in mind that the fetus was producing a lot of insulin to handle all the maternal glucose entering through the placenta. Suddenly, maternal glucose is cut off at delivery, but the high level of fetal insulin continues for a while. The danger of hypoglycemia exists in the first four to six hours after delivery. The baby may be sweaty and appear nervous or even have a seizure. It is necessary to do blood glucose tests on the baby hourly until he or she is stable and to continue testing at intervals for the first 24 hours.

Besides hypoglycemia, the baby may have several other complications right after birth:

- ✔ **Respiratory distress syndrome:** This breathing problem occurs when the baby is delivered early, but it responds to treatment. This condition is rare with good prenatal care.

- ✔ **Low calcium with jitteriness and possible seizures:** Calcium needs to be given to the baby until its own body can take over. This condition is usually a result of prematurity.

- ✔ **Low magnesium:** This complication presents itself like low calcium and is also a result of prematurity.

- ✔ **Polycythemia:** This condition, where too many red blood cells exist, occurs for unknown reasons. Treatment requires removing blood from the baby. The amount is determined by how much extra blood is present.

- ✔ **Hyperbilirubinemia:** This condition is the product of too much break-down of red blood cells. It is treated with light.

- ✔ **Lazy left colon:** Occurring for unknown reasons, this condition presents itself like an obstruction of the bowel but clears up on its own.

If the baby was exposed to high glucose and ketones during the pregnancy, it may show diminished intelligence. This effect is not obvious at birth but is discovered later when the baby is expected to learn something.

The large baby of the poorly controlled mother with diabetes usually loses its fat by age 1. Starting at ages 6 to 8, however, the child has a greater tendency to be obese. Controlling the blood glucose in the mother may prevent later obesity and even diabetes in her offspring.

Identifying Polycystic Ovarian Syndrome

Polycystic ovarian syndrome (PCOS) is responsible for abnormal menstrual function in 5 to 8 percent or more of women during their reproductive years. It tends to run in families. Women with this condition have trouble conceiving a child, and they have increased hair on their faces, arms, legs, and areas of the body that are not usually hairy in women. In addition, they experience acne and obesity.

The surprise finding in PCOS is that these women are also resistant to insulin and have increased blood levels of insulin even when they are not obese. The greater the degree of obesity, however, the more frequent that the metabolic syndrome is present (see Chapter 5). In fact, women with PCOS who do get pregnant have a prevalence of gestational diabetes that is 2 to 3 times that of those women without PCOS.

Another feature that women with PCOS have in common with metabolic syndrome is obstructive sleep apnea. This sleep apnea results in daytime sleepiness and high blood pressure.

The name of the syndrome derives from the fact that early cases of PCOS were associated with multiple ovarian cysts. More recently, the presence of ovarian cysts has not been a prominent feature of the condition, but the name has stuck.

Women with PCOS have increased levels of male-associated hormones called *androgens*. Studies have shown that androgens cause decreased insulin sensitivity when they are given to women who don't have PCOS.

The major health risks for someone with PCOS, besides infertility, are the occurrence of impaired glucose tolerance and type 2 diabetes, as well as gestational diabetes. In addition, just like patients with the metabolic syndrome (see Chapter 5), these women are at greater risk for high blood pressure, abnormal blood fats, and cardiovascular disease.

The most effective treatment for PCOS is lifestyle change. Weight loss and exercise often reverse the condition and prevent the development of diabetes. In very obese women with PCOS, weight loss surgery will reverse PCOS. Oral contraceptives have been used in the past when more treatment is needed, but these don't restore fertility, which is often the main purpose of treatment. They can still be used to control the other symptoms, such as acne and increased hair. Insulin sensitizing drugs, including metformin, and pioglitazone (see Chapter 10), have been very effective for treating all features of the syndrome. In a study reported in *The Journal of Clinical Endocrinology and Metabolism* in April 2005, six months of metformin was much more effective than a drug called clomiphene, a well known inducer of ovulation, in restoring fertility.

Other than oral contraceptives, any treatment that is successful for reducing the acne, hairiness, and decreased insulin sensitivity in PCOS also makes the woman much more liable to get pregnant. If she doesn't want to become pregnant, she and her partner need to take the necessary precautions.

Part III

Managing Diabetes: The "Thriving with Diabetes" Lifestyle Plan

The 5th Wave   By Rich Tennant

@RICHTENNANT

"You know, anyone who wishes he had a remote control for his exercise equipment is missing the idea of exercise equipment."

In this part . . .

Is it possible that you could be healthier with diabetes than your friends who do not have diabetes? This part shows that the answer to that question is yes. While others continue their bad habits leading to illness and perhaps premature death, you can find out exactly what you have to do not just to live with diabetes but to thrive with diabetes. The steps you need to take are simple and basic and involve changes in lifestyle, what and how much you eat as well as your physical fitness. You will probably ask yourself as you're reading, "Why didn't I think of that?"

You will find out how to choose from the vast number of products like glucose meters that help you to manage your disease. You will discover that you can have diabetes and enjoy delicious food. I introduce you to the concept of taking at least 10K (10,000 steps) a day. New medications are appearing regularly and you need to understand how to use them properly. Another function of this part is to show you that lots of people — some of whom you may not have thought of — are out there to provide the information that you need to know.

Chapter 7

Glucose Monitoring and Other Tests

- -

In This Chapter

▶ Monitoring is a must

▶ Choosing a glucose meter

▶ Checking your hemoglobin A1c

▶ Testing for kidney damage

▶ Examining your eyes and feet

▶ Finding your level of cholesterol and other fats

▶ Gauging your blood pressure and weight

- -

*Y*ou may wonder what you have to do to prevent the complications of diabetes that I describe in Chapters 4 through 6 — a fair amount, which I discuss in this chapter. But when you weigh the benefits that add up to a longer quality life against the loss of time and money from preventive care, preventive care wins by a landslide.

With preventive care, you benefit from an explosion of new tests and treatments that have only been available for the last 30 years, beginning with self-testing of blood glucose in 1980 right up to new tests for overall diabetic control and multiple new hardware and software tools made possible by the latest advances in computer and Internet technology.

As Woody Allen points out, "I don't want to achieve immortality through my work; I want to achieve it by never dying." On the other hand, he says, "On the plus side, death is one of the few things that can be done as easily as lying down." Well, I don't want you to take your diabetes lying down. I want to give you the benefit of every important advance. You may not achieve immortality, but you will enjoy every day that you live.

This chapter gives you all the tools you need to detect complications in their earliest stages. And if, by chance, you are reading this section for the first time and complications have already developed, this chapter also shows you how to measure the progression or, hopefully, regression of your complications.

Testing, Testing: Tests You Need to Stay Healthy

A number of tests and measurements should be done on a regular basis. To best make sure that you get your tests done regularly, you can use the chart in Figure 7-1. This form lists the tests and you can list the results underneath. Simply copy the one in Figure 7-1 and keep it up to date. Don't expect your doctor to keep this chart updated for you. He has too much on his mind and too many patients to get it exactly right for each one.

Date	Hemoglobin A1c	GlycoMark	Eye Exam	Filament	TSH	Ualb	Chol	LDL	HDL	TG

Figure 7-1: A sample testing chart that you can copy to track your testing results.

Certain procedures should be done by your doctor (and you, if feasible) according to the following schedule:

✔ Evaluate your blood glucose measurements at each visit. (See the section "Monitoring Blood Glucose: It's a Must," later in this chapter.)

✔ Obtain hemoglobin A1c four times a year if you take insulin and twice a year if you don't. (See the section "Tracking Your Glucose over Time: Hemoglobin A1c," later in this chapter.)

✔ Check for microalbuminuria once a year. (See the section "Testing for Kidney Damage: Microalbuminuria," later in this chapter.)

✔ Have a dilated eye examination by an ophthalmologist or optometrist once a year. (See the section "Checking for Eye Problems," later in this chapter.)

✔ Examine your bare feet at each visit. (See the section "Examining Your Feet," later in this chapter.)

✔ Have an ankle-brachial index performed at least every five years. (See the section "Examining Your Feet," later in this chapter.)

✔ Obtain a lipid panel once a year. (See the section "Tracking Cholesterol and Other Fats," later in this chapter.)

✔ Measure your blood pressure at each visit. (See the section "Measuring Blood Pressure," later in this chapter.)

✔ Measure your weight at each visit. (See the section "Checking Your Weight and BMI," later in this chapter.)

These tests are the *minimum* standards for proper care of diabetes. If an abnormality is found, the frequency of testing increases to check on the response to treatment.

Are we doing the best job of managing diabetes? Government statistics on "Preventive Care Practices" from the Centers For Disease Control and Prevention suggest that we are not. And we don't seem to be getting much better as diabetes becomes a major health problem in the US. The latest statistics compare the annual rates of testing for various abnormalities associated with diabetes between 1994 and 2005. They indicate some improvement but we should be doing a whole lot better.

The results were as follows:

✔ In 1994, 57 percent of people with diabetes had an annual eye examination. By 2005 it had grown to only 60.6 percent.

✔ In 1994, 79 percent of people with diabetes had at least one visit to a doctor in a year. By 2005 the number was up to only 87.7 percent.

✔ In 1994, 48 percent of people with diabetes had a foot examination in the previous year. By 2005 it was only up to 66 percent.

✔ In 2000, 66 percent of people with diabetes had two or more hemoglobin A1c tests in the past year, while in 2005 it had fallen to 64 percent.

✔ In 1994, 38 percent of people with diabetes were doing self-testing of blood glucose. By 2005 it had only risen to 61.5 percent.

✔ In 2000, 62 percent of people with diabetes were examining their own feet. By 2005 it was only 64 percent.

As we have gained knowledge about diabetes, the guidelines for how high various tests should be in people with diabetes have changed. Unfortunately, they seemed to have no effect on the results of clinical practice:

✔ After the Joint National Committee on Prevention, Detection, Evaluation and Treatment of High Blood Pressure lowered its guidelines for blood pressure in people with diabetes in 1997 and again in 2003, there was no better control as late as 2005 according to an article in *Diabetes Care* in January 2007.

✔ The American Diabetes Association lowered its goal for LDL cholesterol (see below) to less than 100 mg/dl in 1998. As late as 2004 there was no indication that patients were meeting the new goal more often than they had in 1994.

There is much to be done. And that's what this chapter is all about.

Monitoring Blood Glucose: It's a Must

Insulin was extracted and used for the first time more than 80 years ago. Since that time, nothing has improved the life of the person with diabetes as much as the ability to measure his or her own blood glucose with a drop of blood.

Prior to blood glucose self-monitoring, testing the urine for glucose was the only way to determine whether your blood glucose was high, but urine testing could not tell at all whether the glucose was low. The urine test for glucose is worthless for controlling blood glucose — it actually provides misinformation. All the thousands of research papers in the medical literature before 1980, which used urine testing for glucose, are of no value and should be burned. (However, testing the urine for other things, such as ketones and protein, can be of value.)

Basically, two kinds of test strips are used today. Both require that glucose in a drop of your blood reacts with an enzyme. In one strip, the reaction produces a color. A meter then reads the amount of color to give a glucose reading. In the other strip, the reaction produces electrons, and a meter converts the amount of electrons into a glucose reading.

One of the first things that was learned when frequent testing of blood glucose became feasible is that a person with diabetes, even a person who works hard to control his glucose, can experience tremendous variation in glucose levels in a relatively short time, as little as 30 minutes. This is especially true in association with food, but variations can occur even in the fasting state before breakfast. For this reason multiple tests are needed.

How often should you test?

How often you test is determined by the kind of diabetes you have, the kind of treatment you're using, and the level of stability of your blood glucose.

- ✔ **If you have type 1 or type 2 diabetes and you're taking before-meal insulin, you need to test before each meal and at bedtime.** The reason for this frequent testing is that you're constantly using this information to make adjustments in your insulin dose. No matter how good you think your control is, you cannot feel the level of the blood glucose without testing unless you're hypoglycemic. In fact, I have had my patients try to guess without testing on numerous occasions and then I test it. They are close less than 50 percent of the time. That degree of accuracy is not sufficient for good glucose control.

  People with type 1 diabetes should occasionally test one hour after a meal and in the middle of the night to see just how high their glucose goes after eating and whether it drops too low in the middle of the night. These results guide you and your physician to make the changes you need.

- ✔ **If you have type 2 diabetes and you're on pills or just diet and exercise, testing twice a day (before breakfast and dinner) gives you the information needed to measure the effect of the treatment.** I'm assuming that you're fairly stable as shown by mostly good blood glucose tests (in the range of 80 to 120 mg/dl) and by the hemoglobin A1c (which I discuss later in this chapter). I even have some of my most stable patients testing only once a day, alternating a pre-breakfast test with a pre-supper test on consecutive days. Any less testing than this minimal amount is not enough to keep you aware of the state of your control.

- ✔ **If you're pregnant, see the testing guidelines I outline in Chapter 6.** I would guess that you're probably willing to test numerous times in a day to keep your developing fetus as healthy as possible.

The blood glucose test can be useful many other times of day:

✔ If you eat something off your diet and want to test its effect on your glucose, do a test.

✔ If you're about to exercise, a blood glucose test can tell you whether you need to eat before starting the exercise or can use the exercise to bring your glucose down.

✔ If your diabetes is temporarily unstable and you're about to drive, you may want to test before getting into the car to make sure that you're not on the verge of hypoglycemia.

You're not being graded on your glucose test results. The human body has too much variation in it to expect that each time you take the same medication, do the same exercise, eat the same way, and feel the same emotionally, you will get the same test result. If the person who reviews your results with you sees your abnormal results as bad, he or she does not understand this point. You may want to consider finding someone who does.

Keep in mind that the occasional blood glucose test done in your doctor's office is of little or no value in understanding the big picture of your glucose control. It is like trying to visualize an entire painting by Seurat (who painted using dots of color) by looking at one dot on the canvas.

Using a lancet

To get the drop of blood you need to perform a glucose test, you have to use a spring-loaded device that contains a sharp lancet. You push the button of the device, and the lancet springs out and pokes your finger.

One product that seems less painful than the others is the Softclix Lancet Device. It allows you to select one of eleven depth settings so that you can penetrate your finger no deeper than necessary. It uses its own type of lancet that is a little more expensive than others on the market. Becton Dickinson makes another lancet, called BDGenie Lancet, that works like a lancet and lancing device all in one. It is less painful and a little less expensive than other devices on the market. Becton Dickinson also makes the thinnest lancets currently available, called the BD Ultra-Fine 33 Lancets.

Although you do not have to use alcohol on your fingers, they should be reasonably clean. (My patients have done millions of finger sticks, and I've never known one of them to have an infection result.) Use the side of your finger to avoid the more sensitive tips that you don't want to hurt, especially if you use a keyboard frequently. Change fingers often so that no finger becomes very sensitive.

Remember never to use a used lancet on someone else. Each lancet lasts for a few pokes and should then be discarded in a special *sharps container* so it can't poke someone else accidentally. Sharps containers are available in drugstores.

How do you perform the test?

If you don't already own a blood glucose meter, be sure to check out the next section. All meters require a drop of blood, usually from the finger. (See the previous section "Using a lancet.") You place the blood on a specific part of a test strip and allow enough time, usually between five seconds and one minute, for a reaction to occur. Some strips allow you to add more blood within 30 seconds if the quantity is insufficient. In less than a minute, the meter reads the product of that reaction, which is determined by the amount of glucose in the blood sample.

Keep the following tips in mind when you're testing your glucose:

- ✔ **If you have trouble getting blood, you can use a rubberband at the point where your finger joins your hand.** You will be amazed at the flow of blood. Take off the rubberband before a major hemorrhage occurs (just joking).

- ✔ **Testing blood from sites other than your fingers is generally reliable, except for an hour after eating or immediately after exercise.**

- ✔ **Some meters use whole blood, and some use the liquid part of the blood, called the *plasma*.** A lab glucose tests the plasma. The whole blood value is about 12 percent less than the plasma value, so it is important to know which you're measuring. The various recommendations for appropriate levels of glucose are plasma values unless specifically stated otherwise. Most of the newer meters are calibrated to give a plasma reading, but check yours to be sure.

- ✔ **Studies have shown that the qualities of test strips, which are loose in a vial, deteriorate rapidly if the vial is left open.** Be sure to cap the vial. Two hours of exposure to air may ruin the strips. Strips that are individually foil-wrapped do not have this problem.

- ✔ **Do not let others use your meter.** Their test results will be mixed in with your tests when they are downloaded into a computer. In addition, a meter invariably gets a little blood on it and can be a source of infection.

Choosing a Blood Glucose Meter

So many meters are on the market that you may be confused about which one to use. One consideration that should play little part in your decision is the cost of the meter. Most manufacturers are happy to practically give you the meter so that you're forced to buy their test strips. Each manufacturer makes a different test strip, and they're not interchangeable in other machines. Some even make a different strip for each different machine that they make.

Because the meters are so cheap and the science is changing so rapidly, you should get a new meter every year or two to make sure that you have state-of-the-art equipment. The cost of test strips is generally about the same from meter to meter, so the cost of strips does not have to play a big role in your meter decision, either.

Another nonconsideration is the accuracy of the various machines. All are accurate to a degree acceptable for managing your diabetes. Keep in mind, though, that they do not have the accuracy of a laboratory. Meters are probably about plus or minus 10 percent compared to the lab.

Factors that may influence your purchase

Your doctor may have a meter that he or she prefers to work with because a computer program can download the test results from the meter and display them in a certain way. This analysis can be enormously helpful in deciding how to alter your therapy for the best control of your glucose.

Any meter you buy should have a memory that records the time and date so you can read that information along with the glucose result. The memory should hold at least 100 glucose values if you test four times a day; 100 values represents 25 days at this testing frequency.

Do not buy a meter without the capability to download the results to a data management system in a computer. Bring your meter with you to your appointments so that your doctor, or one of his or her assistants, can download your glucose test results and evaluate them with the aid of a data management system. Evaluating pages of glucose readings in a log book is virtually impossible. Your insurance company also may mandate a certain meter, in which case you may have no choice.

Ask yourself the following questions when choosing a meter:

- ✔ If a small child is to use it, can the child easily use the meter and strips?
- ✔ Are the batteries common ones, or are they hard to get and expensive?
- ✔ Does the meter have a memory that you and your doctor can check?
- ✔ Is the meter downloadable to a computer program that can manipulate the data?
- ✔ Are the test strips reasonable in cost?

Profiles of different meters

There are more than a dozen companies vying for your meter purchase but there are really four major players in the meter game and a few minor ones. Among them, they produce more than 25 machines. Like everything in business, mergers and acquisitions have occurred and will continue to happen so that the field narrows. You're probably wise to stick with one of the four major companies, which I describe in the following sections, unless a minor company comes out with irresistible features. Strips for the meters produced by the major companies are widely available, and the companies tend to have excellent service should you have a meter problem.

You want to know what I use in my practice? All of my patients use the Accu-Chek Compact Plus meter or one of the other Roche Diagnostics meters that utilizes the same data management system. The Compact Plus uses whole blood, not plasma but the meter converts the result to a plasma value. I like it because it has a drum that contains 17 test strips, which are wrapped up until they are used. That means they are not subject to exposure to air. It also allows you to add blood if the initial drop is not enough. Most importantly, it is very fast and accurate. I like the data management system that the company provides to doctors (or you, if you call the company on the 800 number on the meter) who use its meters.

Abbott Laboratories

Abbott Laboratories purchased the MediSense Company, which first made and sold these meters. This company, which has one of the longest warranties on its meters (four years), is speedy about taking care of problems that arise. The batteries are good for 4,000 tests. They can generally be replaced by you unless otherwise noted. One clue that Abbott is really interested in customer service is that you can find the Owner's Guides for all their meters on the Internet.

✔ **Freestyle Flash:** The manufacturer calls the Freestyle Flash the smallest meter available. It requires a tiny sample of blood and you can add more up to a minute from the first application if you don't have enough on the strip. The Flash works with a data management program called Precision Link Direct Diabetes Data Management System. It will hold up to 250 tests, eliminating the oldest as new ones are added beyond 250, just like all the other meters described in this section. You can see a 1-day average on the screen. You must set the meter to the code that is on the vial of test strips you are currently using. The meter has programmable alarms to remind you to test. It uses CR2032 "coin cell" batteries available at drugstores and grocery stores. You can test away from your finger with this meter.

✔ **Freestyle Freedom:** This meter is identical to the Flash but it is larger with a larger screen for people who have visual difficulties.

✔ **Freestyle Lite:** This meter uses different test strips from the two above and does not require coding. It can remember 400 tests. Otherwise it is similar in its properties to the meters above.

✔ **Precision Xtra:** This meter allows measurement of blood ketones as well as glucose. It uses its own test strips that require calibration of the meter with each new vial. The vial contains a calibration strip that is inserted into the meter before using the test strips in that vial. If you want to do a blood ketone test, you use the calibration strip that comes in that vial before inserting the ketone strip. The meter remembers the last 450 tests that you do and you can view 7-, 14-, and 30-day averages on the screen. It uses the same data management system as the other meters in the Abbott group.

Bayer Healthcare LLC

Bayer Healthcare LLC, which is a branch of Bayer Group (a German company), sells the following two meters in the United States but continues to support several of its old meters (such as the Elite). The meters are accurate and carry the longest warranty in the industry (five years). You can replace the batteries at home. The meters are descendants of some of the first meters available. They both allow testing away from your fingers. No coding of the meters is required.

✔ **Breeze 2:** The Breeze 2 uses a 10-test cartridge that calibrates the meter. It remembers 420 tests. It can provide 1-, 7-, 14-, and 30-day averages. The meter uses WinGLUCOFACTS software for data management.

✔ **Contour:** This meter uses individual test strips that require no coding. It remembers up to 480 tests that can be downloaded and viewed with the same data management system as the Breeze 2. It can provide a 14-day average on the screen. It uses 3-volt lithium batteries.

LifeScan

Johnson & Johnson purchased LifeScan, one of the older meter companies. They have a number of meters in competition with one another. The company is very reliable, taking care of problems within 24 hours. You can replace the batteries in LifeScan meters at home. This company also posts its Owner's Manuals online in case to need to refer to them.

- **One TouchUltra Mini:** This meter is small and portable. It uses a tiny blood sample. Each new vial of Ultra Mini test strips must be coded in the meter. It uses a 3 volt CR 2032 coin cell battery. However it has no way to download test results to a computer and no data management system. Therefore I don't recommend it.

- **One Touch Ultra 2:** This system allows testing away from the fingers. It uses a tiny sample and, therefore, can work with LifeScan's ultrafine lancets. The result is displayed in five seconds, and the blood is drawn up by capillary action. The meter has a 500-test memory that allows averaging on the screen and connects to a data port using One Touch Diabetes Management software. You can see 7-, 14-, and 30-day averages. It uses Ultra test strips. You use buttons on the meter to set the code on the meter to the code on the bottle of test strips. You can add flags to each blood glucose test to specify whether the glucose was taken before or after a meal and whether food or exercise was involved. Testing may be done away from the fingers. It uses 2 3-volt CR 2032 coin cell batteries, one for the meter and one for the backlight. The test is measured from whole blood but expressed in plasma referenced units.

- **One Touch UltraSmart:** This meter has all the features of the One Touch Ultra 2 with the addition of other features. Using "smart buttons, you can enter information about your exercise, health, medication, and food. You are prompted to comment on out-of-range results. You can view charts and graphs that help to analyze your blood glucose on the meter's screen. The UltraSmart uses two AAA batteries. You can see averages for 7, 14, 30, 60, and 90 days. It can store over 3,000 test results. You can also enter test results for hemoglobin A1c, microalbumin, cholesterol, blood pressure, eye exams, foot exams, weight, height and dates of doctor's visits. You can enter the diabetes pills you take and insulin if you use that. Finally, there is a food log book in which you can enter the meal and the calories of fat, carbohydrate and protein. Once the information is in the meter you can get outputs of average insulin used at different times, average carbohydrates at different meals and so forth.

Roche Diagnostics

Roche Diagnostics, which did not sell meters originally, merged with Boehringer Mannheim and now sells its meters. The batteries in these meters are replaceable at home. The meters may be used at alternate sites besides the fingers.

✔ **Accu-ChekAviva:** This meter works with diabetes management software (DMS). It has a very large memory, storing up to 500 blood glucose values, with 7-, 14-, and 30- day averages on-screen. It requires a tiny sample of blood. It comes with Spanish language instructions and a phone number for a Spanish-speaking representative. It has a code key with each new bottle of test strips that are made just for this meter. You can set test reminders for up to 4 times a day with the built-in alarm. It uses a coin cell 2032 battery.

✔ **Accu-Chek Advantage:** This meter also works with DMS and stores 350 blood glucose values. It uses a test strip that takes 27 seconds but does not require cleaning or wiping, and it draws the blood up by capillary action. It uses test strips that come with a code key that is inserted into the meter for that bottle of strips. The strips are Accu-Chek Comfort Curve test strips.

✔ **Accu-Chek Compact Plus:** This meter uses a 17-test drum that requires no test strip handling or calibration. The results are displayed in 5 seconds, and it has a 300-test memory that is downloadable to a DMS. You can see onscreen 7-, 24-, and 30-day averages. It allows testing away from the fingers.

✔ **Accu-Chek Active:** This meter uses a tiny sample of blood and gives a result in five seconds. It has a 200-value memory that is downloadable to a DMS and can show 7- and 14- day averages. It can be used at alternate sites besides the fingers. It uses a new snap-in code key for each new bottle of strips, made just for this meter.

✔ **Accu-Chek Voicemate:** This meter is for the visually impaired. It identifies the type of insulin used, and it audibly takes the user through the glucose test and gives the reading. It also uses the Comfort Curve test strips that draw the blood in by capillary action, and it is downloadable to a DMS.

Roche also makes a software program for people with diabetes called Accu-Chek Compass. It helps patients to better manage their diabetes by providing reports and summaries of the glucose tests.

Two noninvasive meters

Since individual blood glucose measurements represent only a moment in time and blood glucose levels can change in minutes, devices that can measure blood glucose almost continuously, store the measurements, and download them to a computer are being developed. They may replace the above meters once they improve, but for now they often lag behind finger stick measurements, especially after a meal or exercise. Each still requires that you take blood glucose measurements using a finger stick meter to calibrate these continuous meters.

They have their best use when the finger stick results do not correlate well with the hemoglobin A1c measurements, which is especially the case in people with diabetes who take insulin. The doctor, knowing the direction of the blood glucose throughout 24 hours, can adjust the rapid-acting and long-acting insulin more accurately without causing hypoglycemia.

Dexcom STS Continuous Blood Glucose Monitor known as the Seven System. This monitor uses a sensor under the skin that wirelessly transmits glucose readings from the fluid under the skin called the interstitial fluid to a monitor. The monitor collects the information and displays it on a screen. The screen can show 1-hour, 3-hour, and 9-hour trends as well as alert you when the blood glucose goes above or below a set level. Also an alarm sounds when the glucose is below 55 mg/dl. Software called Data Manager 2 helps to display the data on a computer for further understanding of trends. The device is calibrated with a finger stick glucose every 12 hours. It can store up to 30 days of data. It has not been tested in children, adolescents, or pregnant women.

This type of system can be used to design a very accurate program for giving insulin. In the future, it could be hooked up to an insulin delivery device and provide instant responses to changes in blood glucose.

GlucoWatch G2 Biographer

Cygnus, Inc., offers the GlucoWatch G2 Biographer, distributed by the Sankyo Corporation. It is worn like a watch, and glucose readings are taken without pricking the skin. This device can be set to read as often as every 10 minutes for up to 13 hours. It works by passing a tiny electric current through the skin. The current gathers glucose and brings it back to the watch, where it is measured.

This system is meant to supplement but not replace blood glucose testing by detecting trends and tracking patterns. It has a built-in alarm that alerts the wearer if the glucose is too low or too high, based on levels that you set. A finger stick is still required to calibrate the GlucoWatch at the beginning of each 13-hour period. After a two hour warm-up period, you calibrate the meter. The device may not work accurately if it comes in contact with too much perspiration.

It can store up to 8,500 individual readings. It can sometimes cause irritation at the site of the device with redness, itching, and blisters.

As this book was being written, the Animas Corporation, which purchased Cygnus, decided to discontinue production of the GlucoWatch, but continues to support it through July 2008.

Guardian RT Glucose Monitoring System

Like the Dexcom described above, this device has a sensor that is inserted into the skin, a wireless transmitter connected to the sensor and a receiver. It reads the interstitial fluid glucose every 10 seconds and averages them every 5 minutes. By pushing a button you can see the readings. It holds up to 21 days of data that can be downloaded to a computer. It sounds an alarm to alert the wearer to high or low glucose levels but significant abnormalities should always be verified by a finger stick.

How I use my patients' test results

I encourage my patients to keep their own records of their glucose levels so that they can see for themselves how they are doing. I maintain several years of records and can compare and contrast results for each patient. I use software to generate pictures of a patient's diabetic control. The figures in this sidebar show you graphics that depict test results for a typical patient before starting therapy and after insulin treatment had time to work. It is easy to see how helpful the graphic information can be.

The first figure shows the patient's blood glucose levels in three different formats. The top, called the Trendgraph, shows the blood glucoses each day, in this case, between 6/11 and 7/1. The shaded area represents the blood glucoses from 80 to 180 mg/dl. The line below the shaded area is the 50 mg/dl line. Each X represents a distinct blood glucose test. You can see that the glucose is often high, going up to 300, and sometimes low, going down to 50 with large excursions. This graph also shows that the mean of the tests is 159 and that 5 percent of the time, the patient is less than 80; 63.4 percent of the time, she is between 80 and 180; and 31.7 percent of the time, she is above 180.

The next figure, called the Standard Day, puts all those glucose levels in a 24-hour day so that tests taken between certain hours, regardless of the day, appear close to one another. This grouping allows me to see whether the patient has a tendency to be high or low at a given time each day. The software averages out the blood glucose at different times, providing a number to compare to other time periods. This information permits me to adjust her insulin to correct for that particular time.

The bottom figure, called the Pie Chart, clearly shows how much of the time this patient is high, how much of the time she is within the target of 80 to 180, and how much of the time she is below 80.

These three figures provide an excellent picture of the patient's diabetic control and permit me to easily compare it to the result of treatment.

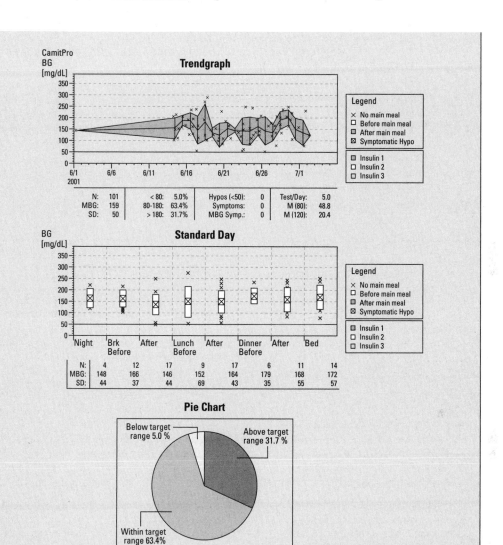

The next set of figures represents tests taken after treatment with a new form of insulin, Lantus, for one week. The results are dramatic. Now almost all the glucoses are in the shaded area, and there is little excursion of the tests. A few X's fall above 180, and a few fall below 80. The Standard Day now shows fairly low averages throughout, except perhaps after lunch. The Pie Chart shows much more in the target range and far fewer above the target range. Comparing the two graphs, the *above target range* area has dropped from 31.7 percent to 6.5 percent.

(continued)

(continued)

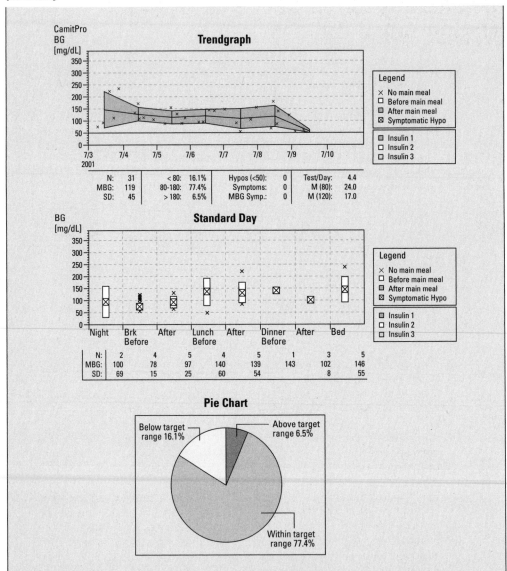

I can print all these graphs and charts. In later visits, I can compare the current control with the way the patient was doing before. When patients can see so clearly how they're improving from time to time, it keeps them motivated to take their medicine and follow their diet and exercise plan.

Tracking Your Glucose over Time: Hemoglobin A1c

Individual blood glucose tests are great for deciding how you're doing at that moment and what to do to make it better, but they do not give the big picture. They are just a moment in time. Glucose can change a great deal even in 30 minutes . What you need is a test that gives an integrated picture of many days, weeks, or even months of blood glucose levels. The test that accomplishes this important task is called the *hemoglobin A1c*. (See the sidebar "How hemoglobin A1c works" for an explanation of the test's function.)

Unfortunately, all labs do not do the hemoglobin A1c test the same way. Some labs report both the hemoglobin A1c and the total *glycohemoglobin* (the amount of glucose attached to hemoglobin). As a result, there are different normal levels depending on how the test was done. You need to know the normal value in the lab where you do the test. Fortunately, each lab usually has a column on its result form showing the normal values for each test. Still, this situation can create confusion.

My medical building has two different labs, each reporting the results differently. As a result of insurance requirements, I have to send patients to one lab or the other. When I get back the result, I have to be sure I know which lab did it. The standard method should be the way it was done in the Diabetes Control and Complications Trial, the study that showed that controlling the blood glucose prevents complications in type 1 diabetes. In that study, a normal level was about 6.05 percent. Figure 7-2 shows you the correlation between the hemoglobin A1c and the blood glucose when this method is used.

As you can see in the figure, a normal hemoglobin A1c of less than 6 percent corresponds to a blood glucose of less than 120, while a fair hemoglobin A1c of 7 percent reflects an average blood glucose of 150.

Large-scale studies have shown that the average hemoglobin A1c in the United States for type 2 diabetes is around 9.4 percent, which means the average blood glucose is 220. The American Diabetes Association recommends taking action to control the blood glucose if the hemoglobin A1c is 8 percent or greater, with the goal being less than 7 percent. The American Association of Clinical Endocrinologists suggests a goal of 6.5 percent or less. While I wish all of my patients would achieve a level of 6.5 percent, I try to get them as low as possible, but still consistent with a decent quality of life, which means few to no severe hypoglycemic episodes.

Blood Glucose Control Chart

Hemoglobin A1c (%)

5	6	7	8	9	10	11	12	13	14

Normal	Good	Fair	Poor

90	120	150	180	210	240	270	300	330	360

Average Whole Blood Glucose (mg/dl)

100	140	170	210	240	280	310	350	380	420

Average Plasma Glucose (mg/dl)

Figure 7-2: Comparison between hemoglobin A1c and blood glucose.

Your physician should test for hemoglobin A1c as follows:

✔ Four times a year if you have type 1 or type 2 diabetes and are on insulin.

✔ Two times a year if you have type 2 diabetes and are not on insulin.

In my own practice, I test all patients every three months. A good hemoglobin A1c is highly motivating to keep up good self-care, while a poor result gives immediate feedback as to the need for tighter control.

How hemoglobin A1c works

Hemoglobin is a protein that carries oxygen around the body and drops it off wherever it's needed to help in all the chemical reactions that are constantly taking place. The hemoglobin is packaged within red blood cells that live in the bloodstream for 60 to 90 days. As the blood circulates, glucose in the blood attaches to the hemoglobin and stays attached. It attaches in several different ways to the hemoglobin, and the total of all the hemoglobin attached to glucose is called *glycohemoglobin.* Glycohemoglobin normally makes up about 6 percent of the hemoglobin in the blood. The largest fraction, two-thirds of the glycohemoglobin, is in the form called *hemoglobin A1c,* making it easiest to measure. The rest of the hemoglobin is made up of hemoglobin A1a and A1b. The more glucose in the blood, the more glycohemoglobins form. Because glycohemoglobin remains in the blood for two to three months, glycohemoglobin is a reflection of the glucose control over the entire time period and not just the second that a single glucose test reflects.

Currently, the National Glycohemoglobin Standardization Program, created by the American Association for Clinical Chemistry, is working to get the hemoglobin A1c test standardized so that a 6 percent result will mean the same thing for every patient. The program might start by doing only one test, the hemoglobin A1c, and calling it by only one name.

A company called Metrika, Inc., has come up with a clever home version of the hemoglobin A1c, called *A1c Now*. You do a finger stick to produce a large drop of blood. The blood is mixed with a solution that is provided, and a sample of that mixture is placed in the testing device. Eight minutes later, the hemoglobin A1c result appears in the device window. The device is then discarded. The device appears to be highly accurate and may save the trouble of going to a lab for this test. Because it's so quick, your doctor can have the test results while you're at his office and can act on them immediately, instead of waiting for a lab to return the test results at a later time. The test kit is available at pharmacies without a prescription.

Another option is to collect your own blood specimen and send it to a company that will run the test and give you and your doctor a result. The companies currently doing this include

- AccuBase A1c Glycohemoglobin (www.diabetestechnologies.com). Each test costs $26.95 and includes lab analysis and reporting.

  Diabetes Technologies, Inc

  P. O. Box 1954

  Thomasville, GA 31799

  Phone 888-872-2443

- A1c at Home (www.flexsite.com) costs $19.95 each including lab analysis and reporting.

  Flexsite Diagnostics, Inc

  3543 SW Corporate Pkwy

  Palm City, FL 34909

  Phone 772-221-9671

- BioSafe A1c Hemoglobin Test Kit (www.ebiosafe.com) costs $24.95 per test.

  Lab 123, Inc

  100 Field Drive, Suite 240

  Lake Forest, IL 60045

  Phone 888-700-8378

Another test similar to the hemoglobin A1c is the *fructosamine*. This test, which measures the glucose combined with protein in the blood, reflects the level of blood glucose for the past three weeks. Fructosamine is a relatively new test that has not seen a lot of use, so its place in diabetes care has not been established. The test should prove very useful for the pregnant woman with diabetes, for example, where you need to know the effect of a treatment change very rapidly. As doctors become more familiar with its use, more fructosamine tests will be ordered.

The Food and Drug Administration has approved a home-testing device called the Duet Glucose Control Monitoring System, which can measure both the blood glucose and the fructosamine. The machine costs around $300, and the test strips are $64 for 8. How useful it will be is yet to be determined.

GlycoMark Test

This test is relatively new in the United States but has been used in Japan for several years. It differs from the hemoglobin A1c test in two important ways:

- Results take two weeks rather than three months to change.
- Better control is marked by a higher rather than a lower number for the GlycoMark test.

The test is based on the normal presence of 1.5 anhydroglucitol (1,5 AG) in the blood. As blood glucose rises and more of it gets into the kidneys, it blocks the return of 1,5 AG to the blood stream and the measured blood level of 1,5 AG falls.

Table 7-1 shows the values for GlycoMark in people without diabetes and at different levels of glucose control.

Table 7-1	GlycoMark Test Results	
GlycoMark (ug/ml)	*Control*	*Glucose (mg/dl)*
12 or higher	Normal	Under 180
10	Well-controlled	185
8	Moderate control	190
6	Poor control	200
4	Very poor control	225

The GlycoMark test has been shown to be an excellent indicator of the blood glucose levels, especially after meals, even when the Hemoglobin A1c test was similar in these patients. It gives the doctor and the patient a much earlier indication of whether therapy is working than does the slow changing hemoglobin A1c. It will see much more use in the future because it is becoming available in most clinical laboratories and it may soon be available as a home test.

Testing for Kidney Damage: Microalbuminuria

The finding of very small but abnormal amounts of protein in the urine, called *microalbuminuria,* is the earliest sign that high glucose may be damaging your kidneys (see Chapter 5). When microalbuminuria is found, you still have time to reverse any damage.

As soon as you are diagnosed with type 2 diabetes, and within five years of being diagnosed with type 1, your doctor must order a urine test for microalbuminuria. If the test is negative, it must be repeated annually. If the test is positive, it should be done a second time to verify the result. If the second test is positive, your doctor should do the following:

- **Put you on a drug called an ACE inhibitor.** After you have been on this drug for some months, the test for microalbuminuria can be repeated to see whether it has turned negative. The ACE inhibitor can be stopped and restarted later if microalbuminuria appears again.

- **Bring your blood glucose under the tightest control possible.** Bringing it under control helps to reverse the damaging process as well.

- **Normalize your body fats so that your cholesterol and triglycerides are made normal.** Elevated cholesterol and triglycerides have been found to damage the kidneys. (See the section "Tracking Cholesterol and Other Fats," later in this chapter.)

Doing this simple little test can protect your kidneys from damage. Ask your doctor about it if you think it has never been done. Show him or her this page if the doctor is unclear as to why it is performed.

Up to 25 percent of patients with diabetes can have ongoing kidney damage without showing an elevated microalbumin. For this reason, the idea that all patients with diabetes should receive an ACE inhibitor may not be far-fetched.

Checking for Eye Problems

All people with diabetes need to have a dilated eye exam done annually by an ophthalmologist or optometrist. No other physician, including the endocrinologist (yours truly excepted, of course), can do the exam properly.

For this exam, the doctor instills drops into your eyes and uses various instruments to examine the pressure, the appearance of your lens, and, most importantly, the retina of your eye.

All kinds of treatments can be done if abnormalities are found, but they must be discovered first. (See Chapter 5 for more information on eye problems.)

This test is something you must demand. Your doctor must refer you to an ophthalmologist or optometrist every year. Better yet, set up the appointment yourself with the eye doctor's nurse at the end of your first visit so that you are reminded about it each year.

Examining Your Feet

Unfortunately, foot problems often end in amputation. An amputation is really evidence of inadequate care. (For more on foot problems, see Chapter 5.) The doctor is not necessarily at fault here. The doctor sees you once in a while. You're with yourself much more often.

If you have any problem sensing touch with your feet, you need to take the following precautions:

✔ You must use your eyes to examine your feet every day.

✔ You must use your hand to test hot water before you step into it so that you do not get burned.

✔ You must shake out your shoes before you step into them to make sure no stone or other object is inside them.

✔ You must not go barefoot.

✔ You must keep the skin of your feet moist by soaking them in water, drying them, and applying a moisturizing lotion.

Your doctor can test your ability to feel an injury by using a 10-gram filament, but, again, that is done only when you have an appointment. You can obtain one of these filaments for yourself. A couple of the places where you can get them include

✔ Center For Specialized Diabetes Foot Care at `www.middelta.com/filamentsinfo.htm`.

✔ Diabetic Care Services at `www.diabeticcareservices.com` under Neuropathy Testing.

✔ Sensory Testing Systems at `www.thetrophyhousebr.com`. Click on STS products.

If you have any suggestion of a loss of sensation, at each visit to the doctor who takes care of your diabetes, you should take off your shoes and socks and have your feet inspected by the doctor.

The other part of a foot examination involves checking the circulation of blood to your feet. To check the cirulation, your doctor does a measurement called an *ankle-brachial index* at least once every five years. The systolic blood pressure is measured in the ankle and the arm. (See the sidebar "The meaning of your blood pressure," later in this chapter, for an explanation of systolic blood pressure.) The value for the ankle is divided by the value for the arm. An index of greater than 0.9 is considered normal. A value between 0.4 and 0.9 indicates peripheral vascular disease (see Chapter 5), while a value less than 0.4 indicates severe disease.

The ankle-brachial index should be done for any person with diabetes over age 50. Patients under 50 require the study if risk factors such as smoking, high cholesterol, and high blood pressure are present.

Tracking Cholesterol and Other Fats

Most people these days know the level of their total cholesterol, but other tests that show levels of various types of fats in the blood are needed as well.

Cholesterol is a type of fat that circulates in the blood in small packages called *lipoproteins.* These tiny round particles contain fat (*lipo,* as in liposuction) and protein. Because cholesterol does not dissolve in water, it would separate from the blood if it were not surrounded by the protein, just like oil separates from water in salad dressing. (That's why you have to shake the salad dressing each time you use it.)

A second kind of fat found in the lipoproteins is *triglyceride.* Triglyceride actually represents the form of most of the fat you eat each day. Although you may eat only a gram or less of cholesterol (an egg yolk has one-third of a gram of cholesterol), you eat up to 100 grams of triglyceride a day. (For more on the place of fats in your diet, see Chapter 8.) The fat in animal meats is mostly triglycerides.

Four types of lipoproteins exist:

- ✔ **Chylomicrons,** the largest fat particles, contain the fat that is absorbed from the intestine after a meal. They are usually cleared from the blood rapidly. Ordinarily, chylomicrons are not a concern with respect to causing *arteriosclerosis* (hardening of the arteries).

- ✔ **Very Low Density Lipoprotein (VLDL)** particles contain mostly triglyceride as the fat. These particles are smaller than chylomicrons.

- ✔ **High Density Lipoprotein (HDL),** known as "good" cholesterol, is the next smallest in size. This particle functions to clean the arteries, helping to prevent coronary artery disease, peripheral vascular disease, and strokes.

- ✔ **Low Density Lipoprotein (LDL),** known as "bad" cholesterol, is the particle that seems to carry cholesterol to the arteries, where it's deposited and causes hardening of the arteries.-

As you might imagine, we need to know which particle your cholesterol comes from in order to understand whether you have too much bad cholesterol (LDL) or a satisfactory level of good cholesterol (HDL).

You do not have to fast to do a test for total cholesterol and HDL cholesterol. However, you do need to fast for eight hours to find out your LDL cholesterol, because the blood has to be cleared of chylomicrons, which rise greatly when you eat.

You should have a *fasting lipid panel* at least once each year. A fasting lipid panel gives you your total cholesterol, your LDL cholesterol, your HDL cholesterol, and your triglyceride levels.

Table 7-2 lists the current recommendations for the levels of these fats in terms of the risk for coronary artery disease.

Table 7-2	Levels of Fat and the Risk for Coronary Artery Disease		
Risk	*LDL Cholesterol*	*HDL Cholesterol*	*Triglycerides*
Higher	Greater than 130	Less than 35	Greater than 400
Borderline	100 to 129	35 to 45	200 to 399
Lower	Less than 100	Greater than 45	Less than 150

You can see from Table 7-1 that the risk goes up as the LDL cholesterol goes up and the HDL cholesterol goes down. A huge study of thousands of citizens of Framingham, Massachusetts, shows that you can get a good picture of the risk by dividing the total cholesterol by the HDL cholesterol. If this result is less than 4.5, the risk is lower. If it's greater than 4.5, you're at higher risk for coronary artery disease. The higher it is, the worse the risk.

In March 2004, the story got a little more complicated. The *New England Journal of Medicine* published results of a study of more than 4,000 men who had just had heart attacks. In the study, some patients' LDL cholesterol was reduced maximally (to a mean of 62) with a large dose of a powerful drug called *atorvastatin.* The result was a major reduction, starting in just 30 days after treatment with the drug, in subsequent heart attacks, chest pain, and strokes compared to a group whose LDL was lowered only to 95. This result calls for a major reappraisal of "normal" for LDL. It may be that the lowest possible LDL level is best and that this applies to everyone, not only people who have just had a heart attack.

Diabetes adds its own complication because of the metabolic syndrome (see Chapter 5). In the metabolic syndrome, the total cholesterol may not be very high, but the HDL cholesterol is low and the triglycerides are elevated. These patients also have a lot of a dangerous form of LDL cholesterol, so they are at higher risk for coronary artery disease. This increased risk must be taken into account in considering treatment for the fats.

In deciding whether and how to treat the fats, you have to consider other risk factors for coronary artery disease. You're at

- ✔ Highest risk if you already have coronary artery disease, stroke, or peripheral vascular disease.
- ✔ High risk if you
  - Are a male over 45.
  - Are a female over 55.
  - Smoke cigarettes.
  - Have high blood pressure.
  - Have HDL cholesterol less than 35.
  - Have a father or brother who had a heart attack before age 55.
  - Have a mother or sister who had a heart attack before age 65.
  - Have a body mass index greater than 30.
- ✔ Low risk if you have none of the preceding risk factors.

The treatment for abnormal fats then depends on your risk category and level of LDL cholesterol (see Table 7-3).

Table7-3	Your Treatment Based on Risk Category	
Risk	*Dietary Treatment if LDL Greater Than*	*Diet and Drug Treatment if LDL Greater Than*
Low	160	190
High	130	160
Very high	100	100

All these decisions depend on obtaining a lipid (fat) panel.

REMEMBER

These treatment guidelines will change as the experts have a chance to evaluate the LDL study of heart attack victims that I discuss in this section.

Measuring Blood Pressure

The United States is experiencing an epidemic of high blood pressure (*hypertension*) similar to the epidemic of diabetes. The reasons are the same:

- ✔ Americans are getting fatter.

- ✔ Americans are storing fat in the center of our bodies, the so-called *abdominal visceral fat.*

- ✔ Americans are getting older as a population. The fastest growing segment of the population is over 75 years of age. Of people age 50 to 55 with diabetes, 50 percent have high blood pressure. Of people older than 75 with diabetes, 75 percent have high blood pressure.

- ✔ Americans are more sedentary than before.

People with diabetes have high blood pressure more often than the nondiabetic population for a lot of other reasons besides the preceding ones:

- ✔ People with diabetes get kidney disease.

- ✔ People with diabetes have increased sensitivity to salt, which raises blood pressure.

- ✔ People with diabetes lack the nighttime fall in blood pressure that normally occurs in people without diabetes.

Doctors generally agree that a normal blood pressure is less than 140/90. For years, the *diastolic blood pressure* (the lower reading) was considered more damaging, and an elevation in that pressure was treated with greater importance than an elevation in the *systolic blood pressure* (the higher reading). Recent studies have shown that the systolic blood pressure, not the diastolic blood pressure, may be more important. (See the sidebar "The meaning of your blood pressure" for more detailed explanations of each type of blood pressure.)

All the complications of diabetes are made worse by an elevation in blood pressure, especially diabetic kidney disease but also eye disease, heart disease, nerve disease, peripheral vascular disease, and cerebral arterial disease (see Chapter 5).

The most recent evidence of the importance of controlling blood pressure in diabetes comes from the United Kingdom Prospective Diabetes Study, published in late 1998. This study found that a lowering of blood pressure by 10 mm systolic and 5 mm diastolic resulted in a 24 percent reduction in any diabetic complication and a 32 percent reduction in death related to diabetes.

Controlling the blood pressure is absolutely essential in diabetes. The goal in diabetes is an even lower blood pressure than in the person without diabetes because studies have shown that lower normal blood pressures result in less diabetic damage than higher normal blood pressures. Your blood pressure should be no higher than 130/80.

How well are doctors doing at controlling blood pressure in people with diabetes? A study has shown that only 15 percent of people with diabetes with hypertension have a blood pressure as low as 140/90, and only 5 percent have a blood pressure down to 130/80.

Your doctor should measure blood pressure at every visit. Better yet, get a blood pressure device and measure it yourself. If you detect an elevation, bring it to the attention of your doctor.

For much more information on every aspect of high blood pressure, see my book *High Blood Pressure For Dummies, 2nd Edition* (Wiley).

Checking Your Weight and BMI

To give you a general idea of how much you ought to weigh, you can use the following formula:

- ✔ If you're a woman, give yourself 100 pounds for being 5 feet tall and add 5 pounds for each inch over 5 feet. For example, if you're 5 feet 3 inches, your appropriate weight should be approximately 115 pounds.

- ✔ If you're a man, give yourself 106 pounds for being 5 feet tall and add 6 pounds for each inch over 5 feet. A 5-foot 6-inch male should weigh around 142 pounds.

The meaning of your blood pressure

What does the blood pressure measurement mean, and what is high blood pressure? When you get a reading, it usually looks something like 120/70 — it has an upper reading and a lower reading.

✔ The upper reading, called the *systolic pressure,* is the amount of force exerted by the heart when it contracts to push blood around the body. A cuff around your arm connects to a column of mercury. You, your doctor, or a machine listens for the first sound you hear on the side of the cuff away from your heart. That sound is the sound of blood finally able to overcome the pressure in the cuff and get through to the other side. The systolic blood pressure is the height of the column of mercury, read in millimeters, just as the blood comes through. (Sometimes the cuff is not connected to a column of mercury but to a gauge that is calibrated so the reading on the gauge is in millimeters of mercury even though no mercury is present.) In our example, the systolic blood pressure reading is 120 mm of mercury.

✔ The lower reading, called the *diastolic blood pressure,* is the pressure in the artery when the heart is at rest. A valve in the heart keeps the blood from flowing backwards so that the pressure does not fall to zero (you hope). When the sound stops, the height of the mercury column gives the diastolic blood pressure, in this case 70 mm of mercury.

Body Mass Index (BMI) is a measurement that relates weight to height. A tall person has a lower BMI than a short person of the same weight. (See Chapter 3 for more on BMI, including instructions for calculating your own BMI.) A person with a BMI under 18.5 is considered slim. A person with a BMI from 18.5 to 24.9 is normal. A person with a BMI from 25 to 29.9 is overweight, and a person with a BMI of 30 or over is obese. By this definition, more than half the people in the United States are overweight or obese.

You cannot step on a scale and get a reading of your BMI, but you can get your weight. This measurement is one of the easiest in medicine. Your doctor should measure your weight at every visit.

The National Heart, Lung and Blood Institute makes it easy for you to know your BMI. Just fill in your weight in pounds and your height in feel and inches, click on compute BMI and you have your result. You can find it on the Internet at http://www.nhlbisupport.com/bmi/.

Maintaining a BMI in the normal range makes controlling your diabetes and blood pressure easier. Also, you must eliminate obesity as a risk factor for coronary artery disease.

Testing for Ketones

When your blood glucose rises above 250 mg/dl (13.9 mmol/L), or if you are pregnant with diabetes and your blood glucose is below 60 mg/dl (3.3 mmol/L), it is a good idea to check for *ketones* — products of the breakdown of fats. Finding ketones means that your body has turned to fat for energy. If you have high glucose and find ketones, you may need more insulin. If you have low glucose and find ketones during pregnancy, you may need more carbohydrates in your diet.

Testing for ketones is done by inserting a test strip into your urine and observing a purple color. The deeper the color, the greater the ketone level. If you find a large amount of ketones, you should contact your physician.

Even better you can use a meter such as the Precision Xtra described earlier to do a blood ketone level.

Testing the C-reactive Protein

C-reactive protein (CRP) is a substance in the blood that is produced by the liver when there is infection or inflammation. It can be measured with a simple blood test. Diabetes is associated with several features that suggest that inflammation plays an important role in the disease. People who develop diabetes have higher C-reactive protein than those who don't. (Other substances associated with inflammation are also elevated in diabetes.)

Drugs that improve diabetes lower the amount of C-reactive protein, which is also considered a marker for coronary artery disease.

Have your C-reactive protein measured with other blood tests about once a year. If the level is elevated, it may serve as a predictor of future diabetes or coronary artery disease. About 90 percent of healthy individuals have CRP levels less than 3, and 99 percent have levels less than 10.

Checking the TSH

Because there is a higher incidence of thyroid disease among people with diabetes and because thyroid disease is often confused with other conditions, a screening test called the thyroid stimulating hormone level is done at the time that diabetes is diagnosed and every five years thereafter if it is normal.

TSH is produced by the pituitary gland in the brain. When the thyroid gland makes the right amount of thyroid hormone, the pituitary produces the right amount of TSH to keep it working properly. The normal level in the blood is 0.5-2.5 microunits per milliliter (mU/ml).

When the thyroid makes inadequate amounts of thyroid hormone, the pituitary increases its production of TSH to stimulate the thyroid and values of 10 or more mU/ml are not uncommon. When the thyroid makes too much thyroid hormone, it causes the pituitary to turn down its production of TSH and values less than 0.5 mU/ml are found.

Too much thyroid hormone leads to insulin resistance, making diabetes worse than before. Too little thyroid hormone increases insulin sensitivity so people with low thyroid function have reduced levels of blood glucose.

Much more about thyroid disease and its treatment can be found in my book *Thyroid For Dummies,* 2nd Edition.

Chapter 8

Diabetes Diet Plan

· ·

· ·

*B*oy, are we big and getting bigger! You would think we were all on steroids. No, that explains professional baseball and football but not us nonprofessionals. The Centers for Disease Control tells us that more than six in ten Americans are overweight or obese. Most adults are 25 pounds heavier than people in the 1960s. And yet more than half of these overweight people think they are at a healthy weight. Something has got to give.

Language specialists claim that the five sweetest phrases in the English language are

   ✔ I love you.

   ✔ Dinner is served.

   ✔ All is forgiven.

   ✔ Sleep until noon.

   ✔ Keep the change.

To that, most people would certainly add, "You've lost weight."

For the diabetic population, most of whom are overweight, appropriate nutrition and weight loss are not an option but a necessity. The Diabetes Control and Complications Trial clearly demonstrated that a person with diabetes who follows a careful nutrition program can reduce his or her hemoglobin A1c (see Chapter 7) by as much as 1 percent compared to the person with diabetes who is careless about diet. The consequence of that lowering is a very significant reduction in both short- and long-term complications of diabetes.

In this chapter, you will find out all you need to know to make your diet work for you, not only to improve your diabetes and control your blood glucose, but generally to feel that you have an improved quality of life.

Considering Total Calories First

Wanda B. Thinner, age 46, was a new type 2 diabetic patient who came to me because of high blood glucose levels, some blurring of her vision, and some numbness in her toes. She was 5 feet 5 inches tall and weighed 165 pounds. She was taking pills for the diabetes, but they were not helping. Her doctor had told her she needed to lose weight but gave no further instructions. I started her on a diet based on the principles in this chapter. She was willing to follow the diet and lost 20 pounds, which she has kept off. Her blood glucose is now in the range of 110 most of the time. She no longer suffers from blurred vision, and her toes are beginning to improve. She is not taking the diabetes medication and feels much better.

No matter how you slice it, your weight is determined by the number of calories you take in, minus the number of calories you use up by exercise or loss of calories in the urine or bowel movements. If you have an excess of calories coming in and have insulin with which to store them, you gain weight. If you have fewer calories in than out, you lose weight. (See Chapter 7 if you're not sure how much you should weigh.) If you are overweight, you will benefit from even a small weight loss:

- ✔ Weight loss markedly reduces the risk of developing type 2 diabetes.
- ✔ Weight loss prevents the progression of prediabetes (see Chapter 2) into type 2 diabetes.
- ✔ Weight loss can reverse the failure to respond to drugs for diabetes that develops after responding at first (see Chapter 10).
- ✔ Weight loss reduces the risk of death from diabetes.
- ✔ Weight loss increases life expectancy in patients with type 2 diabetes.
- ✔ Weight loss has beneficial effects on high blood pressure and abnormal fats (see Chapter 7).

In an article in the *International Journal of Obesity* in June 2006, the authors from the University of Alabama and the University of Wisconsin offered ten other reasons that may be playing a role in our obesity epidemic. They are worth noting and considering for the possible role they play in your over-weight condition:

- **Reduced length of nightly sleep:** There is an inverse relationship between weight and hours of sleep. People are sleeping less than they did before.

- **Hormones and other substances in food:** Substances like estrogens, which are put in animal feed to fatten the animals, do the same to the humans who eat those animals.

- **Decreased exposure to high and low temperatures:** High temperatures cause sweating and low temperatures cause shivering, both of which contribute to weight loss. Modern heat and air conditioning diminish our exposure to extremes of temperature, which is actually good for us.

- **Decreased smoking:** This is a good news, bad news phenomenon. Obviously cigarette smoking is the greatest public health menace that exists, but smokers do tend to be leaner than non-smokers.

- **Use of drugs that cause weight gain:** Many of the drugs used for mental states like depression and high blood pressure cause marked weight gain and even diabetes.

- **Increases in age and ethnic groups that tend to be more overweight or obese:** Hispanic Americans, who are increasing in the population, have a much higher obesity prevalence than Caucasians. At the same time, the general population is older.

- **Increasing age of new mothers:** Older mothers tend to produce more obese children.

- **Effects in the uterus:** Maternal obesity may cause changes in the growing fetus that promote obesity.

- **Heavier women have more offspring:** These offspring, in turn, tend to be heavier.

- **Humans tend to choose heavier mates:** Heavier mates have reproductive advantages.

One or several of these explanations may play a small role in your overweight condition, and several may interact, but the overall effect is a significant increase in weight.

Portion sizes have increased significantly both in restaurants and at home. Here are correct portion sizes for several foods:

- Three ounces of meat is the size of a deck of playing cards.

- A medium apple or peach is the size of a tennis ball.

- One ounce of cheese is the size of four dice.

- One-half cup of ice cream is the size of a tennis ball.

✔ A cup of mashed potatoes is the size of your fist.

✔ A teaspoon of butter or peanut butter is the size of the tip of your thumb.

✔ One-half cup of nuts is the size of a golf ball.

The reason the French, with their much richer diet, may be leaner than us is that they eat significantly smaller portions.

To have an approximate idea of how many *kcalories* (kilocalories) you need each day (not *calories,* which are much smaller), you need to figure your desirable weight. Using the method describe in Chapter 7, a 5-foot 6-inch male with a moderate frame should weigh around 142 pounds. To find the number of kcalories needed:

1. **Multiply your weight times 10.** In our example, this gives a value of about 1,400 kcalories.

2. **Add kcalories for your level of exercise:**

    • A sedentary male adds 10 percent of the basal kcalories.

    • A moderately active male adds 20 percent.

    • A very active male adds 40 percent or more, depending on the length and the degree of exercise.

If the male in our example is moderately active, he needs 1,400 kcalories plus 1,400 times 20 percent (or about 300) more for a total of 1,700 kcalories.

These formulas are true for women as well, but women usually require fewer calories to maintain the same weight as men. Be aware that this is an approximation that differs not only for different people but even for the same person on different days.

Caloric needs are different for people of different ages and different levels of activity. A woman that is pregnant or breastfeeding obviously needs more kcalories. If a person is trying to lose weight, reducing the total kcalories per day can help to accomplish this. I say a lot more about this in the section on weight reduction in this chapter.

After you've calculated your kcalorie needs, you need to try a diet based on those needs, and you need to be willing to modify that diet if you don't have enough energy or aren't maintaining your desired weight. Especially if you are very physically active, your extra caloric needs may be very large and will quickly be noticed because you will lose weight.

When you determine the total kcalories you need, the question becomes how to divide the calories among various foods. Basically, three types of foods contain calories: carbohydrates, proteins, and fats. Within these foods, you have many variables, which I explain in the following sections.

Carbohydrates

There is no more controversial area in nutrition for the diabetic person than carbohydrates. For years, the American Diabetes Association (ADA) told people with diabetes that they should eat 55 to 60 percent of their calories as carbohydrate. Other experts said that amount was too much or too little. The ADA has now modified its recommendation so that it says in the Clinical Practice Recommendations for 2007: "The recommended daily allowance for carbohydrate (130 grams per day) in diabetes management is an average minimum requirement."

In this section, I give you my suggestions for carbohydrate in your diet based on my reading of the medical literature and my clinical experience. You are free to disagree with me and use whatever level of carbohydrate you like as long as it helps to promote a lower blood glucose without increasing your blood fats or weight.

Carbohydrates are the sources of energy that start with *glucose,* the sugar in your bloodstream that is one sugar molecule, and include substances containing many sugar molecules called *complex carbohydrates, starches, cellulose,* and *gums.* Some of the common sources of carbohydrate are bread, potatoes, grains, cereals, and rice.

Physicians know a lot of information about carbohydrate in the body:

- ✔ Carbohydrate is the primary source of energy for muscles.
- ✔ Glucose is the carbohydrate that causes the pancreas to release insulin.
- ✔ Carbohydrate causes the triglyceride (fat) level to rise in the blood.
- ✔ When insulin is not present or is ineffective, more carbohydrate raises the blood glucose higher.
- ✔ If simple sugars are in the diet in increased amounts, they are not harmful as long as the total calorie count is satisfactory. (The major reason to reduce simple sugars in the diet is the harmful effect on dental cavities. Cavities are no more severe or common in people with diabetes than in people without diabetes.)

Although the fat intake of the U.S. population has declined because of the fear of coronary artery disease caused by cholesterol, Americans are getting fatter. In fact, 64 percent of Americans are considered overweight or obese according to the U.S. Department of Health and Human Resources. Because Americans are not eating more protein, the culprit is most likely excess carbohydrate, such as that found in concentrated sweets, such as pastry and candy, as well as the more complex carbohydrate found in bread. Within the body, carbohydrate can be turned into fat and stored. This function was great when everyone lived in caves and got little food for prolonged periods of time, but it doesn't fit today's lifestyle, consisting as it does of abundant food (and minimal foraging for it in the supermarket).

Because carbohydrate is the food that raises the blood glucose, which is responsible for the complications of diabetes, it seems right to recommend a diet that is lower in carbohydrate than previously suggested. Furthermore, a major source of coronary artery disease in diabetes is the metabolic syndrome (see Chapter 5). Because increased carbohydrate triggers increased triglyceride, which is the beginning of a number of abnormalities that lead to increased coronary artery disease, recommending less carbohydrate on this basis as well seems prudent.

My experience has been that a diet of between 40 and 50 percent carbohydrate makes controlling my patients' blood glucose much easier. It also leads to weight loss because you don't tend to substitute protein or fat for the reduced amount of carbohydrate in the diet. My patients on lower carbohydrate diets are able to reduce the amounts of drugs they take, such as insulin, which can cause weight gain and complicate controlling their diabetes. They also have a better fat profile.

Thinking back to our example earlier in this chapter, a man on a diet of 1,700 kcalories should eat about 680 kcalories as carbohydrate. Because each gram of carbohydrate is 4 kcalories, he eats about 170 to 210 grams of carbohydrate a day. This is higher than the minimum recommended above. Translating this into the foods you know and love, this is the same as 13 to 16 slices of whole wheat bread, to 7 cups of oatmeal cereal, or 3 to 4 cups of brown rice a day.

Glycemic index

All carbohydrates are not alike in the degree to which they raise the blood glucose. This fact was recognized some years ago, and a measurement called the *glycemic index* was created to quantify it. The *glycemic index* (GI) uses white bread as the indicator food and assigns it a value of 100. Another carbohydrate of equal calories is compared to white bread in its ability to raise the blood glucose and is assigned a value in comparison to white bread. A food that raises glucose half as much as white bread has a GI of 50, while a food that raises glucose 1½ times as much has a GI of 150.

A recent study reported in the *Archives of Internal Medicine* in November 2007 showed that in a group of Chinese women who tended to eat a lot of high glycemic index rice, there was a significant increase in the risk of developing type 2 diabetes. Another study in the same issue showed that increasing the level of low glycemic cereal in the diet reduced the risk of type 2 diabetes in a group of black women, a group that is getting type 2 diabetes in epidemic numbers.

The point is to select carbohydrates with low GI levels to try to keep the glucose response as low as possible. A glycemic index of 70 or more is high; 56 to 69 is medium; and 55 or less is low.

The following complications have caused the GI to be underutilized:

✔ The GI of a carbohydrate may be different when it is eaten alone or as part of a mixed meal.

✔ The GI of a food may differ if it's processed and prepared differently.

✔ Some low GI foods, like chocolate, contain a lot of fat.

✔ Diabetes educators have been reluctant to teach the concept of the glycemic index because they believe it is hard to understand and will create confusion.

However, good clinical studies have shown that knowledge of the glycemic index of food sources can be very valuable. Evaluation of the diet of people who develop diabetes compared with those who don't shows that, all other things being equal, the people with the highest GI diet most often develop diabetes. After diabetes is present, those who eat the lowest GI carbohydrates have the lowest levels of blood glucose. Patients in these studies have not had great difficulty changing to a low GI diet. The other thing that happens when low GI food is incorporated into a diet is that the levels of triglycerides and LDL (or "bad" cholesterol) fall in both type 1 and type 2 diabetes.

I believe that switching to low GI carbohydrates can be very beneficial for controlling the glucose. You can easily make some simple substitutions in your diet, as shown in Table 8-1.

Table 8-1	Simple Diet Substitutions
High-GI Food	*Low-GI Food*
Whole meal or white bread	Whole grain bread
Processed breakfast cereal	Unrefined cereals like oats or processed low GI cereals
Plain cookies and crackers	Cookies made with dried fruits or whole grains like oats
Cakes and muffins	Cakes and muffins made with fruit, oats, and whole grains
Tropical fruits like bananas	Temperate climate fruits like apples and plums
Potatoes	Pasta or legumes
Rice	Basmati or other low GI rice

Because bread and breakfast cereals are major daily sources of carbohydrates, these simple changes can make a major difference in lowering your glycemic index. Foods that are excellent sources of carbohydrate but have a low GI include legumes such as peas or beans, pasta, grains like barley, parboiled rice and bulgar, and whole grain breads.

Even though a food has a low GI, it may not be appropriate because it is too high in fat. You need to evaluate each food's fat content before assuming that all low GI foods are good for a person with diabetes.

The position of the American Diabetes Association, stated in their position statement in 2007, is that "the use of the glycemic index may provide a modest additional benefit over that observed when total carbohydrate is considered."

And though a food has a high GI, it may still be acceptable in your diet if there is very little total carbohydrate. For example, cantaloupe has a GI of about 70, but the amount of total carbohydrate is so low that it does not raise your blood glucose significantly when you eat a normal portion. This concept is called the *glycemic load* (GL), a number that takes both glycemic index and total carbohydrates into account. A GL of 20 is high; 11 to 19 is medium; and 10 or less is low.

If you want to go into this subject in deeper detail, you can find a listing of many foods by category of food and by level of GI, portion size, and GL on the Web at `http://www.glycemicindex.com/`.

Fiber

Fiber is the part of the carbohydrate that is not digestible and, therefore, adds no calories. Fiber is found in most fruits, grains, and vegetables. Fiber comes in two forms:

- ✔ **Soluble fiber:** This form of fiber can dissolve in water and has a lowering effect on blood glucose and fat levels, particularly cholesterol.

- ✔ **Insoluble fiber:** This form of fiber cannot dissolve in water and remains in the intestine. It absorbs water and stimulates movement in the intestine. Insoluble fiber also helps prevent constipation and possibly colon cancer. This is the fiber called *bulk* or *roughage.*

Before the current trend to refine foods, people ate many sources of carbohydrate that were high in fiber. These were all in plant foods, such as fruits, vegetables, and grains. Animal foods contain no fiber.

Because too much fiber causes diarrhea and gas, you need to increase the fiber level in your diet fairly slowly. The recommendation for daily fiber is 20 to 30 grams. Most Americans eat only about 15 grams daily.

Many of the foods listed in the previous section as having a low glycemic index contain a lot of fiber, which helps to reduce the blood glucose.

The way to eat the right amount of carbohydrate without increasing your blood glucose or triglycerides is to make it a low-glycemic, high-fiber carbohydrate.

Proteins

Excluding vegetable sources of protein like soybeans, legumes, nuts, and seeds, protein in your diet is usually the muscle of other animals, such as chicken, turkey, beef, or lamb. For this reason, people used to believe that you could build your own muscle by eating lots of another animals' muscle. (The truth is that you can build up your muscle only by exercising or weightlifting.) You need little protein to maintain your current level of muscle or increase it for that matter.

Your choice of protein is very important because some is very high in fat while some is relatively fat-free. The following lists can give you an idea of the fat content of various sources of protein. (In the next section, I explain how to integrate fat into your diet.)

One ounce of **very lean** meat, fish, or substitutes has 7 grams of protein and 1 gram of fat. Examples include

- ✔ Skinless white meat chicken or turkey
- ✔ Flounder, halibut, or tuna canned in water
- ✔ Lobster, shrimp, or clams
- ✔ Fat-free cheese

An ounce of **lean** meat, fish, or substitutes has 7 grams of protein and 3 grams of fat. Examples include

- ✔ Lean beef, lean pork, lamb, or veal
- ✔ Dark meat chicken without skin or white meat chicken with skin
- ✔ Sardines, salmon, or tuna canned in oil
- ✔ Other meats or cheeses with 3 grams of fat per ounce

An ounce of **medium-fat** meat, fish, or substitutes has 7 grams of protein plus 5 grams of fat. Examples include

- ✔ Most beef products
- ✔ Regular fat pork, lamb, or veal
- ✔ Dark meat chicken with skin or fried chicken
- ✔ Fried fish
- ✔ Cheeses with 5 grams of fat per ounce, such as feta and mozzarella

High fat meat, fish, or substitutes contain 8 grams of fat and 7 grams of protein per ounce. Examples include

> ✔ Pork spareribs or pork sausage
>
> ✔ Bacon
>
> ✔ Regular cheeses like Cheddar and Monterey Jack
>
> ✔ Processed sandwich meats

You can see that there is a huge difference in kcalories between low-fat sources of protein and high-fat sources. An ounce of skinless white meat chicken contains about 40 kcalories, while an ounce of pork spareribs has 100 kcalories. Because most people eat a minimum of four ounces of meat at a meal, they're eating from 160 to 400 kcalories depending upon the source.

My recommendation is that 20 percent of your kcalories come from protein. This would be about 350 kcalories for the gentleman who weighs 142 pounds and needs 1,700 kcalories each day. Because a gram of protein is 4 kcalories, he can eat 90 grams of protein. Translating that into ounces of meat, because there are 7 grams of protein in each ounce, he can eat about 13 ounces of meat daily. For example, he can eat 6 ounces of flounder at one meal and 5 ounces of dark meat chicken at another, with 2 glasses of milk providing the rest of his protein.

Many authorities suggest less protein in the diet because protein has a damaging effect on the kidneys. Several studies have shown this to be the case, but a very large study in the *Annals of Internal Medicine* in March 2003 came to a different conclusion. It showed that high-protein diets caused increasing damage in kidneys that already had some damage but not in normal kidneys. The jury remains out on this question of lower versus higher protein diets.

Fats

The amount of fat you need is a lot less controversial than the carbohydrate and protein in your diet. Everyone agrees that you should eat no more than 30 percent of your diet as fats. (Currently, the U.S. population eats 36 percent of its diet as fats.)

Keep in mind that some fats are more dangerous in their tendency to promote coronary artery disease than others. These fats should make up less of the dietary fat than the safer fats.

Cholesterol is the fat everyone knows. It has been shown to be the culprit in the development of coronary artery disease, as well as peripheral vascular disease and cerebrovascular disease (see Chapter 5). The recommendation is that no more than 300 milligrams a day of fat come from cholesterol. One egg can take care of that prescription. Most other foods that you eat regularly do not contain a lot of cholesterol, but whole milk and hard cheeses like Jack and Cheddar contain saturated fat, which raises the cholesterol in the body.

The other kind of fat is triglyceride, which comes in several forms:

✔ **Saturated fat** is the kind of fat that usually comes from animal sources. The streaks of fat in a steak are saturated fat. Butter is made up of saturated fat. Bacon, cream, and cream cheese are other examples. Vegetable sources of saturated fat include coconut, palm, and palm kernel oils. Eating a lot of saturated fat increases your blood cholesterol level.

✔ **Trans fatty acid** is produced when polyunsaturated fat (which I describe in the next bullet) is heated and hydrogen is bubbled through it. Fully hydrogenated, it becomes solid fat; partially hydrogenated, it has a consistency like butter and can be used in butter's place. Food manufacturers have used trans fatty acids to replace butter because trans fatty acids are cheaper.

Trans fatty acids may contribute more to the development of heart disease than saturated fats. Keep them out of your diet! Some examples of foods high in trans fats are margarines, some cake mixes and dried soup mixes, many fast foods and frozen foods, baked goods like donuts and cookies, potato chips, crackers, breakfast cereals (even some with seemingly health-conscious names), candies, and whipped toppings. The government now requires food labels to list trans fats, so read those labels!

✔ **Unsaturated fat** comes from vegetable sources like olive oil, canola oil, and margarine. It comes in several forms:

   • **Monounsaturated fat** does not raise cholesterol. Avocado, olive oil, and canola oil are examples. The oil in nuts like almonds and peanuts is monounsaturated.

   • **Polyunsaturated fat** also does not raise cholesterol but causes a reduction in the good or HDL cholesterol. Examples of polyunsaturated fats are soft fats and oils such as corn oil, mayonnaise, and margarine.

Eskimos eat a lot of fat (more than is recommended), and yet they have a low incidence of coronary artery disease. It has been shown that their protection comes from **essential fatty acids.** These acids are found in fish oils, which the Eskimos consume to a great extent. Essential fatty acids reduce triglycerides, reduce blood pressure, and increase the time that it takes for blood to clot, which protects against a blood clot in the heart. You can have the benefits of fish oil by substituting fish for meat two or three times a week in your diet. Pills containing fish oil have not been shown to provide the same benefit. If you don't like fish (which means you have probably never tasted salmon cooked on a barbecue), you can't get this benefit.

Keeping in mind that 30 percent of your total daily calories should come from fat, less than a third of that amount should come from saturated fats. You should also keep your dietary cholesterol under 300 milligrams per day.

For the gentleman who weighs 142 pounds and needs 1,700 kcalories, who is slowly starving waiting for us to figure out how much to feed him, his final 500 kcalories can come from fat. Fat has 9 kcalories per gram, so he can eat about 56 grams of fat daily.

Remember that he has already taken in 40 grams of fat with his flounder and chicken, so he is left with only 16 grams, 8 of which come with his milk. That leaves about a teaspoon of butter from the fat sources.

Getting Enough Vitamins, Minerals, and Water

Your diet must contain sufficient vitamins and minerals, but the amount you need may be less than you think. If you eat a balanced diet that comes from the various food groups, you generally get enough vitamins for your daily needs. Table 8-2 lists the vitamins and their food sources.

Table 8-2	Vitamins You Need	
Vitamin	*Function*	*Food Source*
Vitamin A	Needed for healthy skin and bones	Milk and green vegetables
Vitamin B$_1$ (thiamin)	Converts carbohydrates	Meat and whole grain cereals into energy
Vitamin B$_2$ (riboflavin)	Needed to use food properly	Milk, cheese, fish, and green vegetables
Vitamin B$_6$ (pyridoxine), pantothenic acid, and biotin	All needed for growth	Liver, yeast, and many other foods
Vitamin B$_{12}$	Keeps the red blood cells and the nervous system healthy	Animal foods (for example, meat)
Folic acid	Keeps the red blood cells and the nervous system healthy	Green vegetables
Niacin	Helps release energy	Lean meat, fish, nuts, and legumes
Vitamin C	Helps maintain supportive tissues	Fruit and potatoes

Vitamin	Function	Food Source
Vitamin D	Helps with absorption of calcium	Dairy products, and it is made in the skin when exposed to sunlight
Vitamin E	Helps maintain cells	Vegetable oils and whole grain cereals
Vitamin K	Needed for proper clotting of the blood	Leafy vegetables, and it is made by bacteria in your intestine

As you look through the vitamins in Table 8-2, you can see that most of them are easily available in the foods you eat every day. In certain situations, such as if you are pregnant, you need to be sure that you are getting enough every day, so you take a vitamin supplement. Some evidence also suggests that extra vitamin C protects against colds.

As far as the other vitamins go, the proof just does not exist that large amounts of the vitamins are beneficial, and in some cases, they may be harmful. I do not recommend that you take megadoses of these vitamins.

Minerals are also key ingredients of a healthy diet. Most are needed in tiny amounts, which are easily consumed from a balanced diet. Keep the following in mind:

- ✔ **Calcium, phosphorus, and magnesium build bones and teeth.** Milk and other dairy products provide plenty of these minerals, but evidence suggests that people are not getting enough calcium. Adults should get 1,000 milligrams of calcium every day, and you should get 1,500 milligrams if you are growing up (adolescents) or out (pregnant women). Older people must be sure to eat 1,500 milligrams a day. Increased magnesium in the diet has a protective role in the development of type 2 diabetes.

- ✔ **Iron is essential for red blood cells and is gotten from meat.** However, a menstruating woman tends to lose iron and may need to supplement her food with a pill.

- ✔ **Sodium regulates body water.** You need only about 220 milligrams a day, but you likely take in 20 to 40 times that much, which probably explains a lot of the high blood pressure in the United States. Don't add salt to your food because it already has plenty in it, and you will enjoy the taste a lot more without it.

- ✔ **Chromium is needed in tiny amounts.** No scientific evidence shows that chromium is especially helpful to the person with diabetes in controlling the blood glucose despite reams of articles in health food magazines to the contrary.

✔ **Iodine is essential for production of thyroid hormones.** It is added to salt in order to assure that people get enough of it. In many areas of the world where iodine is not found in the soil, people suffer from very large thyroid glands known as *goiters.*

✔ **Various other minerals, like chlorine, cobalt, tin, and zinc, are found in many foods.** These minerals are rarely lacking in the human diet.

Water is the last important nutrient I discuss in this section, but it is by no means the least important. Your body is made up of 60 percent or more water. All the nutrients in the body are dissolved in water. You can live without food for some time, but you will not last long without water. Water can help to give a feeling of fullness that reduces appetite. In general, people do not drink enough water. You need to drink a minimum of 10 cups, or 2½ quarts, of water a day.

Counting Alcohol as Part of Your Diet

Alcohol is a chemical that has calories but no particular nutritional value; although it has been shown that a moderate amount (a glass or two of wine a day) may reduce the risk of a heart attack. Notice that I call alcohol a *chemical.* That's because alcohol is often taken to excess and does major damage to the body. It wrecks the liver and can lead to bleeding and death.

This book is not the place for a discussion of the social issues that surround the use of alcohol. Suffice it to say that excess alcohol destroys lives and families. In this section, I want to explain the part that alcohol plays in the life of the person with diabetes.

Because alcohol has calories, if you drink some, you must account for it in your diet. The proof of the alcohol is the percentage of alcohol in an ounce of the drink multiplied by 2. Wine that is 12.5 percent alcohol is 25 proof. Beer is 12 proof most of the time. Liquor is often 80 proof. To determine the calories, use the following formula:

Calories = 0.8 8 × proof of the drink × number of ounces

So, for example, for a 12-ounce can of beer, you use the formula 0.8 × 12 8 × 12 for a total of 115 kilocalories.

For a couple of 6-ounce glasses of wine, you use the formula 0.8 8 × 25 8 × 12 to come up with 240 kilocalories.

You can see that the alcohol calories add up pretty quickly. You may even wonder why alcoholics are not often overweight. The answer is that alcohol becomes a staple of their diet, and they develop wasting diseases associated with inadequate intake of protein, carbohydrate, fat, vitamins, and minerals.

In addition to the calories, alcohol plays other roles in diabetes. If alcohol is taken without food, it can cause low blood glucose by increasing the activity of insulin without food to compensate for it. Some alcoholics, even without diabetes, go to bed with several drinks in their systems and are unconscious the next morning because of very low blood glucose. They can have brain damage unless their bodies are able to manufacture enough glucose to wake them up.

If you're having a couple glasses of wine or other alcohol, make sure that you eat some food along with it.

Using Sugar Substitutes

Fear of the "danger" of sugar in the diet has led to a vast effort to produce a compound that can add the pleasurable sweetness without the liabilities of sugar. Interestingly enough, despite the availability of a number of excellent sweeteners, some containing no calories at all, the incidence of diabetes continues to rise. Still, if you can reduce your caloric intake or your glucose response by using a sweetener, doing so has advantages. Sweeteners are divided into those that contain calories and those that do not.

Among the calorie-containing sweeteners are

- ✔ **Fructose, found in fruits and berries:** Fructose is actually sweeter than table sugar (*sucrose*). However, it is absorbed more slowly from the intestine than glucose, so it raises the blood glucose more slowly. It is taken up by the liver and converted to glucose or triglycerides.

- ✔ **Xylitol, found in strawberries and raspberries:** Xylitol is about like fructose in terms of sweetness. It is taken up slowly from the intestine so that it causes little change in blood glucose. Xylitol does not cause cavities of the teeth as often as the other sweeteners containing calories, so it is used in chewing gum.

- ✔ **Sorbitol and mannitol, sugar alcohols occurring in plants:** Sorbitol and mannitol are half as sweet as table sugar and have little effect on blood glucose. They change to fructose in the body. (If you read Chapter 5, you may remember sorbitol. When taken as a food, sorbitol does not accumulate and damage tissues.)

The non-nutritive or artificial sweeteners are often much sweeter than table sugar. Therefore, much less of them is required to accomplish the same level of sweetness as sugar. The current artificial sweeteners include

- ✔ **Saccharin:** This sweetener is 300 to 400 times sweeter than sucrose. It is rapidly excreted unchanged in the urine. Brand names include Sweet 'N Low and Sugar Twin.

- ✔ **Aspartame:** This sweetener is more expensive than saccharin, but many people seem to prefer its taste. It's 150 to 200 times sweeter than sucrose. The brand name is Equal when used as a tabletop sweetener or NutraSweet when used in food and beverages.

- ✔ **Acesulfame:** This sweetener is 200 times sweeter than sucrose and does not leave an aftertaste. It can be used in cooking and is found in numerous foods and beverages, as well as a tabletop sweetener. Its brand name is Sunett or Sweet One. It should not be used by people with a rare genetic disorder called phenylketonuria.

- ✔ **Sucralose:** This sweetener is obtained from sugar and is 600 times sweeter. It is very stable and can be used in place of sugar in any food. It leaves no unpleasant aftertaste. The brand name is Splenda.

- ✔ **Neotame:** Authorized by the FDA in July 2000, neotame has 7,000 to 13,000 times the sweetening power of sucrose. It is not in commercial products yet, but food manufacturers are working with it because it can be used cooked or uncooked with no loss of sweetening. The brand name is not yet determined.

- ✔ **Cyclamate:** Because it has been associated with cancer when given in huge doses, cyclamate is banned in the United States. It is 30 times as sweet as sucrose. The association with cancer has not been substantiated, and this sweetener is awaiting reapproval by the FDA.

- ✔ **Tagatose:** This has been used only in 7-Eleven's Diet Pepsi Slurpees so far. Its production has been put on hold, but it should be available soon again. It has about the same sweetening power as table sugar and is called Naturlose.

For people with diabetes, recommendations regarding using sugar have been changed so that some sugar is permitted. The point is to count the calories eaten as sugar and subtract that from your permissible intake. If you do this, you'll have little use for either the nutritive or the non-nutritive sweeteners.

Eating Well for Type 1 Diabetes

A person with type 1 diabetes takes insulin (see Chapter 10) to control the blood glucose. At this time, doctors and their patients cannot match the human pancreas in the way that it releases insulin just when the food is entering the bloodstream so that the glucose remains between 80 and 120 mg/dl. Therefore, the diabetic patient needs to make sure that his or her food enters as close to the expected activity of the insulin as possible.

Most people with type 1 diabetes take two different types of insulin: one that acts soon after the injection and has a brief period of activity, and a second that acts more slowly and lasts longer. The rapid-acting insulin is meant to cover the food eaten at meals, while the slower acting insulin covers the rest of the time, particularly overnight when a lot of circumstances tend to raise the blood glucose.

Fortunately, you can take a new type of insulin when you start to eat or even in the middle or at the end of a meal. (See Chapter 10 for more information on this insulin.) This insulin overcomes the problem that always previously existed — that the shot had to be taken 30 minutes before eating to give it time to be active. A person with diabetes who had a meal delayed for any reason could easily become hypoglycemic using the old preparation.

The person with type 1 diabetes needs to be very careful when drinking alcohol. Alcohol increases the activity of insulin and can bring the blood glucose way down if food is not taken with it. (See the section on "Counting Alcohol as Part of Your Diet," earlier in this chapter.)

Because the person with type 1 diabetes always has some injected insulin circulating whether food is available or not, this patient should not miss a meal. A midmorning snack, a midafternoon snack, and even a bedtime snack, if necessary, are particularly good ideas.

The person with type 1 diabetes needs to be willing to test the blood glucose frequently. That way, he or she can identify problems in advance. If, for example, blood glucose is low before exercise (see Chapter 9), you can take some nutrition to avoid hypoglycemia.

For much more on this subject see my new book, *Type 1 Diabetes For Dummies* (Wiley).

Eating Well for Type 2 Diabetes

Because most people with type 2 diabetes are overweight, weight control and reduction should be the major consideration. (See the next section for specific techniques to lose weight.)

The benefits of weight loss are rapidly seen, even when relatively little has been lost. The blood glucose falls rapidly. The blood pressure declines. The cholesterol falls. The triglycerides drop, and the good cholesterol (HDL) rises. As I point out in Chapter 5, even a modest reduction of 10 percent of body weight has a significant positive effect on coronary artery disease.

The person with type 2 diabetes has to be very aware of the fats in his or her diet. The metabolic syndrome (see Chapter 5) is commonly found in this type of diabetes. You must pay attention to foods that increase triglycerides, which lead to the production of small, dense LDL particles that are connected to coronary artery disease.

Because hypertension is so prevalent in both types of diabetes and it makes diabetic complications occur earlier, reduction of salt intake is another important consideration.

Reducing Your Weight

Weight reduction is difficult for many reasons. In my experience, most patients do very well initially but tend to return to old habits. There is evidence that this tendency to regain weight is built into the human brain. When fat tissue is decreased or even increased, a central control system in the brain acts to restore the fat to the previous level. If liposuction is done, for example, the remaining cells swell up to hold more fat.

Still, losing weight and keeping it off is possible. At one time, it was calculated that only 1 out of 20 people who lost weight would keep it off. Now the figure is closer to 1 out of 5.

In the next chapter, I cover the value of exercise in a weight-loss program. At this point, you need to realize that successful maintenance of weight loss requires a willingness to make exercise a part of your daily life. If, for some reason, you cannot move your legs to exercise, you can get a satisfactory workout using your upper body alone. A recent study showed that 92 percent of people who maintain weight loss exercise regularly, while only 34 percent of those who regain their weight continue to exercise.

Types of diets

The numerous methods that are available for weight loss certainly suggest that no one method is especially better than all the rest. Some are fairly drastic in the degree to which they cut calories, and weight loss is fairly rapid. But these methods are particularly prone to result in restoration of the original weight. Among the many more drastic diets are the following:

- **Very low calorie diets:** These diets provide 400 to 800 kcalories daily of protein and carbohydrate with supplemental vitamins and minerals. They are safe when supervised by a physician and are used when you need rapid weight loss — for example, for a heart condition. They result in rapid initial weight loss with a fall in the need for medications. Weight restoration commonly occurs, however.

- **Animal protein diets like the Atkins diet:** Food is limited to animal protein sources in an effort to maintain body protein, along with vitamins and minerals. Carbohydrates are strongly discouraged. Patients often complain of hair loss. Weight is rapidly regained when the diet is discontinued. This is not a balanced diet, and I don't recommend it for more than a few weeks. Because the Atkins diet encourages foods that are high in fats, a variation called the *South Beach Diet* was developed that emphasizes decreased carbohydrates along with decreased fats.

✔ **LEARN diet:** The name stands for lifestyle, exercise, attitudes, relationships, and nutrition. It recommends a diet of 55 to 60 percent carbohydrate and less than 10 percent from fat.

✔ **Fasts:** A *fast* means giving up all food for a period of time and taking only water and vitamins and minerals. A fast is such a drastic change from normal eating habits that patients do not remain on the fast for very long, and weight is regained.

Several diets are associated with large organizations and may require that you purchase only their foods. The support given by these organizations seems to be extremely helpful in weight-loss maintenance. In addition, the slower loss of weight and the connection to more normal eating seems to result in a greater tendency to stay with the program and keep the weight off. The leading contenders for this type of diet are

✔ **Jenny Craig:** This organization provides the food that you eat, which you must pay for. It offers some information on behavior modification and has special diets for people with diabetes. In 1997, the government required Jenny Craig to tell its customers that the weight-loss methods may be only temporary, because customers had no way to judge from its advertising that many people regain their weight.

✔ **Weight Watchers:** This organization emphasizes slow weight loss, exercise, and behavior modification. It charges for weekly attendance at its meetings, which are held all over the world. It does not require that you purchase any products, but Weight Watchers foods are available for purchase. Its point program for increasing fiber in your diet may be especially helpful to the person with diabetes.

Do any of these diets have an advantage over the others? Researchers at Stanford University put four groups of overweight women on four different popular diets — Atkins, Ornish, LEARN, and the Zone — for a year. The result was that those people who stuck with the Atkins diet lost significantly more than the women on the other diets, about 12 pounds. Weight loss on the other diets was the same, about five pounds. Does that depress you? It shouldn't, because even that modest weight loss was associated with a 7 to 15 percent reduction of the risk of heart disease. The study was published in the *Journal of the American Medical Association* in March 2007.

The National Weight Control Registry, which has been running since 1993, shows that people can lose a lot of weight and keep it off. The average loss is 60 pounds and is maintained for more than five years. These "losers" do it on their own half the time. They use a combination of a low-fat diet and at least 45 minutes of exercise daily, usually walking, to keep the weight off even though the initial weight loss was accomplished in many different ways like a liquid diet in an organized program, other types of organized programs, or on their own. Most of them (68 percent) eat breakfast every day. The longer they kept the weight off, the easier it became to continue weight maintenance.

Surgery for weight loss

I want to say a few words about surgery for weight reduction. Surgery is used in the most severe and resistant cases of obesity. It has impressive effects, such as correction of high glucose and reduction or discontinuation of glucose-lowering drugs. Results are so successful in some patients that some surgeons consider type 2 diabetes to be a surgical disease. That, I believe, is a little extreme.

Some of the reasons for considering surgery include

✔ You have a body mass index (see Chapter 7) that is greater than 40.

✔ You have an obesity-related physical problem, such as inability to walk.

✔ You have a high-risk obesity-related health problem like heart disease.

Formerly, the best surgical treatment for obesity was the *vertical banded gastroplasty,* where the upper stomach is stapled to create a small, thumb-sized pouch above, a narrow opening, and a larger pouch below. Because the upper pouch is small, you have a feeling of early fullness, and you tend to eat less. The upper pouch is connected to the small intestine so that the lower stomach is bypassed. Patients are forced to eat very small portions and can't eat sugar and other carbohydrates, which cause dizziness and other symptoms. Most of the weight is lost in the first year.

More recently, the *laparoscopic gastric banding* procedure has been used. A constricting band containing an inflatable balloon is placed around the upper end of the stomach to create a small upper pouch and a larger lower pouch. It can be inflated or deflated to control the size of the upper stomach. The usual weight loss is two-thirds of the excess within two years. By removing the band, the procedure can be reversed. This is a simpler operation than gastric bypass and is less likely to result in a surgical complication.

Some of the problems of gastric banding include the following:

✔ The pouch may stretch.

✔ The band may slip.

✔ The reservoir in the constricting band that permits inflation may leak.

✔ Weight loss may not occur (if the patient chooses to overeat).

✔ The patient may experience acid reflux from the stomach into the esophagus.

✔ The patient may experience persistent vomiting.

When you have surgery for obesity, you must be committed to lifelong medical follow-up. You must be willing to give up large meals and be determined to lose weight. There is no question that severely obese patients with type 2 diabetes do well with surgery. As they lose weight, their blood glucose falls, their cholesterol falls, and their blood pressure improves. They sleep better and are less depressed.

As for liposuction and its possible role in the treatment of type 2 diabetes, there are few studies on the subject and they are short-term, but early reports showed some promise. For example, a report in the *Annals of Plastic Surgery* in January 2004 showed a fall in glucose, cholesterol, and insulin secretion after liposuction, but this was only at three weeks after surgery. A report from the *New England Journal of Medicine* later that year in June showed that liposuction did not significantly improve obesity-associated metabolic abnormalities after three months of observation.

Behavior modification

Years of working with obese patients have shown me that weight loss requires more than a commitment to a sound diet and routine exercise; it requires changes in behavior with respect to food. To lose weight and keep it off, you must change your eating behavior to make your diet easier to follow. Some of the best techniques include the following:

✔ Eat according to a schedule to avoid unplanned eating.

✔ Find a single place to eat all food.

✔ Slow down your eating to make the meal last.

✔ Put high calorie foods away. Remove serving dishes and bread from the table.

✔ Don't dispense food to others to avoid exposure for yourself.

✔ Do not clean your plate.

✔ Set realistic goals for weight loss.

✔ When eating out, be careful of salad dressing, alcohol, and bread.

172 Part III: Managing Diabetes: The "Thriving with Diabetes" Lifestyle Plan

✔ Get a ten-pound weight and carry it around for a while to appreciate the importance of losing even that little.

✔ At the market, buy from a list, carry only enough money for the food on that list, and avoid aisles containing loose foods, other than fruits and vegetables, like loose candy.

Incorporate one technique into your life each week (or even longer) until you feel you have mastered it and have added it to your eating style. Then go on and take up another technique.

As you go about this difficult task of losing weight and keeping it off, remember to seek the help of those around you. A loving partner provides great help through the roughest days.

In an effort to lose weight, some people with diabetes skip their insulin shots. If you do so, your body will turn to fat for fuel because glucose can't be used (see Chapter 2), and you will lose weight. However, the result is that you also lose muscle mass, and your blood glucose rises very high. This is a dangerous situation and not a healthy approach to weight loss.

Coping with Eating Disorders

You can't be too rich or too thin. How much damage has this statement done to society, especially the *thin* part? Young people, particularly girls, are preoccupied with their body weight. When this preoccupation becomes too great, it can result in an eating disorder.

Signs of anorexia or bulimia

Young girls with eating disorders (and young boys about a tenth as often) either starve themselves and exercise excessively or eat a great deal and then induce vomiting and/or take laxatives and water pills. Someone who starves herself has *anorexia nervosa,* while someone who binges and purges has *bulimia nervosa.* By themselves, these conditions can result in severe illness and even death when carried to extremes. When combined with diabetes, the danger increases greatly.

Anorexia is usually found in middle- and upper-class girls. They have a distorted body image and are fearful of weight gain. The prevalence may be as high as 1 in 200 in these girls. Their parents are usually very concerned with slimness. The girls may appear unusually thin and do not menstruate. Their malnutrition may be so severe that they die from it.

People with anorexia are in a constant state of starvation. When they have diabetes, their condition is just like that of people with type 1 diabetes before the availability of insulin. They have very low blood glucose levels, so little or no insulin is required (see Chapter 10). They develop problems with their hearts and have low blood pressure and low body temperature. They lose a lot of body musculature once the fat is gone.

If you think you know someone with this disorder, here are some of the clues to look for:

✔ She eats more rapidly than others do.

✔ She eats until uncomfortably full.

✔ She eats large amounts of food even when she is not hungry.

✔ She eats by herself because she is embarrassed.

✔ She feels guilty or disgusted after overeating.

Bulimia involves eating large quantities of easily digested food and then purging it by vomiting and taking laxatives or water pills. These patients are usually not as severely thin as patients with anorexia. However, their backgrounds are often similar to those of anorexia patients: They may represent up to 40 percent of college-age female students. Because their weight is closer to normal, they usually menstruate normally.

Management of diabetes requires a certain amount of routine from day to day. There is no way to achieve such systematization when the amount of food coming into the body is so uncertain.

The girl with severe anorexia may require intravenous feeding until she is stabilized a little bit. This sometimes leads to very high blood glucose levels, necessitating the use of insulin. After the life-threatening starvation is under control, it is possible to achieve good blood glucose control with help from the patient and a therapist who can help her to understand her distorted body image. If she suffers from clinical depression, antidepressant medication may be necessary.

With a bulimic patient, the food intake is extremely variable but less severe than that of an anorexic. Therefore, diabetes is a little easier to treat. However, girls with bulimia are more likely to go on to adult obesity and are harder to treat psychologically. They actually do not do as well with therapy as those with anorexia. They end up with more psychiatric problems later in life.

Sources of help

The Eating Disorder Referral and Information Center provides information and treatment centers online at www.edreferral.com. You can also contact the center at 2923 Sandy Pointe, Suite 6, Del Mar, CA 92014-2052; or call 858-792-7463.

A major source of useful information is the National Eating Disorders Association at 603 Stewart Street, Suite 803, Seattle, WA 98101 (206-382-3587). The association's Web site, containing extensive information on this subject, is www.nationaleatingdisorders.org.

The National Association of Anorexia Nervosa and Associated Disorders provides information online, including referrals to support groups, therapists, and treatment centers, at www.anad.org. You can also contact the association at P.O. Box 7, Highland Park, IL 60035; or call 847-831-3438.

Chapter 9

Keeping It Moving: Exercise Plan

● ●

In This Chapter

▶ Understanding the importance of exercise

▶ Tailoring exercise for type 1 and type 2 patients

▶ Determining how long and how hard to exercise

▶ Choosing your activity

● ●

More than 60 years ago, the great leaders in diabetes care declared that diabetes management has three major aspects:

✔ Proper diet

✔ Appropriate medication

✔ Sufficient exercise

Since then, millions of dollars and man (and woman) hours have been spent to define the proper diet and the right medication, but exercise has rarely received its proper place in the triad of care. I am writing this chapter to correct that omission.

Exercise has become so central to diabetes care, especially type 2 diabetes that authors of articles on diabetes have titles, such as:

✔ "Make Your Diabetic Patients Walk," *Diabetes Care,* June 2005

✔ "Walking to Work Is an Independent Predictor of Incidence of Type 2 Diabetes in Japanese Men," *Diabetes Care,* September 2007

✔ "Exercise Training Improves Glycemic Control in Long-Standing Insulin-Treated Type 2 Diabetic Patients," *Diabetes Care,* October 2007

✔ "Exercise Is Required for Visceral Fat Loss in Postmenopausal Women with Type 2 Diabetes," *Journal of Clinical Endocrinology and Metabolism,* March 2005

✔ "Increase in Physical Activity Energy Expenditure Is Associated With Reduced Metabolic Risk Independent of Change in Fatness and Fitness," *Diabetes Care,* August 2007

These titles should tell you, before I even write another word, how central exercise is to your health. And not just if you have diabetes. Grab your spouse, significant other, child, parent, grandparent, or great grandparent, and start walking!

Getting Off the Couch: Why Exercise Is Essential

When the diabetes experts wrote their recommendations for proper care, the isolation and administration of insulin had just recently begun, and they were focusing specifically on how to control type 1 diabetes. Since that time, many studies have shown that exercise doesn't normalize the blood glucose or reduce the hemoglobin A1c (see Chapter 7) in type 1 diabetes. Many other studies have shown that exercise does normalize blood glucose and reduce hemoglobin A1c in type 2 diabetes.

But while exercise cannot replace medication for the type 1 diabetic, its benefits are crucial for patients with both types of diabetes.

Preventing macrovascular disease

The major benefit of exercise for both types of diabetes is to prevent *macrovascular disease* (heart attack, stroke, or diminished blood flow to the legs). Macrovascular disease affects everyone, whether they have diabetes or not, but is particularly severe in people with diabetes. Exercise prevents macrovascular disease in numerous ways:

- ✔ Exercise helps with weight loss, which is especially important in type 2 diabetes.
- ✔ Exercise lowers bad cholesterol and triglycerides, and it raises good cholesterol.
- ✔ Exercise lowers blood pressure.
- ✔ Exercise lowers stress levels.
- ✔ Exercise reduces the need for insulin or drugs.

Taking charge of your health

John Plant is a 46-year-old male who has had type 1 diabetes for 23 years. He takes insulin shots four times daily and measures his blood glucose multiple times a day. He follows a careful diet.

Prior to developing diabetes, he was a very active person, participating in vigorous sports and doing major hiking and mountain climbing. At the time, his doctor warned him that he would have to give up many of the most strenuous activities because he would never know his blood glucose level and it might drop precipitously during heavy exercise. He ignored this advice and continued his active way of life. He found that he could do with much less insulin than his doctor prescribed and rarely became hypoglycemic. He has been able to continue these activities without limitation. His blood glucose level is generally between 75 and 140. His last hemoglobin A1c was slightly elevated at 5.7 (see Chapter 7). A recent eye examination showed no diabetic retinopathy (see Chapter 5). He has no significant microalbuminuria in his urine and no tingling in his feet (see Chapter 5).

Is John lucky? You bet he is. But like most "luck," his is based on a self-realization that the human body is made up of both a mind and a body. If humans were meant to spend their lives munching potato chips in front of a TV set, why would they have all these muscles?

When a new diabetic patient enters my office, I give him a bottle of 50 pills. I instruct him not to swallow the pills but to drop them on the floor three times daily and pick them up one at a time. The condition a person is in can be judged by which thing he or she takes two at a time: pills or stairs.

Understanding your body mechanics during exercise

The feeling of fatigue that occurs with exercise is probably due to the loss of stored muscle glucose.

With exercise, insulin levels in nondiabetics and people with type 2 diabetes decline, because insulin acts to store and not release glucose and fat. Levels of glucagon, epinephrine, cortisol, and growth hormone increase to provide more glucose. Studies show that glucagon is responsible for 60 percent of the glucose, and epinephrine and cortisol are responsible for the other 40 percent. If insulin did not fall, glucagon could not stimulate the liver to make glucose.

You might wonder how insulin can open the cell to the entry of glucose when insulin levels are falling. In fact, two things are at work here. Glucose is getting into muscle cells without the need for insulin, and the rapid circulation that comes with exercise is delivering the smaller amount of insulin more frequently to the muscle. The muscle seems to be more sensitive to the insulin as well. This is exactly what the person with type 2 diabetes hopes to accomplish when insulin resistance is the major block to insulin action.

One way to preserve glucose stores is to provide calories from an external source. Any marathoner knows that additional calories can delay the feeling of exhaustion. The timing is important. If the glucose is given an hour before exercise, it will be metabolized during the exercise and increase endurance. However, if it's given 30 minutes before exercise, it may decrease stamina by stimulating insulin, which blocks liver production of glucose.

Fructose can replenish you when you're doing prolonged exercise. This sweetener can replace glucose because it is sweeter but is absorbed more slowly and does not provoke the insulin secretion that glucose provokes. Fructose is rapidly converted into glucose inside the body. (See Chapter 8 for more on fructose.)

Reaping the benefits

As your body becomes trained with regular exercise, the benefits for your diabetes are very significant. Your body starts to turn to fat for energy earlier in the course of your exercise. At the same time, the hormones that tend to raise the blood glucose during exercise are not produced at the same high rate because they aren't needed. Because you don't require as much insulin, your insulin doses can be reduced, and it's much easier to avoid hypoglycemia during exercise.

Exercising When You Have Diabetes

If you have diabetes and have not exercised previously, you should check with a doctor prior to beginning a new exercise program, especially if you're over the age of 35 or if you've had diabetes for ten years or longer. You should also check with a doctor if you have any of the following risk factors:

- ✔ The presence of any diabetic complications like retinopathy, nephropathy, or neuropathy (see Chapter 5)
- ✔ Obesity
- ✔ A physical limitation
- ✔ A history of coronary artery disease or elevated blood pressure
- ✔ Use of medications

You need to discuss these issues with your doctor in order to choose the appropriate exercises. I say more about the choice of exercise in the section "Is Golf a Sport? Choosing Your Activity," later in this chapter.

When you begin to exercise, whether you have type 1 or type 2 diabetes, you can take many steps to make your experience safe and healthful. Some important steps to take include the following:

- ✔ Wear an ID bracelet.
- ✔ Test your blood glucose very often.
- ✔ Choose proper socks and shoes.
- ✔ Drink plenty of water.
- ✔ Carry treatment for hypoglycemia.
- ✔ Exercise with a friend.

And here are some things to avoid when you exercise:

- ✔ Don't assume that you have to buy lots of special clothing to exercise. The right shoes and socks are essential, but other than that, you need special clothing only if your sport demands it (such as soft pants for the cyclist).
- ✔ Don't expect to lose certain "spots" by repetitively exercising them.
- ✔ Don't exercise to the point of pain.
- ✔ Don't get too focused on using exercise gadgets, like belts or other objects, that do not require you to move.

Working out with type 1 diabetes

The person with type 1 diabetes depends on insulin injections to manage the blood glucose. He or she does not have the luxury of a "thermostat" that automatically shuts off during exercise and turns back on when exercise is finished. After an insulin shot is taken, it is active until it is used up.

The person with type 1 diabetes has to avoid overdosing on insulin before exercise, which can lead to hypoglycemia, or underdosing, which can lead to hyperglycemia. If the body does not have enough insulin, it turns to fat for energy. Glucose rises because it is not being metabolized but its production is continuing. If exercise is particularly vigorous in a situation of not enough insulin, the blood glucose can rise extremely high.

Reducing your insulin dosage prior to exercise helps prevent hypoglycemia. One study showed that an 80 percent reduction of the dose allowed the person with diabetes to exercise for 3 hours, while a 50 percent reduction forced the person with diabetes to stop after 90 minutes due to hypo-glycemia. Each person with diabetes varies, and you must determine for yourself how much to reduce insulin by measuring the blood glucose before, during, and after exercise.

What are aerobic and anaerobic exercise?

Aerobic exercise is exercise that can be sustained for more than a few minutes, uses major groups of muscles, and gets your heart to pump faster during the exercise, thus training the heart. I give you many examples of aerobic exercise throughout this chapter.

Anaerobic exercise, on the other hand, is brief (sometimes a few seconds) and intense and usually cannot be sustained. Lifting large weights is an example of an anaerobic exercise. A 100-yard dash is another example.

Another way to prevent hypoglycemia, of course, is to eat some carbohydrate (see Chapter 8). You need to have some carbohydrate (which quickly raises blood glucose) available during exercise.

In addition, the site of the insulin injection is important because this determines how fast the insulin becomes active. If you are running and inject insulin into your leg, it will be taken up more quickly than an injection into the arm.

You can exercise whenever you will do it faithfully. If you like to sleep late and you schedule your exercise at 5:30 a.m., you probably won't consistently do it. Your best time to exercise is probably about 60 to 90 minutes after eating because this is when the glucose is peaking, providing the calories you need; if you exercise at this time you avoid the usual post-eating high in your blood glucose, and you burn up those food calories.

Working out with type 2 diabetes

Other than the insulin discussion, many of the suggestions for the type 1 patient in the previous section apply to type 2 patients as well.

With sufficient exercise and diet, some people with type 2 diabetes can revert to a nondiabetic state. This does not mean that they no longer have diabetes, but it certainly means that they will not develop the long-term complications that can make them so miserable later in life (see Chapter 5).

Determining How Much Exercise to Do

Unless you have a physical abnormality, there is no limitation on what you can do. You need to select an activity that you enjoy and will continue to perform.

Checking the value of your exercise

Measuring your pulse during exercise (or even at rest) may be hard for you. Instead, you can use the Perceived Exertion Scale. Exercise is given a descriptive value from *very, very light* to *very, very hard* with *very light, fairly light, somewhat hard,* and *very hard* in between. You want to exercise to a level of *somewhat hard,* and you will be at your target heart rate in most cases. As you get into shape, the amount of exertion that corresponds to *somewhat hard* will increase.

Here is a description of these various levels of exercise:

✔ **Extremely light exercise** is very easy to do and requires little or no exertion.

✔ **Very light exercise** is like walking slowly for several minutes.

✔ **Light exercise** is like walking faster but at a pace you can continue without effort.

✔ **Somewhat hard exercise** is getting a little difficult but still feels okay to continue.

✔ **Very hard exercise** is difficult to continue. You have to push yourself, and you're very tired. At this level, you have trouble talking. The very hard level of exercise is most beneficial.

✔ **Extremely hard exercise** is the most difficult exercise you've ever done.

Do not continue exercising if you have tightness in your chest, chest pain, severe shortness of breath, or dizziness.

Exerting enough effort

In the recent past, exercise physiologists said that you needed to make sure that you monitored your exercise intensity by periodically checking your heart rate. Your exercise heart rate was supposed to be based on your age. The usual formula to figure this out is to take the number 220, subtract your age, and multiply that number by 60 to 75 percent to get the recommended exercise heart rate for aerobic exercise. (See the sidebar "What are aerobic and anaerobic exercise?" if you're not sure what aerobic exercise is.)

Now studies have shown that people can sustain aerobic exercise at higher heart rates. Perhaps the best way to know whether you're meeting your exercise goals is to use the "Perceived Exertion Scale" described in the sidebar "Checking the value of your exercise."

The younger you are, the faster your exercise heart rate may be. Like everything in this book, your exercise heart rate is an individual number. If you are a world-class athlete training for your ninth marathon, your exercise heart rate may be higher. If you have some heart disease, your exercise heart rate may be significantly lower.

Devoting an hour a day

When you know your maximal exercise heart rate, you can choose your activity and use the "Perceived Exertion Scale" to be sure that you achieve that level during exercise. I must repeat that the best choice of exercise for you is an exercise you enjoy and will continue to perform.

The choices are really limitless. The number of kcalories you use for any exercise is determined by your weight, the strenuousness of the activity, and the time you spend actually doing it. In the past it was suggested that in order to have a positive effect on your heart, you need to do a moderate level of exercise for 20 to 45 minutes at least three times a week. In 2002, the Institute of Medicine (the medical division of the National Academies) recommended that in order to maintain health and a normal body weight, you need to do one hour of exercise a day.

An hour (not an apple) a day keeps the doctor away! Moderate aerobic exercise done for an hour every day provides enormous physical, mental, and emotional benefits.

You need to warm up and cool down for about five minutes before and after you exercise. Stretching is one possibility for both warm-up and cool-down. I am not going to discuss stretching in detail because the place of stretching for the healthy exerciser is not clear. One study showed that a group of runners who did not stretch did better than a group who did. Most doctors agree that stretching after an injury is appropriate, but whether all the advice about stretching before exercise for an uninjured person is much ado about nothing is yet to be determined. If you do stretch, do not stretch to the point that it hurts. This is where muscle tears occur. See the excellent book *Fitness For Dummies,* 3rd Edition, by Suzanne Schlosberg and Liz Neporent, M.A. (Wiley), for more about stretching.

Making moderate exercise your goal

Moderate exercise has a moving definition. If you're out of shape, moderate exercise for you may be slow walking. If you're in good shape, moderate exercise may be jogging or cross-country skiing. Moderate exercise is simply something you can do and not get out of breath. For ideas on the types of exercise you can do, see the following section.

How long can you stop exercise before you start to decondition? It takes only about two to three weeks to lose some of the fitness your exercise has provided. Then it takes up to six weeks to get back to your current level, assuming that your holiday from exercise does not go on too long.

When you need support

The Diabetes Exercise and Sports Association is an organization that you can turn to for help, instruction, and friendship as you add exercise to your good diabetes care. You can reach this organization by writing P.O. Box 1935, Litchfield Park, AZ 85340, or by calling 800-898-4322. They know all about diabetes and sports and are eager to share the information with you. They have a newly reconstructed Web site at `http://www.diabetes-exercise.org/about.asp`.

Is Golf a Sport? Choosing Your Activity

The following factors can help you determine your choice of activity:

- ✔ Do you like to exercise alone or with company? Pick a competitive or team sport if you prefer company.

- ✔ Do you like to compete against others or just yourself? Running or walking are sports you can do alone.

- ✔ Do you prefer vigorous or less vigorous activity? Less vigorous activity over a longer period is just as effective as more vigorous activity.

- ✔ Do you live where you can do activities outside year-round, or do you need to go inside a lot of the year? Find a sports club if weather prevents year-round outside activity.

- ✔ Do you need special equipment or just a pair of running shoes?

- ✔ What benefits are you looking for in your exercise: Cardiovascular, strength, endurance, flexibility, or body fat control? You should probably look for all these benefits, but you may have to combine activities to get them all in.

Perhaps a good starting point in your activity selection is to focus on the benefits. Table 9-1 gives you some ideas.

Table 9-1	Match Your Activity to the Results You Want
If You Want to . . .	*Then Consider . . .*
Build up cardiovascular condition	Vigorous basketball, racquetball, squash, cross-country skiing, handball
Strengthen your body	Low-size, high repetition weight lifting, gymnastics, mountain climbing, cross-country skiing

(continued)

Table 9-1 *(continued)*

If You Want to ...	Then Consider ...
Build up muscular endurance	Gymnastics, rowing, cross-country skiing, vigorous basketball
Increase flexibility	Gymnastics, judo and karate, soccer, surfing
Control body fat	Handball, racquetball, squash, cross-country skiing, vigorous basketball, singles tennis

You can tell from Table 9-1 that living in the mountains where you have plenty of snow is helpful because cross-country skiing is on almost every list. On the other hand, so is vigorous basketball, so you don't have to give up exercise if you live in a warm climate like Florida.

The special needs of many of these sports may turn you off to exercise. The curious thing is that the best exercise that you can sustain for life is right at your feet. A brisk daily walk improves heart function, adds to muscular endurance, and helps control body fat. So many people drive their cars to the gym and try to park as close as possible so that they can get to the building with as little effort as possible. Seems a little strange, doesn't it?

Of course, the social benefits of exercise are very important. You are together with people who are concerned with health and appearance. These people usually share many of your interests. The person who likes to jog often likes to hike and climb and camp out. Many lifetime partnerships begin on one side of a tennis court (and some end there as well).

Cross-training, where you do several different activities throughout the week, is a good idea. Cross-training reduces the boredom that may accompany doing one thing day after day. It also permits you to exercise regardless of the weather because you can do some things indoors and some outside.

Table 9-2 lists a variety of activities, including some that don't exactly fit into the category of *exercise* but offer some interesting comparisons. Next to each activity, I include the amount of kcalories that you burn in 20 minutes.

Table 9-2	**Calories Burned in 20 Minutes at Different Body Weights**	
Activity	*Kcalories Burned (125 pounds)*	*Kcalories Burned (175 pounds)*
Standing	24	32
Walking, 4 mph	104	144

Activity	Kcalories Burned (125 pounds)	Kcalories Burned (175 pounds)
Running, 7 mph	236	328
Gardening	60	84
Writing	30	42
Typing	38	54
Carpentry	64	88
House painting	58	80
Baseball	78	108
Dancing	70	96
Football	138	192
Golfing	66	96
Swimming	80	112
Skiing, downhill	160	224
Skiing, cross-country	196	276
Tennis	112	160

Everything you do burns calories. Even sleeping and watching television use 20 kcalories in 20 minutes if you weigh 125 pounds.

Your choice of an activity must take into account your physical condition. If you have diabetic neuropathy (see Chapter 5) and cannot feel your feet, you do not want to do pounding exercises that may damage them without your awareness. You can swim, bike, row, or do armchair exercises where you move your upper body vigorously. One of my favorite relatively new machines that give you a good workout without trauma to your joints is the elliptical trainer, but you may have to join a club to get at one unless you buy one for home.

If you have diabetic retinopathy (see Chapter 5), you won't want to do exercises that raise your blood pressure (like weight lifting), cause jerky motions in your eyes (like bouncing on a trampoline), or change the pressure in your eyes significantly (like scuba diving or high mountain climbing). You also should not do exercises that place your eyes below the level of your heart, such as when you touch your toes.

Patients with nephropathy (see Chapter 5) should avoid exercises that raise the blood pressure for prolonged periods. These exercises are extremely intense activities that you do for a long time, like marathon running.

Some people have pain in the legs after they walk a certain distance. This may be due to diminished blood supply to the legs so that the needs of the muscles in the legs cannot be met. Although you need to discuss this problem with your doctor, you do not need to give up walking. Instead, determine the distance you can walk up to the point of pain. Then walk about three-quarters of that distance and stop to give the circulation a chance to catch up. After you have rested, you will find that you can go about the same distance again without pain. By stringing several of these walks together, you can get a good, pain-free workout. You may even find that you are able to increase the distance after a while because this kind of training tends to create new blood vessels.

Is there a medical condition that should absolutely prevent you from doing exercise? Short of chest pain at rest, which must be addressed by your doctor, the answer is no. If you cannot figure out an exercise that you can do, get together with an exercise therapist. You will be amazed at how many muscles you can move that you never knew you had.

Walking 10K a Day

The idea of walking 10,000 steps a day may seem like a huge, unattainable goal to you, but you may be surprised. This is certainly a goal worth striving toward because, as I discuss previously in this chapter, walking is one of the most beneficial exercises you can do.

The first step toward reaching this goal is to buy a *pedometer,* a device that you wear on your waist that counts each step you take. Don't buy a fancy one with a lot of bells and whistles. All you need is to be able to count your steps and, if you want, to convert the steps into miles. To do this, you need to know how far you walk each time you take a step. Walk ten steps, measure the distance, and divide by ten to get your stride length. Input this number in the appropriate place in the pedometer, and it will give you the miles that correspond with the steps you walk.

Accusplit pedometers work very well. The model I like is the Accusplit Eagle, which does nothing but record your steps. You can find it at `www.accusplit.com/product.html`. You also can find pedometers at sporting goods stores.

Begin by doing your usual amount of exercise each day. Remember to record the steps at the end of the day and reset the button on the pedometer to zero. After seven days, add up the steps and divide by seven to get your daily count. You will probably find that you are doing between 3,000 and 5,000 steps a day.

Next, you want to build up your daily number. Here are some tips to help:

- ✔ Get a good pair of walking shoes or sneakers and replace them when they begin to wear out.
- ✔ Leave your car parked. If you can make a trip in an hour or less by foot, save your gas money and add substantially to your daily step count.
- ✔ Try to add a few hundred steps a week. Begin by identifying a baseline day in your first week when you did the most steps, and make every day like that one. Each week add a few hundred more.
- ✔ Find an exercise buddy to walk with you. It's much more fun.
- ✔ Keep a record of the number of steps involved in various walks you take, so you can easily get the steps you are missing on any given day.
- ✔ Use stairs instead of the elevator, whether you're going up or down.
- ✔ Take a walk at lunchtime daily.
- ✔ Stop if you feel pain, and check with your doctor before continuing.

If you don't have a pedometer, or if you want to count other types of exercise toward your walking goal, use the following conversions:

- ✔ 1 mile = 2,100 average steps
- ✔ 1 block = 100 average steps
- ✔ 10 minutes walking = 1,200 steps on average
- ✔ Biking or swimming = 150 steps per minute
- ✔ Weight lifting = 100 steps per minute
- ✔ Rollerskating = 200 steps per minute

 If you like tangible rewards for what you do (besides the reward of a lower blood glucose, a lower cholesterol, a lower blood pressure, and possibly a lower weight), join the President's Challenge at `www.presidents challenge.org`. It provides a place to record your activity, and it offers all kinds of information on activities for every age. You choose what you like to do, and every time you do it you record your progress. It gives you points towards awards.

 If you prefer to follow an actual trail, take a virtual walk on the American Discovery Trail, a 5,048-mile walk across America from Delaware to California. You can find it at `http://www.discoverytrail.org`. Every time you walk, convert your steps into miles and see how far they take you along that trail. The page has links to all the sights you will see. If you have trouble converting your steps into miles, just use the steps and eliminate the last two digits (so 10,000 steps becomes 100 miles).

A study in the *Archives of Internal Medicine* in June 2003 provides the best evidence for the benefits of walking. Diabetics who walked at least 2 hours a week had a 40 percent lower death rate than inactive diabetics.

The study that I mentioned at the beginning of the chapter entitled "Make Your Diabetic Patients Walk" followed 179 patients with type 2 diabetes who were divided into six groups and followed for two years. The groups differed in the amount of increased exercise they did. For example the first group did a little more exercise by the end of the study while the last group did much more exercise by the end of the study. The other groups fell in between those extremes. The results were that the highest exercisers had the lowest blood pressure, greatest weight loss, greatest reduction in total cholesterol and bad cholesterol and increase in good cholesterol, greatest reduction in blood glucose, and greatest reduction in money spent on drugs. While the people who did the least exercise had no change in the cost of their annual medications, the highest exercisers had a reduction of $660 per year. What are you waiting for? Take the first steps!

Lifting Weights

Weight lifting is a form of anaerobic exercise. (See the sidebar earlier in this chapter if you're not sure what anaerobic exercise is.) It involves the movement of heavy weights, which can be moved only for brief periods of time. It results in significant muscle strengthening and increased endurance.

Doctors are looking for drugs that can increase insulin sensitivity (see Chapter 10). You need look no further. Lifting weights has been shown in several studies to accomplish this. Writing in *Diabetes Care* in September 2007, a group of investigators from the Centers for Disease Control showed that muscle-strengthening activity significantly increased insulin sensitivity, thereby lowering the blood glucose and the hemoglobin A1c in 4,500 adults between the ages of 20 and 70.

Older adults from age 50 and above who were given only eight weeks of flexibility and resistance training had substantial improvement in strength and flexibility while their glucose levels improved as well.

Because weight lifting causes a significant rise in blood pressure as it is being done, people with severe diabetic eye disease should not do it.

Weight training, which uses lighter weights, can be a form of aerobic exercise. Because the weights are light, they can be moved for prolonged periods of time. The result is improved cardiovascular fitness along with strengthening of muscles, tendons, ligaments, and bones. Weight training is an excellent way to protect and strengthen a joint that is beginning to develop some discomfort.

I recommend that you do seven different exercises with light weights every other day, or daily if possible. Choose weights that permit you to do each exercise ten times in a row for three sets of ten with a rest in between. You should need only five to ten minutes to complete all seven, and the benefits will be huge. These exercises are the bicep curl, shoulder press, lateral raise, bent-over rowing, good mornings, flys, and pullovers.

Figure 9-1 shows the bicep curl. To do this exercise:

1. **Hold the dumbbells along the sides of your body, palms facing forward.**

2. **Raise the dumbbells until your elbows are fully bent.**

3. **Slowly lower the dumbbells to the original position.**

Figure 9-1:
Bicep curl.

Figure 9-2 shows the shoulder press. To do this exercise:

1. **Hold the dumbbells with your palms facing each other and your elbows bent.**

2. **Raise the dumbbells over your head, turning your palms to face forward.**

3. **Lower the dumbbells to the original position.**

Figure 9-2:
Shoulder
press.

Figure 9-3 shows the lateral raise. To do this exercise:

1. **Hold the dumbbells along the sides of your body, palms facing each other.**

2. **Lift the dumbbells out to the sides, palms facing the floor until they are above your head.**

3. **Lower the dumbbells down to your sides.**

Figure 9-4 shows bent-over rowing. To do this exercise:

1. **Hold a dumbbell in each hand, arms hanging down, legs straight, and back parallel to the floor.**

2. **Raise the dumbbells up to your chest.**

3. **Lower the dumbbells back to the floor.**

Figure 9-5 shows good mornings. To do this exercise:

1. **Hold the ends of one dumbbell above your head, arms straight.**

2. **Lower the dumbbell forward as you bend your back parallel to the floor.**

3. **Raise the dumbbell to the original position.**

Figure 9-3:
Lateral
raise.

Figure 9-4:
Bent-over
rowing.

Figure 9-5:
Good
mornings.

Figure 9-6 shows flys. To do this exercise:

1. **Lie on your back and hold the dumbbells out to each side at the shoulder.**

2. **Lift the dumbbells together until they are above your head.**

3. **Lower them to the sides again.**

Figure 9-7 shows pullovers. To do this exercise:

1. **Lie on your back holding one dumbbell with both hands straight up above your head.**

2. **Lower the dumbbell with your arms straight to the floor behind your head.**

3. **Raise the dumbbell back above your head.**

Older people in nursing homes who are given weights of just a few pounds have shown excellent return of strength to what appeared to be atrophied muscles. The benefits for you will be that much greater.

Figure 9-6:
Flys.

Figure 9-7:
Pullovers.

Weight training may be good for the days that you do not do your aerobic exercise, or you can add it for a few minutes after you finish your activity. Weight training is also good for working on a particular group of muscles that you feel is weak. Very often, these muscles are in the back. Weight-training exercises can isolate and strengthen each muscle.

If you do a lot of aerobic exercise that involves the legs, you may want to use upper body weight training only. I can tell you from personal experience that you not only feel a stronger upper body, but your ability to do your usual exercise is enhanced as well.

Chapter 10

Medications: What You Should Know

*Y*ou don't know how lucky you are (but I'm about to tell you). You are the beneficiary of the greatest advances in diabetes medications in the history of the disease. From 1921, when insulin was isolated and used for the first time, to 1955, when a class of glucose-lowering drugs called *sulfonylureas* became available, insulin was the only option for treating diabetes. For another 40 years, nothing new showed up in the United States — until 1995. Now five newer classes of drugs, each in its own way, lower blood glucose. In Chapter 16, I show you even more drug options that are coming soon.

Since the last edition of this book new medications have been introduced and older medications have run into trouble. You will find the latest information on all those changes in this chapter.

If you have diabetes and diet and exercise are not keeping your blood glucose under control, you need to see your doctor about taking medication. In this chapter, you find out all you need to know to use diabetes medications effectively and safely.

This chapter helps you become an educated consumer. Not only can you find out about the medication you're taking and how it works, but you discover when to take it, how it interacts with other medications, what side effects it may cause, and how to use several medications together, if necessary, to normalize your glucose. Right now, today, you have all the tools needed to control your diabetes, and there is more to come. In the immortal words of the great entertainer Al Jolson, "You ain't seen nothin' yet."

Taking Drugs by Mouth: Oral Agents

For years, insulin shots were the only treatment available for diabetes. Most people do not care for shots. You may be an exception, but I doubt it. Fortunately, drugs that can be taken by mouth have been available for some time. One thing you should know about these pills: You can take them or leave them, but they work much better if you take them.

Sulfonylureas

Scientists discovered sulfonylureas accidentally when they noticed that soldiers who were given certain sulfur-containing antibiotics developed symptoms of low blood glucose. When scientists began to search for the most potent examples of this effect, they came up with several different versions of this drug. Sulfonylureas all have the following characteristics:

- They work by making the pancreas release more insulin.

- They are not effective in type 1 diabetes where the pancreas is not capable of releasing any insulin.

- Sometimes they don't work when first given (primary failure), but almost always they stop working within a few years after you start them (secondary failure). Sulfonylureas continue to be used because, for most people, they improve glucose control for at least those first few years.

- They are all capable of causing hypoglycemia.

- When you use any of a class of antibiotics called *sulfonamides,* the glucose-lowering action of the sulfonylureas is prolonged.

- They should not be taken by a pregnant woman or a nursing mother.

- They can be fairly potent when given in combination with one of the other classes of oral agents.

The original sulfonylureas from the 1950s, the first-generation sulfonylureas, are not used as initial treatment as much anymore but are actually just as useful as the newer, second-generation sulfonylureas. The old ones are just as potent, but more milligrams are required for the same effect. All the first-generation drugs are available in a generic form, which makes them less expensive. The first-generation sulfonylureas include:

- **Tolbutamide,** brand name Orinase. This is the only short-acting sulfonylurea. Because it is rapidly broken down in the liver, tolbutamide begins to work in one hour and is gone from the body in ten hours. It is available in 250 and 500 mg strength. Tolbutamide is usually given before each meal, but some patients require only one or two doses a day. Because it lasts for such a short time, tolbutamide is much safer in elderly people. The maximal dose is 3 grams daily (six 500 mg pills).

✔ **Tolazamide,** brand name Tolinase. This agent is absorbed more slowly than other sulfonylureas, so it takes 4 or more hours to notice its effects, and its activity lasts up to 20 hours. Tolazamide is available in 100, 250, and 500 mg. When more than 500 mg is needed, the dose is divided. The maximum dose is 1,000 mg. This drug is changed in the liver, but the new products produced by this change have the ability to lower the blood glucose just like tolazamide. Because the new products are then disposed of in the urine, a person with kidney disease should be careful about taking this medication.

✔ **Acetohexamide,** brand name Dymelor. Acetohexamide begins to work about 1 hour after it's taken and lasts for 12 hours. It comes in 250 and 500 mg strength. Acetohexamide is given in one or two doses daily, and the maximum useful dose is 1.5 grams (three 500 mg tablets). Acetohexamide is inactivated and excreted just like tolazamide, so it requires the same precautions as kidney problems.

✔ **Chlorpropamide,** brand names Diabinase and Glucamide. Chlorpropamide is the longest acting of the first-generation sulfonylureas and was responsible for many cases of hypoglycemia in the past. It is active for 24 hours or longer. Chlorpropamide causes a very prolonged hypoglycemia that sometimes requires treatment with intravenous glucose for several days. It comes in 100 and 250 mg sizes. The maximum recommended dose is 750 mg. It is broken down into other chemicals, which are also active and are slowly eliminated in the urine, so any kidney problem will greatly lengthen its time of activity. This drug is taken only once a day because it lasts so long.

Chlorpropamide has several unique side effects. It causes water retention that sometimes results in low levels of sodium in the blood. If a person on chlorpropamide drinks alcohol, his or her face flushes shortly after taking the alcohol, lasting for ten minutes. Other sulfonylureas do not cause this flushing.

In making a choice among the first-generation drugs, tolbutamide, acetohexamide, and tolazamide are considered less potent, and chlorpropamide is felt to be the most potent. If the first three (of which tolbutamide is the mildest) do not work, then chlorpropamide is tried. If chlorpropamide doesn't lower the blood glucose sufficiently, then the second-generation drugs are used.

Too often, doctors today do not try the first-generation drugs and go right to the second-generation pills. For many people, the second-generation pills are too potent, and hypoglycemia becomes a problem. For others, the second-generation drugs provide no greater benefit than the earlier ones. All these drugs — both first- and second-generation — suffer from the fact that, sooner or later, they no longer control the blood glucose.

Three second-generation sulfonylureas now exist:

- ✔ **Glyburide,** brand names Micronase, Diabeta, and Glynase. Among the foreign brand names for glyburide are Antibet, Azuglucon, Betanase, Gliban, Glibil, Gluben, and Orabetic. Pretty confusing, huh? Glyburide comes in 1.25, 2.5, and 5 mg strengths. The usual starting dose is 2.5 to 5 mg with breakfast, and the maintenance dose is 1.25 to 20 mg. Glyburide leaves the body equally in the bowel movement and the urine, so patients with either liver or kidney disease are at greater risk for low blood glucose. Glyburide is carried around the bloodstream bound to proteins, so if other drugs that bind to proteins are taken, such as aspirin, the activity of glyburide may increase. When these drugs are withdrawn, the activity of glyburide may decrease. Other than hypoglycemia, the incidence of negative effects is very low.

  Glynase is a form of glyburide that is slightly more active because it is absorbed better, so less is required for the same effect. The starting dose is 1.5 mg, and it's available in 1.5, 3, or 6 mg tablets with a maximum dose of 12 mg.

  You can take either form of glyburide once a day in the morning, but sometimes it works better when given twice a day.

- ✔ **Glipizide,** brand names Glucotrol and Glucotrol XL. Among the foreign brand names are Digrin, Glibenase, Glican, Glyco, Glynase (which is the same name as glyburide in the United States!), Mindiab, Napizide, and Sucrazide. Glipizide is similar to glyburide but slightly less potent so that it comes as 5 and 10 mg pills. You take it 30 minutes before food. The starting dose is 5 mg. Up to 40 mg can be given daily in several doses. Because it's less potent, glipizide is preferred in the elderly.

  Glucotrol XL is an extended release form of glipizide that lasts for 24 hours, so it usually is given as 5 or 10 mg once a day.

- ✔ **Glimepiride,** brand name Amaryl. This drug also lasts a longer time and is fairly potent, so it is given once a day. It comes in 1, 2, and 4 mg sizes with a maximum daily dose of 8 mg.

Choosing among the second-generation sulfonylureas, I generally select glimepiride because of its long duration of action. However, the other two are available as generic preparations and are, therefore, less expensive.

Metformin

Metformin, brand name Glucophage, is an entirely different kind of glucose-lowering medication. Outside the United States, it's called Benoformin,

Dextin, Diabex, Diaformin, Fornidd, Glucoform, Gluformin, Metforal, Metomin, and Orabet.

More than 20 years ago, the United States banned a sister medication called *phenformin* because of an association with a fatal complication. Metformin has been used in Europe for years without much trouble and was finally approved in this country in 1995. Metformin is rarely, and perhaps never, associated with the fatal complication *lactic acidosis* that caused phenformin to be banned. A study reported in the *Archives of Internal Medicine* in November 2003 stated that no evidence exists to date that metformin therapy leads to lactic acidosis.

Metformin has the following characteristics:

✔ It lowers the blood glucose mainly by reducing the production of glucose from the liver (the *hepatic* glucose output).

✔ It works for both type 1 and type 2 diabetes, because (unlike the sulfonylureas) it does not depend on stimulating insulin to work.

✔ Used by itself (*monotherapy*), it does not cause hypoglycemia.

✔ It may increase the sensitivity of the muscle cells to insulin and slow the uptake of glucose from the intestine.

✔ It must be taken with food because it causes gastrointestinal irritation, but this side effect declines with time.

✔ It's available in 500 mg, 850 mg, and 1,000 mg tablets.

✔ A relatively inexpensive generic form is available, which is just as good as any of the brand name forms.

✔ The maximum dose is 2,500 mg taken in divided doses with each meal.

✔ It's often associated with weight loss, possibly from the gastrointestinal irritation or because of a loss of taste for food.

✔ It's not recommended when you have significant liver disease, kidney disease, or heart failure.

✔ It's usually stopped for a day or two before surgery or an x-ray study using a dye.

✔ It's not recommended for use in alcoholics.

✔ It's not recommended for use in pregnancy or by a nursing mother.

✔ When given in combination with the sulfonylureas, hypoglycemia can occur. If low blood glucose is persistent, the dose of sulfonylurea is reduced.

Metformin can be a very useful drug, especially when *fasting hyperglycemia* (high blood glucose upon awakening) is present. Metformin has some positive effects on the blood fats, causing a decrease in triglycerides and LDL cholesterol and an increase in HDL cholesterol. About 10 percent of patients fail to respond to it when it is first used, and the secondary failure rate is 5 to 10 percent a year. It occasionally causes a decrease in the absorption of vitamin B$_{12}$, a vitamin that is important for the blood and the nervous system.

Bristol-Myers Squibb, the maker of the brand name of metformin, Glucophage, and other drug makers have come up with new preparations of metformin, which, they believe, have some advantages over the original drug:

- ✔ **Glucophage XR:** The original preparation of metformin has to be taken at each meal. Glucophage XR lasts for 24 hours and comes in a 500 mg strength. Its longer lasting effects help overcome the problem of patients not taking their medication the required multiple times a day. Glumetza is the same drug by Biovail Phamaceuticals.

- ✔ **Glucovance:** This pill combines glyburide (a sulfonylurea described in the previous section) with metformin at a dose of 250 or 500 mg. The various combinations are 1.25 mg of glyburide with 250 mg metformin, 2.5 mg glyburide with 500 mg metformin, and 5 mg glyburide with 500 mg metformin. The advantage is the convenience of having to take only one pill instead of two. Glyburide/metformin is the generic form.

- ✔ **Metaglip:** Made by Bristol-Myers Squibb, combines metformin 250 mg and glipizide 2.5 mg. Glipazide/metformin is the generic form that also comes in 500 mg/5 mg.

- ✔ **Avandamet:** This drug is a combination of 4 mg of Avandia (which I describe in the section "Rosiglitazone," later in this chapter) and 500 mg of metformin. This is a potent combination of two drugs that act differently to improve insulin sensitivity. Avandia has been associated with increased heart attacks. I do not recommend this combination.

- ✔ **ACTOsplus Met:** Combines 500 or 850 mg metformin with 15 mg Actos, discussed under the section "Pioglitazone." It is made by Takeda.

- ✔ **Janumet:** Combines 500 or 1000 mg metformin with 50 mg sitagliptin, a member of a new class of drugs called DPP-4 inhibitors (see below). It is made by Merck.

In my experience, the combination drugs work better than giving two drugs separately. This may reflect the greater compliance that results when a single pill is given compared to two separate pills. If you are already taking both of the drugs separately that are available in a combination pill, ask your doctor about getting the single pill that contains both.

Alpha-glucosidase inhibitors

These are drugs that block the action of an enzyme in the intestine that breaks down complex carbohydrates into simple sugars that can be absorbed. Taking alpha-glucosidase inhibitors results in a slowing of the rise in glucose after meals. The carbohydrates are eventually broken down by bacteria lower down in the intestine, producing a lot of gas, abdominal pain, and diarrhea — the main drawbacks of these drugs.

There are two alpha-glucosidase inhibitors currently being used:

✔ **Acarbose,** brand name Precose. This drug seems to have much greater popularity in Europe than it does in the United States. It was the first alpha-glucosidase inhibitor on the market. Its main characteristics are

- It's supplied in 25, 50, and 100 mg strengths.

- The recommended starting dose is 25 mg at the beginning of each meal. This dose can be increased to 50 or 100 mg three times daily, depending on the blood glucose. The highest dose is not given unless the patient weighs more than 130 pounds.

- It does not require insulin for its activity, so it works for both type 1 and type 2 diabetes.

- It does not cause hypoglycemia when used alone but does in combination with sulfonylureas. If hypoglycemia is persistent, the dose of sulfonylurea is decreased.

- It should not be used by people with intestinal disease.

- Many people do not like it because of the gastrointestinal effects.

- The lowering of glucose and hemoglobin A1c is modest at most.

✔ **Miglitol,** brand name Glyset. This was the second alpha-glucosidase inhibitor introduced. Its characteristics are identical to acarbose. It comes in 25, 50, and 100 mg. Curiously, the manufacturer is the same for both drugs: Bayer.

Because these drugs block the breakdown of complex carbohydrates, hypoglycemia occurring with acarbose or miglitol and sulfonylurea combinations must be treated with a preparation of glucose, not more complex carbohydrates.

In my own practice, I have not found a use for either drug. I tried acarbose on a number of patients, and even though they started at a low dose and gradually built up to a more effective level, they complained about the gas and abdominal pain and asked me to take them off the drug. Because I was not seeing much change in the blood glucose, I did not object. I see no reason to expect that miglitol would be any different.

Thiazolidinediones (the glitazones)

This is the first group of drugs for diabetes that directly reverses insulin resistance.

Troglitazone

Troglitazone, brand name Rezulin (called Prelay outside the United States), was the first oral agent for type 2 diabetes that actually reversed the basic lesion in this disease, namely the insulin resistance. It does this by causing changes within the muscle and fat cells where the insulin resistance resides. These changes take several weeks to occur, and if the patient stops taking troglitazone, they take several weeks to subside.

In March 2000, because of continuing occurrences of severe liver disease sometimes leading to death in a small number of patients taking troglitazone, the FDA removed troglitazone from the market. The other glitazone drugs currently on the market — rosiglitazone and pioglitazone — have not had this problem, although the FDA requires monitoring the patient's liver function when these drugs are first used.

Rosiglitazone

Rosiglitazone was the second thiazolidinedione to be approved by the FDA. It is marketed by Glaxo SmithKline as Avandia. The characteristics of rosiglitazone are:

- ✔ It's available as 2, 4, and 8 mg tablets.
- ✔ Tablets are taken with or without food once a day.
- ✔ The recommended starting dose is 4 mg, and 8 mg is the maximum recommended dose. Increases in the dose are made no more often than every two to four weeks. Rosiglitazone may take three months or longer to have its maximum effect.
- ✔ Because it improves insulin resistance, this drug has its greatest effect on the blood glucose after eating, rather than the first morning glucose.
- ✔ By itself, rosiglitazone does not cause hypoglycemia. It results in hypoglycemia only when combined with insulin or sulfonylurea.
- ✔ If rosiglitazone is given to a patient on sulfonylurea or metformin, those drugs must not be stopped when the rosiglitazone is started because it takes so long for the rosiglitazone to begin to work.

✔ Rosiglitazone is *insulin-sparing,* meaning the body does not have to make as much insulin to control blood glucose when this drug is given.

✔ The drug is eliminated from the body almost entirely through the bowels, so no adjustment of the dose is needed when the kidneys are poorly functioning.

So far, secondary failure, where the drug works initially but stops working later, does not seem to be a problem. A major advantage is that rosiglitazone needs to be taken only once a day, which greatly helps with one of the major problems in all medicine, namely compliance.

However, rosiglitazone does have some problems:

✔ Although rosiglitazone has not been shown to cause severe liver damage, the FDA requires that liver testing be done before starting treatment, every two months for the first year, and periodically thereafter. If the specific liver test called ALT rises more than three times the upper limit of normal, the drug must be stopped. So far, I have had no such problem after treating several hundred patients with this drug.

✔ Rosiglitazone causes water retention and swelling of the ankles, especially in the older population, which some people do not find tolerable. Occasionally the drug is stopped for this reason. This water retention may also be responsible for a mild decrease in red blood cells called *anemia.* The drug should not be used in people with heart failure.

✔ It should not be taken during pregnancy or by a nursing mother.

Rosiglitazone has been associated with an increased incidence of heart attacks. *I do not recommend it.* I have switched all my patients on roziglitazone to pioglitazone or other drugs.

Rosiglitazone has been found to have unexpected effects in women of child-bearing age — specifically, unintended pregnancies due to improved fertility. Many women with type 2 diabetes have reduced fertility as a result of insulin resistance. When these women take rosiglitazone, their fertility may improve, and they may become pregnant.

Pioglitazone

Pioglitazone, manufactured by Eli Lilly and Takeda in the United States, was the third thiazolidinedione to come to market. The brand name is Actos, and its properties are the same as rosiglitazone with the following differences:

✔ The initial dose is 15 mg once a day with or without food, but most patients require 30 or even 45 mg. It comes in all three sizes.

✔ In addition to restoring fertility in some women who are infertile due to insulin resistance, pioglitazone reduces estrogen levels in women taking estrogen and may result in making hormone-based contraception, such as the Pill or Depo-Provera, less effective.

✔ Pioglitazone has been shown to reduce bad (LDL) cholesterol particles in people with or without diabetes (as reported in *Diabetes Care*, September 2003).

✔ Pioglitazone has been shown to be associated with increased osteoporosis in women.

✔ Pioglitazone has not been shown to be associated with a higher incidence of heart attacks.

✔ It is authorized for use alone, with insulin, with metformin, or with a sulfonylurea.

Pioglitazone 30 mg has been combined with glimepiride 2 or 4 mg in a pill called Duetact made by Takeda.

Meglitinides

Each of these drugs, although they are chemically somewhat different, has about the same activity. They are chemically unrelated to the sulfonylureas but work by squeezing more insulin out of the pancreas just like the sulfonylureas do. They are taken just before meals to stimulate insulin for only that meal.

There are two drugs in this class:

✔ **Repaglinide,** brand name Prandin. This was the first meglitinide. The characteristics of repaglinide include:

- It is available as 0.5, 1, and 2 mg tablets and is taken just before or up to 30 minutes before meals.

- The starting dose is 0.5 mg with a mild elevation of blood glucose or 1 or 2 mg if the initial blood glucose is higher. The dose may be doubled once a week to a maximum of 4 mg before meals.

- Because it acts through insulin, repaglinide can cause hypoglycemia.

- It's not recommended in pregnancy or for nursing mothers.

- It's not used with the sulfonylureas but can be combined with metformin. Use in combination with rosiglitazone has not been studied.

- Repaglinide lowers the blood glucose and the hemoglobin A1c effectively when used in combination with metformin.

- It's mostly broken down in the liver and leaves the body in the bowel movement. Therefore, if liver disease is present, the dose has to be adjusted downward.

- Despite the lack of excretion through the kidneys, increases in the dose have to be made more carefully when kidney impairment is present.

Experience with repaglinide has shown that it causes no problems when given with nondiabetes medications. It's bound to protein in the blood, so medications like aspirin (which also bind to protein) may, theoretically, increase its activity. I have not seen this as a problem with my patients who are on this medication.

✔ **Nateglinide,** brand name Starlix. This drug is very similar to repaglinide in its activity. However, it comes in 60 and 120 mg sizes. The starting dose is usually 120 mg before each meal; if a meal is skipped, no dose is taken. If hypoglycemia occurs, the dose is lowered to 60 mg. The features of repaglinide also apply to nateglinide, other than the dosage. A report in *Diabetes Care* in July 2003 showed that repaglinide combined with metformin is a more potent combination than nateglinide with metformin.

DPP-4 inhibitors

This new class of drugs has a different mechanism from any of the previous classes of oral agents. There is a hormone called glucagon-like peptide-1 (GLP-1) which is made in the small intestine and has a number of positive effects for people with diabetes:

✔ It slows the movement of food in the intestine.

✔ It reduces the production of glucagon from the pancreas. Glucagon raises the blood glucose.

✔ It increases insulin levels.

✔ It decreases food intake leading to weight loss.

✔ It normalizes the blood glucose in many patients.

The only problem with GLP-1 is that it's rapidly broken down by an enzyme called DPP-4. Therefore, under usual circumstances, GLP-1 is not around long enough to have these effects in a major way.

This class of drugs called DPP-4 inhibitors block the rapid breakdown of GLP-1 and prolong its actions. There are currently two DPP-4 inhibitors, only one of which is available for patients:

✔ **Sitagliptin:** This drug has the brand name Januvia, is made by Merck and comes in 25, 50 and 100 mg. The dose is 100 mg daily. Since it is excreted by the kidneys, people with kidney disease must take lower doses. It can cause stomach discomfort.

The problem with sitagliptin is that the amount of lowering of the hemoglobin A1c is less than 1 percent. In addition, it does not result in weight loss, which, I believe is the major advantage of GLP-1. Finally, it has been tested in only a few thousand patients. We don't know what unexpected side effects will show themselves once millions of people start to use it. Therefore, I am using it sparingly if at all in my practice until we know more about it, particularly since it doesn't have a major effect on blood glucose.

✔ **Vidagliptin:** This drug with the brand name Galvus is very similar in its effects to sitagliptin. It has not yet been authorized for sale by the FDA. It is made by Novartis.

Combining oral agents

Taking one oral agent alone often does not control the blood glucose sufficiently to prevent complications of diabetes. (A hemoglobin A1c of less than 7 percent is the goal; see Chapter 7.) In this section, I explain how you can use two or more of these drugs together.

You should never take a drug, or a combination of drugs, as a convenient way of avoiding the basic diet and exercise that are the keys to diabetic control. (See Chapters 8 and 9 for more information on these crucial points.)

I currently start all new type 2 patients who are mildly out of control onpioglitazone. I give this medication at least eight weeks to work. Many patients need no more treatment than this in addition to their diet and exercise. I usually begin with a 15 mg dose and increase to 30 mg if the blood glucose is still elevated after four weeks. I check liver function before starting this drug and every two months thereafter.

If 30 mg of pioglizone does not control the patient's blood glucose, it's often the first morning glucose that is still elevated — the *fasting blood glucose.* Metformin is an excellent second drug to add at this point, usually at a dose of 500 mg with breakfast and supper, but most patients need 1,000 mg twice daily to achieve sufficient glucose reduction. Several articles in the medical literature have shown that the combination of pioglitazone and metformin is highly effective and safe.

When a patient is taking these two drugs but still has slightly elevated blood glucose, I add a sulfonylurea. I like to use a longer-acting form, such as glimepiride, because I always prefer a drug that can be taken only once a day to drugs that require multiple dosing. That's one of the reasons I like pioglita-zone so much, in addition to its effectiveness. I have found that 2 to 4 mg of glimepiride combined with the other drugs is all the treatment needed to achieve the goal.

A few patients will still have elevated blood glucose and hemoglobin A1c levels, even with the preceding treatments. For them, repaglinide in place of the sulfonylurea usually does the trick. Starting with a dosage of 1 mg before each meal, those patients have found this medication to be very helpful.

If low blood glucose starts to be a problem, the dose of the sulfonylurea or repaglinide is lowered because the other medications are not responsible for hypoglycemia.

Many diabetes specialists believe that the pancreas gradually fails to make insulin in type 2 diabetes and that most patients need to take insulin sooner or later (see the sidebar "Combining insulin and oral agents in type 2 dia-betes"). My experience is that this is not necessarily true and that the modern medications, particularly the glitazones and metformin, can delay or eliminate the need for insulin. Certainly, numerous people with diabetes are well controlled with only a small dose of an oral medication. And I have seen many others who used insulin when nothing else was available but have since stopped taking it and do not appear as though they will ever need it again. Some people need no drugs at all.

New injectable drugs

The discussion of DPP-4 inhibitors mentioned that these drugs work by blocking the breakdown of the natural hormone GLP-1. Amylin Pharmaceuticals and Eli Lilly have been able to extract a substance from the venom of a lizard called the Gila Monster that acts like GLP-1 but does not break down nearly as fast, which they call exenatide. They have also been able to produce a second injectable substance called pramlintide with many similar properties.

Exenatide

Exenatide, which the companies call Byetta, is a powerful form of GLP-1 that lasts for several hours. It is taken within an hour before breakfast and supper. It may only be used in type 2 diabetes and comes in vials containing either 5 or 10 micrograms per dose. It may be used with metformin, a sulfonylurea or pioglitazone or combinations of those drugs. It can sometimes cause sub-stantial weight loss and eliminate the need for all of those drugs. It is associ-ated with nausea and, rarely, can't be used because the nausea is so severe. Hypoglycemia is frequent when it is used with a sulfonylurea. At present it is not supposed to be used with insulin.

A long-acting version of Byetta is soon to be available. It will require taking only one shot a week. Studies have shown it controls glucose even better than twice daily Byetta.

This drug has proved to be very valuable in the treatment of type 2 diabetes. It is sometimes necessary to use more than the maximum recommended dose of 20 micrograms a day.

Pramlintide

Pramlintide (brand name Symlin) is an extract from the same beta cells of the pancreas that produce insulin. It has a number of valuable properties for type 1 and type 2 diabetes. Among them are:

- It blocks the secretion of glucagon, a major hormone that tends to raise blood glucose (see Chapter 2 for details).
- It slows the emptying of the stomach so that glucose is absorbed more slowly.
- It causes loss of appetite and weight loss.

Amylin, therefore, has an important effect on the rate at which glucose appears in the blood after eating. These effects occur when amylin reaches certain centers in the brain.

Because amylin comes from the same cells that make insulin, it's absent in type 1 diabetes just as insulin is absent in type 1 diabetes. It was thought that providing amylin to a patient with T1DM may improve the blood glucose. However, naturally occurring amylin has chemical properties that make it unusable as a pill or an injection. Mainly, it couldn't be made to dissolve in any liquid. A small change in the chemical structure made it possible to dissolve the new chemical while retaining all the properties of amylin.

Pramlintide is taken before meals that contain at least 30 grams of carbohydrate or 250 kilocalories. It does not mix with insulin. Since pramlintide is so potent, the insulin dose must be reduced by half. It can cause nausea and hypoglycemia.

The starting dose of pramlintide is 15 micrograms before meals and this is increased by 15 micrograms every 3 days. The maximum daily total dose is 120 micrograms.

Pramlintide has not been studied in pregnancy and while breast feeding so it should not be used for these conditions. Children may use it.

You should probably not use pramlintide if you have hypoglycemia unawareness (see Chapter 4) or a form of diabetic neuropathy called gastroparesis (see Chapter 5), which makes the stomach empty slowly.

Insulin

If you have type 1 diabetes, insulin is your savior. If you have type 2 diabetes, you may need insulin late in the course of your disease. Insulin is a great drug, but most people take it through a needle, and that is the rub (or the pain). Inventors have come up with many different ways to administer insulin, but using a syringe and a needle has been the standard for so long that most patients continue to do so. In this section, I tell you about the newer methods, which you should at least consider because they are easier and possibly more accurate than the old method. However, the new syringes and needles are just about painless.

Until a few years ago, insulin could be obtained only by extracting it from the pancreas of a cow, pig, salmon, or some other animal. This was not entirely satisfactory because those insulins are slightly different from human insulin. Using them resulted in an immune reaction in the blood and certain skin reactions. The preparation was purified, but tiny amounts of impurities always remained. In 1978, researchers were able to trick bacteria called *E coli* into making human insulin. Almost all insulin is now perfectly pure human insulin. Soon, no insulin besides human insulin will be available.

Previously, insulin came in two different strengths, U40 and U80, which meant 40 units per milliliter or 80 units per milliliter. This was confusing, especially if the wrong syringe was used — you had to use a U40 syringe for U40 insulin. To eliminate confusion, all insulin in the United States is now U100 or 100 units per milliliter, and all syringes are U100 syringes. This standardization does not necessarily apply in Europe or elsewhere, so check the insulin strength and the markings on the syringe.

In the human body, insulin is constantly responding to ups and downs in the blood glucose. No simple device is currently available to measure the blood glucose and give insulin as the pancreas does. In order to avoid having to take many shots a day, forms of insulin were invented to work at different times. These forms of insulin include:

✔ **Rapid-acting lispro insulin:** Lispro insulin (called *Humalog insulin* by its manufacturer, Eli Lilly) begins to lower the glucose within five minutes after its administration, peaks at about one hour, and is no longer active by about three hours. Lispro is a great advance because it frees the person with diabetes to take a shot just when he or she eats. With the previous short-acting insulin (regular insulin), a person had to take a shot and eat within 30 minutes or hypoglycemia might occur. Because its activity begins and ends so quickly, lispro does not cause hypoglycemia as often as the older preparations.

Novo Nordisk has come out with *insulin aspart* (called NovoLog), which has characteristics indistinguishable from lispro insulin.

Sanofi-Aventis produces insulin glulisine (called Apidra), which is similar in its properties to the other two rapid-acting insulins.

✔ **Short-acting regular insulin:** Regular insulin takes 30 minutes to start to lower the glucose, peaks at 3 hours, and is gone by 6 to 8 hours. Until Humalog, NovoLog, and Apidra came along, patients used this preparation before meals to keep their glucose low until the next meal.

✔ **Intermediate-acting NPH or Lente insulins:** Both begin to lower the glucose within 2 hours of administration and continue their activity for 10 to 12 hours. They can be active for up to 24 hours. The purpose of this kind of insulin is to provide a smooth level of control over half the day so that a low level of active insulin is always in the body. This attempts to parallel the situation that exists in the human body.

✔ **Long-acting Ultralente insulin:** This insulin begins to act within 6 hours and provides a low level of insulin activity for up to 26 hours. It was invented to provide a smooth, basal level of control requiring only one shot a day. It can act differently in different people, looking more like intermediate insulin in some patients.

✔ **Long-acting insulin glargine and detemir:** Aventis sells an insulin called *insulin glargine* or Lantus. Studies have shown that insulin glargine has its onset in 1 to 2 hours after injection, and its activity lasts for 24 hours without a specific peak time of activity, which is exactly what is needed to control the blood glucose over an entire day. Insulin glargine is released in a smooth fashion from the site of injection, and it doesn't matter what part of the body is injected. Because of its smooth and predictable activity, insulin glargine does not tend to cause low blood glucose at night, which often happens with NPH insulin. I have used this insulin in a number of my patients with type 1 diabetes and have been extremely pleased with the results. I now use it with all new type 1 diabetes patients. One disadvantage of insulin glargine is that it can't be mixed with other insulins in one syringe.

Insulin detemir or Levemir has similar properties to glargine but does not last quite as long. It is a product of Novo Nordisk.

If you do not have good diabetic control (defined as hemoglobin A1c of 7 percent or less) with NPH insulin, ask your doctor to consider using insulin glargine or detemir.

✔ **Premixed insulins:** Several mixtures are available: one with 70 percent NPH insulin and 30 percent regular; one with a 50–50 mix of NPH and regular; one with a 75–25 mix of NPH-like insulin and lispro insulin; and one with a 70–30 mix of NPH-like insulin and insulin aspart. These insulins are helpful for people who have trouble mixing insulins in one syringe, have poor eyesight, or are stable on a preparation that does not change.

Combining insulin and oral agents in type 2 diabetes

Sometimes the characteristics of the currently available oral agents do not provide the tight control needed to avoid complications. This is particularly true after many years of type 2 diabetes. Then insulin may be required. Insulin may be added in a number of ways, but often a shot of glargine insulin at bedtime is all that is needed to start the day under control and continue it with oral agents. For example, pioglitazone may control the daytime glucoses very well after eating, but the first morning glucose may need the overnight shot of glargine insulin. By gradually increasing the dose of glargine, most patients with type 2 diabetes on oral agents can be controlled so that their hemoglobin A1c is 7 or below.

As type 2 diabetes progresses, the oral agents may be less effective, and insulin is taken more often. Two shots a day of intermediate and short-acting insulin may do the trick. Usually you take two-thirds of the dose in the morning and one-third before supper because you need short-acting insulin to control the supper carbohydrates. This is a situation where 75 percent protamine lispro (like NPH) and 25 percent lispro insulin may be useful, allowing the patient to measure from only one bottle. This combination is especially valuable in the older person with diabetes, where the tightest level of control is not being sought because the expected lifespan of the patient is shorter than the time necessary to develop complications. In this patient, doctors want to prevent problems like frequent urination leading to loss of sleep or vaginal infections, so they give enough to treat this but not so much that a frail, elderly patient is having hypoglycemia on a frequent basis.

You need to know a few things that are common to all insulins:

- ✔ Insulin may be kept at room temperature for four weeks or in the refrigerator until the expiration date printed on the label. After four weeks at room temperature, the insulin should be discarded.

- ✔ Insulin does not take too well to excessive heat, such as direct sunlight, or excessive cold. Protect your insulin against these conditions.

- ✔ You can safely give an insulin shot through clothing.

- ✔ If you take less than 50 units in a shot, there are ½ cc syringes that make it easy to measure up to 50 units. If you take less than 30 units, you can use ³⁄₁₀ cc syringes.

- ✔ Shorter needles may be more comfortable, especially for children, but the depth of the injection helps to determine how fast the insulin works.

- ✔ You can reuse disposable syringes a couple of times.

- ✔ Used syringes and needles must be disposed of in a puncture-proof container that is sealed shut before being placed in the trash.

Shooting yourself

Whatever type of insulin you use, chances are you'll be taking it by syringe and needle. (I discuss other delivery options later in the chapter, in the sections "Delivering insulin with a pen," "Delivering insulin with a jet injection device," and "Delivering insulin with an external pump.")

Drawing insulin up is done in the same way no matter which type of insulin is involved. If you look at the syringe in Figure 10-1, you see that it's lined. Starting at the needle end of the syringe, you'll find nine small lines above the needle, followed by a tenth longer line where the number 10 may be found. Each line is one unit of insulin. Above the 10-unit line, you'll find a succession of four small lines followed by a larger line representing 15, 20, 25, and so on.

Figure 10-1:
The insulin syringe and bottle.

If the insulin is lispro or regular, it should be clear and you do not have to shake the bottle. The other kinds of insulin are cloudy, and you need to shake the bottle a few times to suspend the tiny particles in the liquid. A new bottle has a cap on the top, which you break off and discard. When you're ready to take insulin, wipe the rubber stopper in the top of the bottle with alcohol.

Pull up the number of units of air that corresponds to the number of units of insulin you need to take. Turn the insulin bottle upside down and penetrate the rubber stopper with the needle of the syringe. Push all the air inside and pull out the insulin dose you need. Because air replaces the insulin, the pressure inside the bottle is unchanged, and no vacuum is created. Check to make sure that you have the right amount of the right insulin and no air bubbles in the syringe.

To give the injection, use alcohol to wipe off an area of skin on your arm, chest, stomach, or wherever you're injecting it. Insert the needle at a right angle to the skin and push it in. When the needle has penetrated the skin, push the plunger of the syringe down to zero to administer the insulin.

If you're taking two kinds of insulin at the same time (but not insulin glargine), you can mix them in one syringe, thus avoiding two shots. Here's how you do that:

1. **Wipe both bottles with alcohol.**

2. **Draw up the total units of air corresponding to the total insulin you need.**

3. **Push the units of air into the longer-acting insulin bottle that corresponds to the number of units of longer-acting insulin you need, and withdraw the needle.**

4. **Push the rest of the units of air into the shorter-acting insulin bottle, and withdraw the correct units of insulin.**

5. **Go back to the longer-acting bottle and withdraw the correct units of insulin from there.**

By doing this, you do not contaminate the shorter-acting insulin with the additive in the longer-acting insulin.

ANECDOTE

Carbohydrate counting to maximum health

To find out how you can accomplish carbohydrate counting in everyday life, take a typical type 1 patient. Salvatore Law is a 41-year-old who has had type 1 diabetes for 31 years. He has been well controlled because he follows a good diet, does lots of exercise, and takes his insulin appropriately. He takes 30 units of insulin glargine at bedtime.

Law has a list of dosages of lispro insulin that tells him to take 1 unit of insulin for each 20 grams of carbohydrate he eats. He is about to have breakfast and knows that it will contain 80 grams of carbohydrate. Therefore, he needs four units of lispro insulin. He measures his blood glucose before breakfast and finds that it is 202 mg/dl. His doctor has told him to take an extra unit of lispro insulin for each 50 mg/dl above 100 mg/dl. He adds two more units for a total of six units of insulin taken just before breakfast.

At lunch, his blood glucose measures 58. He is about to have a lunch of 120 grams of carbohydrate, so he needs 6 units for that. However, he reduces it by 1 unit for the glucose measurement that is approximately 50 mg/dl lower than 100, so his final dose is 5 units.

Before supper, Law's blood glucose measures 120. His supper contains only 60 grams of carbohydrate, so he needs 3 units for that. He does not have to adjust the dose because the glucose is close to 100, so he takes only 3 units.

At bedtime, his blood glucose is 108, so he is doing very well. Unless the blood glucose is 200 or greater, he does not need to take any bedtime lispro because he is taking insulin glargine to control his glucose overnight.

Where you inject the insulin helps determine how fast it works. Insulin injected into the abdomen is most rapidly absorbed, followed by the arms and legs and then the buttocks. You may use these differing rates of uptake of the insulin to get faster action when your blood glucose is high. If the body part that gets the insulin is exercised, the insulin enters more quickly. If you use the same injection site repeatedly, the absorption rate slows down, so rotate the sites.

The timing of your insulin injections helps to determine the smoothness of your glucose control. The more regular you are in your injections, your eating, and your exercise, the smoother your glucose level.

Conducting intensive insulin treatment

Intensive insulin treatment is essential in type 1 diabetes if you hope to prevent the complications of the disease. This means measuring your blood glucose at least before each meal and at bedtime, plus using both short-acting and longer-acting insulin to keep the blood glucose between 80 and 100 before meals and less than 140 after eating. How you do this is the subject of this section.

In a person who doesn't have type 1 diabetes, a small amount of circulating insulin is always present in the bloodstream and, after eating, insulin increases temporarily to control the glucose in the meal. Intensive insulin treatment attempts to mirror the activity of the normal human pancreas as much as possible.

In intensive insulin treatment, you usually take a certain amount of longer-acting insulin at bedtime. I prefer insulin glargine because it produces a smooth basal level of glucose control over 24 hours. In addition, you take a dose of rapid-acting insulin before each meal. I prefer lispro because it is more convenient and less hypoglycemia occurs. The dose of lispro is determined by the expected grams of carbohydrates in the meal you're about to eat, as well as by your blood glucose at that moment. Your doctor should provide you with a list of how much insulin to take for a given situation. Each patient is different, and the dosage must be individualized.

Using the carbohydrates in a meal to determine your insulin dose is called *carbohydrate counting*. The key to this system is to know the carbohydrates in your food. Here is where you make use of your friendly dietitian, who can go over your food preferences and show you how many carbohydrates are in them. The dietitian can also show you where to find carbohydrate counts for any other foods that you might eat.

You also need to know how many grams of carbohydrate are controlled by each unit of insulin you take. This is determined by checking your blood glucose an hour after eating a known amount of carbohydrate. For example, one person may need 1 unit to control 20 grams of carbohydrate, while another person needs 1 unit to control 15 grams of carbohydrate. If both of them eat a breakfast of 75 grams of carbohydrate, the first person might take 4 units of lispro, while the second person takes 5 units of lispro. Then additional units are added for the amount that the blood glucose needs to be lowered. A typical schedule is to take 1 unit for every 50 mg/dl that the blood glucose is above 100 mg/dl. Insulin can also be subtracted if the blood glucose is too low. For every 50 mg/dl that the glucose is below 100, subtract 1 unit. (To see how carbohydrate counting works in practice, see the sidebar "Carbohydrate counting to maximum health.")

By measuring your blood glucose frequently, you can find out how different carbohydrates affect your blood glucose. By using the carbohydrate sources that have a low glycemic index, you will need to use less insulin to control them. (See Chapter 8 for more on carbohydrates.)

As you attempt to help your body mirror normal insulin and glucose dynamics, you often have to deal with a greater frequency of hypoglycemia. The best way to handle hypoglycemia is by eating slightly smaller meals and using the unused calories as between-meal snacks. This technique smoothes out the ups and downs.

At what point do you adjust your insulin glargine? If you find that several mornings in a row your fasting blood glucose is too high, you might add a unit or two to your bedtime glargine. If it's too low, you might reduce your insulin glargine by a unit or two or try eating a small bedtime snack. A high blood glucose level throughout the day is an indication to raise the glargine. Getting a lot of hypoglycemia at different times of day is a reason to lower the glargine. These adjustments are best done in consultation with your doctor. If, however, you're unable to see your doctor, you can put your knowledge to use and make these adjustments on your own.

Adjusting insulin when you travel

If you're traveling between time zones, you may wonder if you need to change your insulin routine while you're gone. Time changes of less than three hours require no modifications, but changes above three hours require progressively more. You should probably discuss these changes with your physician before you go.

Say that you're taking the red-eye flight at 10 p.m. from San Francisco, arriving at 6 a.m. at Kennedy Airport in New York. If you are taking insulin glargine, you do not have to change your dose. Just start using lispro at the beginning of your meals (which you'll be eating three hours earlier than usual because of the time change).

When you return to California, you add three hours to your day. In this case, you need to take an extra measurement of your blood glucose. If it's around 150, you need do nothing, but if it's 200 or more, take a couple of units of lispro insulin to bring it down. If your blood glucose is much below 100, eat a small snack. Again, you do not have to adjust your insulin glargine.

Delivering insulin with a pen

Several manufacturers, including Eli Lilly, Owen Mumford, Diesetronic, Novo Nordisk, Sanofi-Aventis, and Becton Dickinson, have sought ways to make delivering insulin easier. The insulin pen, shown in Figure 10-2, is one useful tool. The pen doesn't eliminate the need for needles, but it does change the way you measure your insulin. Either the pen comes with an insulin cartridge already inserted, or the cartridge is placed inside the pen just like ink cartridges used to be put in pens and replaced when it runs out.

Figure 10-2:
The insulin
pen.

Each cartridge contains 1.5 or 3.0 milliliters of insulin — either NPH, regular, lispro, aspart, a mixture of NPH-like lispro and lispro (such as 75 percent NPH-like lispro and 25 percent lispro), or a mixture of NPH-like aspart plus aspart. You can then dial the amount of insulin that you need to take. Each unit (sometimes two units) is accompanied by a clicking sound so the visually impaired can hear the number of units. The units also appear in a window on the pen. If you draw up too many units, one of the pens forces you to waste the insulin by pushing it out of the needle, while others allow you to reset the pen and start again. Depending on the pen, you can deliver from 30 to 70 units of insulin. You screw on a new needle as needed.

A number of different companies make pens for their own insulin. Available pens include the following:

- ✔ Autopen, which is available in four different models. Two contain a 1.5-ml cartridge, and two contain a 3-ml cartridge. Within each size, one pen delivers insulin in 1-unit increments, and the other pen delivers insulin in 2-unit increments.

- ✔ Humalog Mix 75/25, Humalog Mix 50/50, Humalog Pen, Humulin Mix 70/30, and Humulin N, all of which are prefilled, disposable pens containing 3 ml of the particular kind of insulin you use.

- ✔ HumaPen Luxura HD, used for Humalog insulin when half-unit doses are needed, particularly in children.

- ✔ HumaPen Memoir, a new pen that remembers the 16 most recent doses, their times, and dates; and is used with 3-ml lispro cartridges.

- ✔ Levemir FlexPen, a prefilled disposable pen containing 3 ml of Levemir insulin.

- ✔ NovoLog FlexPen and NovoLog 70/30 FlexPen, which are prefilled disposable insulin syringes containing 3 ml of insulin.

- ✔ NovoPen Junior, which takes NovoLog cartridges containing 3 ml of insulin and can be measured in half-unit doses.

- ✔ NovoPen 3, which holds NovoLog 3-ml cartridges.

- ✔ SoloStar, a disposable pen that contains 3 ml of Lantus insulin.

- ✔ Opticlix, which uses 3 ml glargine or glulisine cartridges.

Insulin pens require needles, and you must match the pen with the proper needle in order for the pen to work properly. If the needles don't come with the pen, the instructions with the pen tell you which needle to use.

Should you shift from your syringe and needle to a pen? If you're comfortable with the syringe and needle and feel your technique is accurate, you probably have no reason to do so. If you're new to insulin, have some visual impairment, or feel that you're not getting an accurate measurement of the insulin, a pen may be the solution for you.

Delivering insulin with a jet injection device

Jet injection devices (see Figure 10-3) are for the person who just can't stick a needle into his or her skin. At around $1,000 or more, they're expensive, but they last a long time and replace the syringe and needle.

Figure 10-3:
A jet
injection
device.

Jet injection devices are made by at least two different manufacturers:

- ✓ Advanta Jet, which delivers ½ to 50 units of all types and mixes of insulin
- ✓ Advanta Jet ES, which is useful when the skin is particularly tough
- ✓ Adveanta Jet's Gentle Jet, which is a low-power version for children of the two Advanta Jet
- ✓ Medi-Jector Vision, which delivers all types of insulin from 2 to 50 units in 1-unit increments

A large quantity of insulin is taken into the injection device, enough for multiple treatments. The amount of insulin to be delivered is measured, usually by rotating one part of the device while the number of units to be delivered appears in a window. The device is held against the skin. With the press of a button, a powerful jet of air forces the insulin through the skin into the subcutaneous tissue, usually with no pain perceived by the patient. The devices come in a lower power form for smaller children. These devices can deliver up to 50 units at one time.

Should you try an insulin jet injector? If you have no trouble with the syringe and needle or find the pen to be an easy substitute, you don't need a jet injector. If you hate needles or need to give frequent shots to a small child who is very resistant to them, a jet injector may solve your problems.

Delivering insulin with an external pump

For some people — and you may be one of them — the external insulin pump (see Figure 10-4) is the answer to their prayers. These devices are as close as you currently can come to the gradual administration of rapid-acting insulin that is normally taking place in the body. They're expensive, costing more than $4,000, but the insulin pump may be the answer for patients who simply cannot achieve good glucose control with syringes, pens, or jet injectors.

Figure 10-4:
The insulin
pump with
its infusion
set.

Currently, five companies — Animas, DANA Diabecare, Deltec, Medtronic MiniMed, and Nipro Diabetes Systems — sell these pumps, which are the size of a pager. Inside the pump is a motor. A syringe filled with short-acting insulin is placed within the pump, with the plunger against a screw that slowly pushes it down to push insulin out of the syringe. The end of the syringe is attached to a short tube, which ends in a needle pushed into the skin of the abdomen. Insulin is slowly pushed under the skin.

The rate at which insulin slowly enters the abdomen is called the *basal rate.* It can be set, by way of computer chips, to vary as often as every half hour to an hour. For example, from 8 a.m. to 9 a.m., the pump may deliver 0.8 units, while from 9 a.m. to 10 a.m., the pump may deliver 1.0 units, depending upon the needs of the patient. This amount is determined, of course, by measuring the blood glucose with a meter (see Chapter 7).

When the patient is about to eat a meal, he or she can push a button to deliver extra insulin, called a *bolus* of insulin. (The amount is determined by carbohydrate counting, which I explain earlier in this chapter.) You can get extra insulin if the blood glucose is too high at any time.

Pump usage has its advantages:

✔ It's flexible because the bolus is taken just before meals.

✔ It often smoothes out the swings of glucose during the day because the insulin is administered slowly and in small doses.

✔ It can be rapidly disconnected and reconnected to take a shower or swim. (However, it can take a little getting used to when worn to bed.)

✔ It's safe from overdosage because it has built-in protective devices to prevent this occurrence.

However, pump usage has definite disadvantages besides the high cost:

- ✔ Infections of the skin are frequent because the infusion set is left in place for several days. These infections are usually mild, however.
- ✔ Overall diabetic control is not necessarily better with the pump than with other ways of delivering insulin, especially with the new insulin glargine. The latest proof of this was an article published in *Diabetes Care* in September 2003.
- ✔ Because the patient receives only short-acting insulin, if insulin stops entering, ketoacidosis may come on rapidly (see Chapter 4).
- ✔ Some patients are allergic to the tape that holds the infusion set onto the abdomen.
- ✔ Blood glucose must be measured often to adjust the pump for optimal control.

Pump usage is definitely not treatment to be done on your own at the beginning. You need a diabetologist to help with dosages, a dietitian to help you calculate amounts of boluses based upon carbohydrate intake, and someone from the manufacturer to teach you how to set the pump and to be available to fix any malfunctions.

If you use a pump and your blood glucose rises above 250 mg/dl, take the following steps:

1. **Take a bolus of insulin with the pump to bring it down. (The amount is determined by your sensitivity to insulin.)**
2. **Recheck your glucose in an hour.**
3. **If the glucose is still above 250 mg/dl, use a syringe to take more insulin.**
4. **Check your infusion set.**
5. **Check the ketones in your urine and report to a doctor if the amount is moderate to large.**
6. **Recheck your glucose every two hours and use more insulin as needed.**

Is an insulin pump for you? If you're willing to invest the time and effort at first, if your schedule is very uncertain particularly with respect to meals, and if your glucose control has not been good with other means, you should look into this option.

My patients who use the pump have generally had positive experiences. Now that they have it, none of them are willing to give up the pump. Occasionally, they disconnect the pump to allow their skin to heal. They have generally shown improved glucose control and a better hemoglobin A1c.

Do I recommend using an insulin pump? With the new form of insulin called insulin glargine, you can accomplish a continuous basal control of the blood glucose much like the pump does. The pump proponents say that you need to be able to alter the basal dose for different conditions throughout the day and you can't do that with a single shot of insulin. Although this is true, I am not sure that it makes a great difference in the course of controlling the blood glucose.

Is one pump better than another? All seem to have excellent mechanical features, and all provide you with the ability to adjust your insulin in several ways. They all have alarms for any eventuality like blockage of the tube, an electrical failure, and so forth. They try to differentiate themselves by offering different options for how the insulin is delivered, but you may find that you need the help of a rocket scientist to figure those differences out.

One pump that does deserve special mention, because it is the wave of the future, is the Medtronic MiniMed Paradigm 512. This pump is sold with the Paradigm Link Blood Glucose Monitor. Readings taken by the monitor are wirelessly sent to the pump, which uses a software program to calculate the bolus of insulin to be given, taking into account the food about to be eaten, which must be entered into the pump. The wearer must accept the bolus before it is delivered. This product is just short of the so-called *closed loop system,* where the blood glucose determines the amount of insulin to be given, just as the normal pancreas is constantly doing. The pump chooses the boluses, but it does not constantly alter the basal level of insulin, because there is no continuing information about the current blood glucose level. The wearer must test the blood glucose with his or her meter in order for the pump to know glucose levels.

For an extensive discussion of the various types of insulin pumps that are available, their pros and cons and much more about using a pump to deliver insulin, see my new book, *Type 1 Diabetes For Dummies* (Wiley).

Utilizing aids to insulin delivery

For those of you still using the old needle-and-syringe method, I want you to be aware of numerous aids that can make it easier for you to take insulin:

- ✔ **Spring-loaded syringe holders:** You place your syringe in the holder, hold it against the skin, and press a button. The needle enters, and you've administered the insulin.

- ✔ **Syringe magnifiers:** These help the visually impaired person administer insulin.

> ✔ **Syringe-filling devices:** You can feel and hear a click as you take up insulin.
>
> ✔ **Subcutaneous infusion sets:** A catheter is placed under the skin, and injections are made into the catheter instead of the skin to reduce punctures.
>
> ✔ **Needle guides:** You can use these guides when you can't see the rubber part of the insulin bottle to insert the needle to take up the insulin.

Call your local American Diabetes Association branch or look in the back of the ADA's *Diabetes Forecast* magazine to find sources for these products.

If you take a drug that makes you prone to hypoglycemia, you need to wear a medical bracelet or necklace that identifies you as a person with diabetes who may be hypoglycemic. Numerous companies make these products.

Using Other Medications

Most of this chapter is devoted to medications that lower the blood glucose, but diabetes involves more than elevated blood glucose levels. People with diabetes often have high blood pressure and high cholesterol, and they suffer more sickness when exposed to influenza or pneumonia. It is important to consider this fact in the overall management of your disease.

If you have high blood pressure (see Chapter 7), lifestyle changes, including weight loss and physical activity, may be all you need to control the condition. However, if lifestyle changes alone don't work, numerous medications are available that control blood pressure. See my book *High Blood Pressure For Dummies, 2nd Edition* (Wiley) for a complete discussion of this subject. Controlling blood pressure is as important as controlling blood glucose in preventing diabetic complications.

Most people with diabetes also have elevated levels of LDL or "bad" cholesterol (see Chapter 7). Excellent drugs are available to manage this problem if lifestyle changes don't suffice. See *Controlling Cholesterol For Dummies* (Wiley) by Carol Ann Rinzler and Martin W. Graf for the answers to your questions on this topic. Cholesterol control is another cornerstone of excellent diabetic care. A study published in the *New England Journal of Medicine* in March 2004 indicates that when it comes to LDL cholesterol, the lower, the better. Talk to your doctor about this.

People with diabetes, especially those whose glucose is poorly controlled, are prone to become sicker when they develop influenza or pneumonia. Excellent vaccinations for these illnesses are available. Flu vaccine is given annually, and pneumonia vaccine is given once if you are older than 65 and received a previous vaccination more than five years ago.

Finally, aspirin has been shown to reduce sickness and death due to coronary artery disease (which I discuss in Chapter 5). Because coronary artery disease is such a prominent feature of diabetes, many doctors recommend that all patients with diabetes take a daily aspirin tablet. Diabetics may need more than the usual dose of a baby aspirin to reduce their risk of heart attacks; a full adult pill may be necessary.

Avoiding Drug Interactions

Studies have shown that some patients with diabetes are taking as many as four to five drugs, including their diabetes medications. These drugs often interact, and the cost of treating harmful drug interactions is more than $4 billion. Sometimes (believe it or not) even your doctor is not aware of the interactions of common drugs. You need to know the names of all the drugs you take and whether they affect one another.

Many common medications used for the treatment of high blood pressure also raise the blood glucose, sometimes bringing out a diabetic tendency that might otherwise not have been recognized:

- **Thiazide diuretics** often raise the glucose by causing a loss of potassium. Among these drugs are Diuril, hydroDiuril, Oretic, and Zaroxolyn.

- **Beta blockers** reduce the release of insulin and include such drugs as Inderal, Lopressor, and Tenormin.

- **Calcium channel blockers** also reduce insulin secretion and include Adalat, Calan, Cardizem, Isoptin, Norvasc, and Procardia.

- **Minoxidil** can raise blood glucose.

Drugs used for other purposes can also raise blood glucose:

- **Corticosteroids,** even in topical use, can raise blood glucose. (See Chapter 2 for more on corticosteroids.)

- **Cyclosporine,** used to prevent organ rejection, can raise the blood glucose by poisoning the insulin-producing beta cell.

- **Diphenylhydantoin,** known as Dilantin, is a drug for seizures and blocks insulin release.

- ✔ **Oral contraceptives** were previously accused of causing hyperglycemia when the dose of estrogen was very high, but current preparations are not a problem.

- ✔ **Nicotinic acid and niacin,** used to lower cholesterol, can bring out a hyperglycemic tendency.

- ✔ **Phenothiazines,** such as Compazine, Serentil, Stelazine, and Thorazine, can block insulin secretion and cause hyperglycemia.

- ✔ **Thyroid hormone,** in elevated levels, raises the blood glucose by reducing insulin from the pancreas.

Many common medications, either on their own or by doing something to make the oral drugs that lower blood glucose more potent, also lower the blood glucose. The most important of these include the following:

- ✔ **Salicylates and acetaminophen,** known as aspirin and Tylenol, can lower the blood glucose, especially when given in large doses.

- ✔ **Ethanol,** in any form of alcohol, can lower the blood glucose, particularly when taken without food.

- ✔ **Angiotensin converting enzyme inhibitors,** used for high blood pressure, such as Accupril, Captopril, Lotensin, Monopril, Prinivil, Vasotec, and Zestril, can lower the blood glucose, though the mechanism is unclear.

- ✔ **Alpha-blockers,** another group of antihypertensives that includes Prazosin, lower the glucose as well.

- ✔ **Fibric acid derivatives** like Clofibrate, used to treat disorders of fat, cause a lowering of blood glucose.

If you start a new medication and suddenly find that your blood glucose is significantly higher or lower than usual, ask your doctor to check for the possibility that the new medication has a definite glucose-lowering or glucose-raising effect.

Finding Assistance Obtaining Drugs

Diabetes can be expensive, especially if you need several drugs to control your blood glucose. The pharmaceutical companies understand, and several offer programs to provide medication for a period of time. Table 10-1 tells you what you need to know about these companies.

Table 10-1	How You Can Get Drug Supplies	
Company	*Program Name*	*Phone Number*
Bayer Corporation (acarbose)	Indigent Patient	800-998-9180
Bristol-Myers Squibb (metformin)	Patient Assistance	800-437-0994
Eli Lilly and Company (all insulin preparations)	Lilly Cares	800-545-6962
Sanofi-Aventis (glyburide, glimepiride, Lantus)	Patient Assistance	800-221-4025
Novo Nordisk (insulin preparations)	Indigent Program	800-727-6500
Pfizer (glipizide, glipizide extended release, chlorpropamide)	Pfizer Prescription Assistance	800-438-1985

All these programs require you to get a prescription from your doctor. The doctor usually fills out forms that state that the patient meets the financial requirements and needs the drug. Not all companies give away free drugs for life. If you cannot afford to buy a drug that you're taking, do not hesitate to call the company and ask whether it has a patient-assistance program.

Chapter 11

Diabetes Is Your Show

. . . .

In This Chapter

▶ Preparing for your role as author, producer, director, and star

▶ Tapping into the talents of your physicians

▶ Welcoming other professionals to your crew

▶ Inviting your family and friends — your captivated and caring audience

▶ Making use of the Internet

. . . .

Shakespeare said it: "All the world's a stage." That quote applies to diabetes beautifully. You have many roles in life, and one of them is the role of a person with diabetes. As with any role, you're not expected to play it alone. You have a large cast and crew, all of whom are eager to help you, but you must be willing to ask for their help and know how to use them so that they can give you their best. Believe me, as a member of that crew, everyone wants to give you their best.

The question is, do you want your play to be a comedy or a tragedy? Because you hold all the major positions, the choice is entirely up to you. And remember, as with all plays, life goes on offstage. Your role as a person with diabetes is one of many, including brother or sister, mother or father, boss or employee, and so on. Fortunately, the life skills that you discover as someone with diabetes are applicable to all your other roles.

One of the new kids on the block is the Internet (perhaps not so new). The resources it offers deserve mention in this chapter on using all the tools available to manage your diabetes.

Your Role as Author, Producer, Director, and Star

Being the author, the producer, the director, and the star may seem like a lot of responsibility — and it is. Unlike many short-term illnesses where the doctor knows what has to be done, instructs you to do it, writes a prescription, and you're cured, diabetes is your daily companion for life. No one, not even your mother or spouse, can be with you all of the time. Therefore, you're the one who writes the script and the action. You decide whether you'll take your medication or exercise regularly. You determine whether you'll follow a diet that will control your weight and your blood glucose.

You're the one who needs to gather the resources needed to play the role properly. In this sense, you're the producer. You need your props and your theater, the equipment, the medications, and the environment in which to manage your diabetes. Your environment may be a comfortable home where you can eat the proper diet and a good exercise facility where you can burn up calories while you strengthen your heart. Or it may be the sidewalk where you can safely walk or jog.

After you have the resources, you need to direct your cast and crew to make your play come out the way you envision it. You're the one who sees to it that the primary physician obtains a hemoglobin A1c (see Chapter 7) every three or four months and that he or she sends you to the eye doctor at least once a year. The physician is dealing with many patients each day and can easily forget your specific needs. You must let the doctor know what your needs are and not expect the doctor to read your mind. You may be dealing with other doctors who treat your heart, your lungs, and other parts of you. Each doctor needs to know all the medications you take.

Finally, you're the star of the show. That role is both an honor and a responsibility. Although you may wish that you had never been chosen for this particular role, there it is. You can make of it what you will. You can learn all your lines (understand your disease) and speak them fluently (take your medications, follow your diet, and so on), or not. Obviously, not studying your lines is a lot easier, but in that case, the result can be a tragedy. Take proper care of yourself, and the smile on your face and that of all your fellow cast members and crew will clearly indicate that you have written, produced, directed, and starred in a comedy.

The Primary Physician — Your Assistant Director

Your primary physician takes on a new role in diabetes, where he or she becomes a facilitator. In the United States, where you can find numerous specialists, only 8 percent of people with diabetes are regularly seen by a specialist. The other 92 percent are in the hands of more general doctors who have to deal with many other illnesses besides diabetes. This is a consequence of the large size of the diabetic population and the requirements of a healthcare system with limited resources.

While using a primary physician instead of a specialist may seem not conducive to the best care, I can say many good things about it. Remember, you're a person who has diabetes. Other things can go wrong, and the primary physician can handle them as well. Your mild heart disease may not require a cardiologist, and your primary physician can also manage your bronchitis very well.

You should expect your primary physician to have a decent working knowledge of diabetes. Chapter 7 describes the proper way to follow a person with diabetes. The various tests are essential to your health, and the primary physician must know which ones to order and when to send you to a specialist because your needs are beyond his or her expertise.

The Diabetologist or Endocrinologist — Your Technical Consultant

An *endocrinologist* should have the most in-depth knowledge of the management of diabetes. She has had advanced training for several years (on top of the years of training in general internal medicine) and devotes his or her practice to taking care of people with diabetes, plus patients with problems of the thyroid, adrenals, or other glands. A *diabetologist* is an endocrinologist who takes care of only diabetic patients.

If you have type 1 diabetes, you will certainly see an endocrinologist sooner or later. If you have type 2 diabetes and get into trouble with complications or control, the endocrinologist will be called in for consultation. You have the right to expect that this physician will be able to answer most questions that arise during the care of diabetes.

This doctor will be up on the newest treatments for diabetes, so if you have questions about the future of diabetes care, ask him. This doctor should also have the best understanding of all the drugs currently used for diabetes, how they interact with each other, their side effects, and other drugs that interact with them.

If you're not satisfied with the answers you're getting from your primary physician, ask for a referral to a specialist. Many health plans today try to steer you away from the specialist because this doctor orders more expensive tests and costs more to see by virtue of the extra years of specialty training. Do not take no for an answer. If your primary doctor will not refer you, find one who will.

If your endocrinologist or diabetologist makes any changes to your treatment, report those changes to your primary physician. One of the big problems in medicine is the lack of communication between medical care providers of all types, not just doctors.

For your own sake, make sure that all your medical care providers know what the others are doing for you. Carry a list of your medications and show it each time you have a doctor visit. You might even carry the actual medications so the doctor can verify that you are getting the medications in the strengths that she thinks you are getting.

The Eye Doctor — Your Lighting Designer

The eye doctor (*ophthalmologist* or *optometrist*) ensures that your diabetes does not damage your vision. This doctor has had advanced training in diseases of the eye. Your primary care physician must see (no pun intended) to it that you have an examination by this specialist at least once a year and more often if necessary.

An ophthalmologist or optometrist must dilate the pupils of the eyes in order to do a proper examination.

The eye doctor examines you for the conditions I outline in Chapter 5. He or she must send a report to your primary care physician. He or she should also take the opportunity to educate you about diabetic eye disease.

Sometimes the good deed of restoring vision leads to unexpected, negative consequences. One ophthalmologist I talked to told me that he restored the vision of a diabetic patient, only to have the patient buy a gun and nearly shoot someone with whom he had a grievance.

The Foot Doctor — Your Dance Instructor

The foot doctor or *podiatrist* is your best source of help with the minor (and some of the major) foot problems that all people suffer. You should go to him with such problems as toenails that are hard to cut, corns and calluses, and certainly any ulcer or infection of your foot. This is especially true if you have any neuropathy (see Chapter 5). In that case, you're better off not trying to cut your toenails by yourself.

Foot doctors I spoke with emphasized that the earlier you see a podiatrist, the less likely that a minor problem will be converted into a major disaster. For example, an infected toe that would respond to soaking by the person without diabetes may need antibiotics, special shoes, and surgical removal of dead tissue in the person with diabetes.

The doctor can tell you which preparations you should not use on your skin. He or she can show you how important it is that you give lesions time to heal and not to rush to put weight on your injured feet. Many podiatrists also give you a list of dos and don'ts for the proper care of your feet, such as conducting daily inspections, avoiding extreme heat, and so on. Chapter 5 details all the things you need to do to preserve good foot health.

The Dietitian — Your Food Services Provider

This person serves one of the most important roles in your care. Because most diabetes is type 2, and type 2 is greatly worsened by obesity, a good dietitian can really help you to control your blood glucose both by eating the right foods and amounts and helping you to lose weight. The dietitian can also show you which foods belong to which energy source — carbohydrate, protein, and fat. (See Chapter 8 for more on your diet.)

The person with type 1 diabetes needs to know how food interacts with the insulin injections that are mandatory. The dietitian can teach you to count carbohydrates so that you know how much insulin to take for your meals. (See Chapter 10 for more on carbohydrate counting.)

A good dietitian usually holds up a mirror to you, showing you not only what you eat but how you eat as well. When do you consume most of your calories, and where do they come from? All ethnic foods can be adjusted so that you enjoy the foods you have always eaten while you stay within the bounds of a diabetic diet. A good dietitian is the best source for this kind of information.

The dietitian can also show you what a portion of food really means. This demonstration is an eye-opener in most cases. You usually find that you have been eating portions much larger than necessary. Unfortunately, when it comes to a diabetic diet, you can't have your cake and eat it, too. But you can see in Appendix A, which offers gourmet recipes for people with diabetes, that every culture makes delicious food that is actually good for the person with diabetes. For even more information on this important topic, see my book *Diabetes Cookbook For Dummies, 2nd Edition* (Wiley).

One thing you want to be sure of is that the dietitian is flexible in her approach to food. There are a few rules about where your calories should come from, but you have plenty of room for variation within those rules. The diet you are ultimately given should take into account your preferences as well as the fact that the amount of carbohydrate, protein, and fat is different for different individuals. Any dietitian who simply hands you a printed diet and says "Go follow it" is doing you no favor.

The Diabetes Educator — Your Researcher

Every person in your play is actually an educator in addition to his other role, but this person is especially trained to teach you what you need to know about every aspect of diabetes so that you properly take care of yourself. He should have CDE (Certified Diabetes Educator) after his name. A CDE has taken extensive courses in diabetes and has passed an examination.

A diabetes educator teaches you how to take your insulin or pills, how to test your blood glucose, and how to acquire any of the other skills you need. You can find many diabetes educators in a Diabetes Education Program. Once you have gotten over the shock of having diabetes, asking your primary physician to refer you to such a program is a good idea. After you have gone through the program, go back and update yourself. New drugs and new procedures are constantly being discovered. The diabetes educator can be a wonderful source of information about these, while making sure that you continue in your good diabetic habits.

The Pharmacist — Your Usher

The role of the usher may not sound important, but how will you enjoy the play if you cannot find your seat? The pharmacist is your guide to all the medications and tools required to control your blood glucose and manage any complications that you develop. He or she ushers you into the use of all these strange and new products. You may see your pharmacist more often than you see any other of your cast and crew who are actually in the medical field.

Each time you start a new medication, a good pharmacist checks to make sure that it does not conflict with other medicines you are taking. The pharmacist tells you about side effects and makes sure that your doctor is checking you for adverse drug reactions or interactions. The pharmacist may give you a printout that you can take home and refer to, telling you all you need to know about your new medication.

Many pharmacists also prepare a list of medications that you take, telling you each drug's strengths and dosage frequency. You can carry this around in case any doctor ever needs to know what you take.

Modern pharmacists are also doing a lot of education. Posters in the pharmacy explain diseases and drugs. Pharmacists can tell you about helpful over-the-counter drugs that your doctor doesn't prescribe. They are also often aware of new drugs and treatments before they become well known. Some pharmacies have blood pressure devices that you can use for free, as well as glucose meters.

The Mental Health Worker — Your Supporting Actor

Your mental health worker may be a psychiatrist, a psychologist, or a social worker, or your primary physician may play this role. This person comes in handy whenever you have days when you feel you just can't cope. (See Chapter 1 for more about dealing with the emotional aspects of diabetes.) The mental health worker is there at those times to support you and get you going again. Diabetes certainly proves the fact that all disease is both physical and emotional.

Your Family and Friends — Your Captivated and Caring Audience

Your audience is the people you live with, eat with, and play with. Your family and friends can be a tremendous source of help, but you must clue them to the fact that you have diabetes. If you have type 1 diabetes, you can teach them how to recognize when your glucose is too low, in case you're ever too ill to take care of yourself. If you have type 2, ask them to moderate their diet so that you can follow yours. A diabetic diet is good for anyone. Complying with your diet is difficult enough, and you don't need your family exposing you to high-calorie foods.

A family member or friend can also become your exercise partner. Sticking to a program is a lot easier when a partner is counting on you to show up to work out. Your family and friends can also accompany you when you visit the doctor and remind you to ask the doctor a question or to follow the instructions you received.

Let these people know about your diabetes and buy them a copy of this book so that they better understand what you are going through and how they can best help you.

The Internet: Your Potential Partner in Lifestyle Change

Type 2 diabetes is a lifestyle disease. Some harmful choices for your lifestyle contributed to your development of type 2 diabetes and some helpful choices will help you control it or prevent it if you don't have it yet. Unlike the people in your life, who can hardly be there with you 24 hours a day, the Internet is only a mouse click away at any time. On the Internet you can find help for the two key aspects of your lifestyle that affect diabetes, diet and exercise.

Because weight loss is the main preoccupation of millions of Americans, there are numerous sites that promise incredible results. Probably the single most important feature of the site that will help you to succeed is continued feedback. If you get regular new advice (at least weekly) and peer support in the form of bulletin boards where you can interact with others, you will lose three times as much as with sites that provide only Internet-based diet and exercise information.

Sites for diet and weight loss

Some of the better sites for diet and weight loss include:

- ✔ **Ediets.com,** which gives you a choice of many different diets and will provide the food as well as weekly updates and suggestions. There are more than 22 diet plans, one of which is sure to appeal to you.

- ✔ **Diet.webmd.com** uses a questionnaire to develop a "diet just for you". The diet is called a nutritional plan rather than a diet. It is personalized and nutritionally sound. You fill out a daily nutritional journal that the people at webmd comment upon. They analyze your progress and nutritional needs each week.

✔ **Shapeup.org** is the web address of Shape Up America, a site that was founded by C. Everett Koop, M. D. It offers lots of information about nutrition and a place where you can tell your story or read the story of others. If you are running into difficulty, you can e-mail the site and get feedback from others who have been successful.

Sites for exercise programs

Some of the better sites for these types of programs include:

✔ **Freetrainers.com** offers individualized fitness programs with individual advice and message boards for reading the experiences of others and offering your own.

✔ **Workoutsforyou.com** offers personalized fitness programs. You get weekly email tips and unlimited email consultations. There are lots of member testimonials in case you want to read the experience of others.

✔ **Global-fitness.com** is the address for Global Health and Fitness, a site that offers a large amount of information on fitness with lots of feedback from trainers. Judging by the successful clients they show on the site, they get some fairly good results.

None of these sites tell you about the people who did not do so well or even the ratio of successful to unsuccessful clients. Don't spend a lot of money up front until you are sure the program is what you need and what works for you. Good luck!

Finding reputable Web sites

Not everything that you find on the Internet is true, let alone reputable. The Health on the Net Foundation has established a set of principles that any site on the Internet can adhere to. From its Web site at www.hon.ch, you can search for medical sites that follow these HONcode principles:

✔ **Principle 1:** Any medical or health advice provided and hosted on this site will be given by medically trained and qualified professionals unless a clear statement is made that a piece of advice offered is from a non-medically qualified individual or organization.

✔ **Principle 2:** The information provided on this site is designed to support, not replace, the relationship that exists between a patient/site visitor and his/her existing physician.

✔ **Principle 3:** Confidentiality of data relating to individual patients and visitors to a medical/health Web site, including their identity, is respected by this Web site. The Web site owners undertake to honor or exceed the legal requirements of medical/health information privacy that apply in the country and state where the Web site and mirror sites are located.

✔ **Principle 4:** Where appropriate, information contained on this site will be supported by clear references to source data and, where possible, have specific HTML links to that data. The date when a clinical page was last modified will be clearly displayed (e.g. at the bottom of the page).

✔ **Principle 5:** Any claims relating to the benefits/performance of a specific treatment, commercial product or service will be supported by appropriate, balance evidence in the manner outlined in Principle 4.

✔ **Principle 6:** The designers of this Web site will seek to provide information in the clearest possible manner and provide contact addresses for visitors that seek further information or support. The Webmaster will display his/her e-mail address clearly throughout the Web site.

✔ **Principle 7:** Support for this Web site will be clearly identified, including the identities of commercial and non-commercial organizations that have contributed funding, services, or material for the site.

✔ **Principle 8:** If advertising is a source of funding, it will be clearly stated. A brief description of the advertising policy adopted by the Web site owners will be displayed on the site. Advertising and other promotional material will be presented to viewers in a manner and context that facilitates differentiation between it and the original material created by the institution operating the site.

If a site agrees with these principles, you can bet the information on it is very reliable. I describe many of the HONcode sites in Appendix C.

Chapter 12

Putting Your Knowledge to Work for You

*I*f you read every word in Part III of this book, you now know as much as the experts. But knowing is often quite a distance from doing. If this fact were not the case, the world would be a much better place to live in because most people know what needs to be done. They just don't do it.

The key thing is to get going on improving your health now. Don't wait another day to begin to do the things that can prolong your life and increase its quality at the same time. You don't want to regret your life the way poor George Burns did. When a beautiful girl walked into his hotel room and said, "I'm sorry, I must be in the wrong room," he told her, "No, you're not in the wrong room. You are just 40 years too late."

Delaying or Preventing Diabetes

There are a number of things you can do to delay or prevent your development of diabetes. Among the key things are

✔ **Lifestyle modification:** Lose weight or don't allow yourself to gain weight. Start an exercise program and exercise for 30 to 45 minutes every day.

✔ **Monitoring:** Make sure your doctor checks for diabetes with a blood glucose test every year, especially if you have prediabetes (see Chapter 3).

✔ **Drugs:** Although there are drugs that have been shown to delay the onset of diabetes, they are associated with side effects and are not currently recommended.

Developing Positive Thinking

Studies have shown fairly conclusively that if you start with a positive frame of mind, your body can work with you and not against you. Even when things go wrong, if you're optimistic, you can pick yourself up and move forward. If you're pessimistic, you can become depressed and believe that nothing will help you. That kind of attitude is not conducive to good control of your blood glucose and avoidance of complications.

I have a patient who came to me to improve his glucose control just after having a toe amputated. This is a patient who sees a lot of manure and knows there is a beautiful horse in the area. He refuses to believe that a temporary setback is a permanent defeat. I got him on a program of tight diabetic control with the newer oral medications. His eyes have gotten better and his neuropathy (see Chapter 5) has improved. He believes in his ability to control his blood glucose, and all his actions are directed toward doing just that. The result has been an amazing turnaround in his hemoglobin A1c (see Chapter 7). With his attitude, he is willing to make the changes necessary because he knows they will pay big dividends for his health.

Achieving a positive attitude has a lot to do with how you interpret problems. If you see them as permanent and unchangeable because of a flaw in your own character, you will have trouble being positive. If you see them as temporary and the result of something you can change given enough time, you will be much more optimistic and able to solve most problems.

Monitoring and Testing

Many of my patients ask me about a cure for diabetes. One doesn't exist yet, but the future looks very promising. So far, doctors don't have a portable machine that can measure the blood glucose and respond with the right amount of insulin. Such a gadget would not be of much use for the people who take pills anyway. Therefore, you have to use your brain to make the calculation that your pancreas would do automatically if it could. The calculation is, of course, how much medicine to take for a given glucose. To make the calculation, you need to know the glucose. This is where monitoring comes in.

Without fail, you should have one of the monitors that I describe in Chapter 7. If you have type 1 diabetes, you need to monitor at least before meals and at bedtime. If you have type 2 diabetes, you can get away with a couple of tests daily and sometimes even less if you're stable.

Chapter 10 is where you can find what you should do in response to your test results. If you or your doctor is computer literate, you will do much better with a meter that can be downloaded into a computer. What you look for are trends, and the computer makes it simple to see trends. It can look at dozens of tests at once on a screen, compared to turning pages of a booklet containing your blood glucose readings.

Remember, however, that blood glucose tests reflect only a moment in time. What you need to know is whether you are in control 24 hours a day. That is where the hemoglobin A1c comes in. Your doctor should order this test at least every four months if you're stable and every three months if not. If you have close to normal results in this test, you do not have to worry about long-term complications (see Chapter 5) and will probably not be suffering from short-term complications (see Chapter 4) either.

Even with near-normal hemoglobin A1c results, you still want to be checked for any sign of complications. That means regular eye examinations, regular blood and urine tests for kidney damage, and regular tests for sensation in your feet. Your doctor should do this on schedule, and, if not, you have to remind the doctor.

Great treatment exists for every diabetic complication, and the earlier the treatment is started, the less likely the complication will lead to serious damage. Routine monitoring and testing allow you to discover the problem as early as possible.

Using Medications

Medications can be tricky. Some of them are very potent, but none of them work if you don't take them. Doctors use the word "noncompliance" when they talk about the tendency of patients not to take their medications. Some of the things you need to know when you take your medications include

✔ Are you taking the right dose at the right time?

✔ Are you taking it with or without food depending upon the medication?

✔ Does it mix with your other medications?

✔ Are you aware of side effects, and are they being monitored?

✔ Can the desired effect sometimes be too strong?

✔ Do you have an antidote to its effect available if necessary?

✔ Do you need to adjust the dose when you're not feeling well?

Starting metformin along with lifestyle changes early in the development of type 2 diabetes is recommended by many doctors. Discuss this with your physician as early as you can.

Your doctor, your pharmacist, and your diabetes educator can all help you with your medications, but you're on your own when it comes to taking them. If you have trouble remembering, get yourself a plastic case containing seven sections with a day of the week above each section and fill them with each day's pills. These are available in pharmacies. You can easily see whether you took them or not.

For more on medications, see Chapter 10.

Following a Diet

If you look at Appendix A and its gourmet recipes, it should be clear to you that you're not sacrificing very much by following an appropriate diabetic diet, unless you consider avoiding becoming overweight to be a sacrifice. You can enjoy delicious food that provides plenty of energy for your needs.

In years past, people often focused on reducing fat in their diets, especially cholesterol and saturated fat (see Chapter 8). That's important, but the attention now being paid to carbohydrate intake is especially helpful for diabetics. And it doesn't hurt to know something about the quality of the carbohydrate as well as the quantity. Try to choose low glycemic index carbohydrate, like basmati rice instead of white rice. Any carbohydrate with lots of fiber will be a low glycemic source. You will have a lower blood glucose as a result and require less insulin to control it. Not only does that mean better diabetic control, but your fats, particularly triglyceride, are also lower, and this will decrease the severity of the metabolic syndrome (see Chapter 5) if you have type 2 diabetes.

Most people can make changes in their diet in the short term, but maintaining these changes over the long term is difficult. The best way to accomplish a long-term change is to have a plan and stick to it. The times when you are in unplanned situations are probably the most damaging to your diabetic control. For example, when you enter a restaurant, you're presented with a menu. The job of the author of that menu is to entice you by the description of the food to order that dish, just as the pictures on the food boxes in stores entice you to buy that food. If you have in mind what is good for your diabetic diet, you tend to order what helps you, not what messes up your control.

One of the things I encourage restaurants to do is to devote a section of their menus to delicious diabetic meals so that you can more easily avoid temptation. Restaurants are just starting to do this, and it will take a long time to get a lot of them to offer it. Some restaurants probably never will (especially in Paris). Until they do, you must go out to eat prepared to order appropriately.

The same holds true when you eat at someone else's home. If they know you have diabetes, hopefully they will prepare something you can eat. If they do not, you must select with great care. Do not be afraid to say no. Your friendly dietitian can give you a lot of help on what to select and what to reject.

One thing that helps a lot in diabetes is if you have a fair amount of order in your life. If your life is disorganized, controlling your diabetes will be much more difficult. You must take your medications at about the same time each day and eat at about the same time. You must test at about the same time and exercise at about the same time. But you don't have to eat the same thing all the time. An endless variety of delicious foods is available to you.

For more on your diet, see Chapter 8.

Exercising Regularly

The more you exercise regularly, the better you can control your blood glucose. This holds true for your weight as well. If you have type 2 diabetes, exercising regularly translates into needing less or no medication. If you have type 1 diabetes, you need less insulin. Your exercise choices are unlimited (see Chapter 9). Yes, even a game of golf is exercise, though most people (who are not professional golfers) do not play the sport more than once or twice a week.

If you're having trouble exercising, follow these tips:

- **Do something daily, if possible, but no less than three or four times a week.** If you can't do it regularly on your own, get an exercise partner. You do not need a sports club to find step aerobics. Just walk up a few flights of stairs where you work. Go for a walk outside if the weather permits for at least 20 minutes.

- **Set up a program with goals so that you do not stay stuck in a low level of exercise.** If you do not know how to do this yourself, check with an exercise physiologist or personal trainer. If you're older than 40 and have not exercised and are overweight, check with your doctor before beginning a strenuous program.

- **Don't limit yourself to aerobics.** A little weight lifting a few days a week can make an amazing difference in your strength, your stamina, and your physique. If your sport is tennis, you may find that you can play that third set with much greater ease once you start on a weight program. All other sports benefit from weight lifting in a similar fashion.

Exercise is definitely a way to get high without drugs. It is good for depression or any unhappy state of mind. Don't take my word for it. Get out and find out for yourself. See Chapter 9 for more on exercise.

Using Expertise Available to You

People are usually eager to help you with your diabetic condition. (See Chapter 11 to find out more about your supporting cast.) So much knowledge is out there, just waiting to be tapped. Insurance companies recognize the value of these resources, such as dietitians and diabetes educators, and are usually willing to pay for them.

Diabetes self-management education is another program that you should attend early in your diagnosis and at regular intervals of every three to five years thereafter. Who knows what great advances may have taken place since your last educational program? Sometimes even your doctor is unaware of them.

You can get lots of free information from your friendly pharmacist, the Internet, and other people with diabetes. You may want to be careful of these last two groups, however. A lot of misinformation is shared on the Internet and among diabetic patients. Before you make a major alteration in your treatment on the basis of uncertain information, check with your physician. (You can find out about some of the most common bits of misinformation in Chapters 17 and 19.)

Every time you have a question about your diabetes, write it down and save it for your next office visit with your doctor, unless it is urgent. If you don't know whether something is urgent, call your doctor and let the doctor determine the urgency of your problem.

Don't neglect your family and friends as a helpful source. These are the people who love you and know that you would help them if the tables were turned. The problem is that they cannot help you if they do not know what you're dealing with. Tell them that you have diabetes and the risks, such as hypoglycemia, that you face. Tell them how to help you if the need arises. You will find that the result will be a much closer relationship.

Part IV
Special Considerations for Living with Diabetes

The 5th Wave   By Rich Tennant

"Since discovering Lamar's diabetes, I've used the exchange system when preparing meals. I exchanged my deep fryer for a steam basket, and my candy thermometer for a melon baller."

In this part . . .

Two groups of people, children and the elderly, have special needs that the average adult does not have to deal with. Children are growing and developing sexually, while the elderly are often coping with other illnesses as well. Both groups have emotional problems that are unique. The child is learning to fit in with peers while separating from parents. The elderly are losing friends and relatives at the same time that their mental processes are declining. This part explains their special problems and how to tackle them.

The middle-aged adult has specific problems to cope with as well, relating to insurance (both life and health) and employment. Fortunately, the barriers for adults with diabetes are rapidly coming down, but you still need to know about possible pitfalls. Discrimination cannot be tolerated, and you can find out what to do about it here.

Finally, I tell you about the huge number of new developments in diabetes, putting them into perspective as to usefulness and appropriateness. I also expose false promises. So many things have been proposed for diabetes care without benefit of careful evaluation. The scientific evidence for and against each is presented so that you can make up your own mind.

Chapter 13

Your Child Has Diabetes

*W*hen I wrote the first edition of this book in 1998, almost all diabetes in children was type 1 diabetes. Today there has been a vast change in this situation. The incidence of type 2 diabetes is rapidly approaching the incidence of type 1 diabetes in children. The culprits to blame for this huge increase in the population of children with type 2 diabetes are obesity and lack of exercise. I will have a lot more to say about this in the section on type 2 diabetes in children later in this chapter.

There are still plenty of new cases of type 1 diabetes in children. This chapter contains basic information about their care but for a full discussion of type 1 diabetes see my book *Type 1 Diabetes For Dummies* (Wiley).

Children with diabetes present special problems that adults with diabetes do not have. Not only are they growing and developing from babies to adults, but they have problems of psychological and social adjustment. Diabetes can add complications to a period of time that is not exactly smooth, even without it.

Many doctors believe that if a child has diabetes, the whole family really has the disease because everyone must adjust to it. Because diabetes is the second most common chronic disease in children after asthma, it is no small problem.

In this chapter, you find out how to manage diabetes in your child at each stage of growth and development. You need to remember that your child is first a child and then a child with diabetes. And you also need to remember that you are not to blame for your child's diabetes. Diabetes is not a form of retribution for your sins. It's also important to remember that your child is not to blame either.

Your Baby or Preschooler Has Diabetes

If your infant or preschooler is diagnosed with diabetes, you may feel overwhelmed. The information in this section can help you understand that this diagnosis isn't the end of the world — it's the beginning of many years of special care for your child.

Nurturing a diabetic infant

Although type 1 diabetes does not usually show up in babies, it can, and you should know what to expect when it does. Obviously, your baby is not verbal and cannot tell you what is bothering him or her. For this reason, you may miss the fact that the baby is urinating excessively in his or her diaper. The baby will lose weight and have vomiting and diarrhea, but this may be ascribed to a stomach disorder rather than diabetes. When the diagnosis is finally made, the baby may be very sick and require a stay in a pediatric intensive care unit. Do not blame yourself for not realizing that your baby was sick with diabetes.

After the diagnosis is made, the hard work begins. You must learn to give insulin injections and to test the blood glucose in a child who will be reluctant to have either one done. You have to learn when and what to feed the baby, both to encourage growth and development and to prevent low blood glucose.

At this stage, you don't need to be as worried about tight glucose control as you will be later on. There are several reasons for this. First, the baby's neurological system is still developing. Frequent, severe low blood glucose damages this development, so the glucose is permitted to be higher now than later on. Second, studies show that changes associated with high blood glucose leading to diabetic complications do not begin to add up until the prepubertal years, so you have a grace period during which you can allow less tight control.

On the other hand, a small baby is very fragile. He or she has less of everything, so small losses of water, sodium, potassium, and other substances lead more rapidly to a very sick baby. If you keep the baby's blood glucose around 150 to 200 mg/dl (8.3 to 11.1 mmol/L), you are doing very well.

Taking care of a toddler with diabetes

Diagnosing diabetes in your preschooler may be just as difficult as it is in the baby. The child may still be preverbal and running around in diapers.

A preschooler is beginning the process of separating from his parents and starting to learn to control the environment (by becoming toilet-trained, for example). This separation process makes it more difficult for you, the parent, to give insulin injections and test the glucose. You must be firm in insisting that these things be done. You'll need to do them yourself because a small child neither knows how to do them nor understands what to do with the information generated by the glucose meter.

Because a toddler's eating habits may not be very regular, the use of very short-acting insulin like lispro is especially helpful (see Chapter 10). Very soon, people with diabetes should have a way of measuring the blood glucose in a painless fashion, which will be of great assistance in monitoring these children.

Becoming an educated caregiver

For a time of variable duration — a so-called "honeymoon period" — your child will have seemingly regained the ability to control his or her blood glucose with little or no insulin. (See the nearby sidebar "The honeymoon period.") This period always ends, and it isn't your fault that it does. When it ends, you have to work with your child's doctor, dietitian, and diabetes educator to find out how to control diabetes with insulin.

To give your child appropriate care, you need to know how to do the following things:

- ✔ **Identify the signs and symptoms of hyperglycemia, hypoglycemia, and diabetic ketoacidosis (see Chapters 4 and 5).** Each child has a particular way of expressing low or high blood glucose, for example, by becoming quiet or loud. Learn the signs for your child, and let anyone else who cares for the child know them.

- ✔ **Administer insulin (see Chapter 10).** Thanks to rapid-acting insulin, you can wait to see how much the baby is eating before you decide on the amount of insulin.

- ✔ **Measure the blood glucose and urine ketones (see Chapter 7).** Very frequent blood glucose measurements are essential. The more information you have, the better the control and the less frequent the hypoglycemia. Most children need between four and seven blood glucose measurements a day to achieve excellent control.

  Toddlers who are toilet-trained may have accidents when their glucose is high, because high glucose causes a large quantity of urine.

- ✔ **Treat hypoglycemia with food or glucagon (see Chapter 4).** Children this young require half the adult dose of glucagon. Glucagon may cause a toddler to vomit, but it still raises the blood glucose.

> ✔ **Feed your diabetic child (see Chapter 8).**
>
> ✔ **Set an example for lifelong exercise for your child by exercising with her.**
>
> ✔ **Know what to do when your child is sick with another childhood illness.** If your child must go to the hospital, approach this as a positive experience — a chance to get a tune-up.

Your responsibilities as the parent of a diabetic baby or preschooler are extensive and time-consuming. Training your usual helpers to take over, even for a short time, is especially difficult. Unless you hire a professional to take over for a while, you may not get very much time away from your diabetic infant.

Placing your child in preschool is a difficult decision. You can do so only if you are sure that the adult supervisors are fully aware of your child's needs and willing to provide them.

Your other children may resent the attention that you pay to this one child. If your other children start to misbehave, this may be the reason.

Your Primary School Child Has Diabetes

The division of children into type 1 and type 2 diabetes begins around age 10. Important differences exist in the way type 1 and type 2 are recognized and treated. Therefore, I discuss each separately in this section. In 1990, less than 4 percent of children diagnosed with diabetes had type 2. In 2003, the figure had risen to more than 30 percent. In 2007 almost one of every two children with diabetes had type 2 diabetes. For a discussion of why that number has grown so rapidly, see the section "Obesity and Type 2 Diabetes in Children," later in this chapter.

Coping with type 1 diabetes

In some ways, type 1 diabetes care gets a little easier with a primary school child, but in other ways, it gets more difficult. Your child can finally tell you when he or she has symptoms of hypoglycemia, so this is easier to recognize and treat. But you must begin to control the blood glucose more carefully because your child is reaching the stage where control really counts.

The honeymoon period

Given its name because it represents a period of improvement in type 1 diabetes that does not last, the honeymoon period occurs in most patients. After the disease has been diagnosed and treated so that the blood glucose levels are close to normal, the child may require little or no insulin for a time. This is a period of remission in the disease and means there is still some function in the beta cell of the pancreas (see Chapter 2). Longer remissions are seen when:

✔ The age at onset of diabetes is older.

✔ The initial presentation of the disease is milder.

✔ The amount of islet cell antibody (see Chapter 2) is lower.

This is a temporary remission and ends with a sudden or slowly increasing requirement for insulin. Within three years after the diagnosis, young children experience a complete loss of insulin production. Older children may have some preservation of function.

You still have a child who is growing and developing, so nutrition remains critical. You must provide enough of the right kinds of calories to fuel the growth process. A snack such as four ounces of apple juice and a graham cracker between breakfast and lunch, between lunch and supper, and at bedtime can help smooth out glucose control and avoid hypoglycemia.

Your child is going to do more to separate from you. He or she may insist on giving insulin shots and doing blood tests. Studies again indicate that this is not a good time for you to give up these tasks, certainly not completely. Your child may not be physically capable of performing them and, in an attempt to hide the disease from peers, may not perform them at all during school. Diet may also suffer at school as the child tries to fit in and not stand out by eating the things that diabetes requires.

Managing hypoglycemia

Because you are beginning to tighten the level of glucose control, hypoglycemia is more of a risk, especially at night. At this stage (and from now on), you can avoid hypoglycemia by taking any or all of the following steps:

✔ Give a bedtime snack regularly.

✔ Give cornstarch at bedtime. Cornstarch is slowly broken down so that it provides glucose over a longer period of time. There is even a commercial product, called NightBite, that contains cornstarch and can be given before bedtime.

✔ Measure and treat a low blood glucose before bedtime.

✔ Occasionally check the blood glucose at 3 a.m.

✔ Ask about symptoms of nighttime low blood glucose, such as nightmares and headaches.

✔ Be sure your child does not skip meals.

✔ Have your child eat carbohydrates before exercising.

At least one member of your family must be able to administer glucagon by injection to treat hypoglycemia should you be unable to get your child to eat or drink.

Handling school issues

When your child goes to school or a daycare setting, you need to address new problems. One issue is that he interacts with other children, wants their approval, and wants to fit in. Your child may consider diabetes a stigma and be very reluctant to share it with other children. A plan of treatment that interferes with school and friendships may be very unwelcome.

Other issues may arise regarding the school's willingness to participate in your child's care. To best handle these issues, you must be aware of your rights.

Federal laws, especially the Diabetes Education Act of 1991, specify that diabetes is a disability and that it's unlawful to discriminate against children with diabetes. If a school receives federal funding or is open to the public, it has to reasonably accommodate the special needs of the diabetic child.

Any school receiving federal funds must develop a *Section 504 plan* to meet the needs of the disabled child. This refers to Section 504 of the Rehabilitation Act of 1973. The plan takes every need of the child into account from the moment she is picked up in the morning by a bus driver (who must know how to help the child with a diabetic problem) until she arrives back home at the end of the day. The plan includes the child's self-care abilities, and it lists trained personnel by name and responsibility.

If you plan to send your child to a private school that receives no federal funds, before enrolling, insist on a plan of care for your child identical to a 504 plan.

The law requires that a diabetic child participate fully in all school and after-school activities. This means provisions must be made for blood glucose testing, for treatment with insulin, and for taking snacks or going to the bathroom as needed.

To accomplish this, the written Section 504 treatment plan is developed by your doctor, you, and the school nurse, and relevant people in the school have assigned roles. The plan must include

✔ Blood glucose monitoring

✔ Insulin administration

✔ Meals and snacks

✔ Recognition and treatment of hypoglycemia

✔ Recognition and treatment of hyperglycemia

✔ Testing of urine ketones as indicated

As the parent, you are responsible for providing all supplies for testing and treatment. The school provider has a responsibility to understand and treat hypoglycemia, to test the blood glucose and treat when the level is outside certain parameters, to coordinate meals and snacks, and to permit excused appointments to the doctor as well as restroom use. There is no reason that your child should not participate fully in school.

You have to provide a kit every day for school that contains everything the child needs to test the blood glucose and, if necessary, the urine for ketones. The kit must also include any necessary insulin and syringes. A list of signs and symptoms of high and low blood glucose is another useful addition to this kit. A source of food must be available to the child throughout the school day, both for snacks and prevention of hypoglycemia during exercise. The teachers need to know to remind the child to eat. The child must be free to eat when necessary and not have to request food from the teacher.

These kits and food sources also have to go with the child whenever the child leaves school — for example, for a fire drill or a field trip.

Recognizing and treating type 2 diabetes

A number of clues point to a child having type 2 diabetes rather than type 1:

✔ The child is overweight rather than underweight at diagnosis.

✔ Symptoms, such as thirst and increased urination, are mild or not present at all; if they are present, they have been going on a long time (often months).

✔ The child has a strong family history for diabetes.

✔ The child's glucose level at diagnosis is usually lower than the glucose of a patient with type 1.

✔ The child belongs to an ethnic group at increased risk for type 2, such as African American, Hispanic, Asian, or Native American.

✔ The child has *acanathosis nigricans,* dark patches on the skin between the fingers and toes, on the back of the neck, and on the underarms. These patches are present in 90 percent of type 2 patients.

✔ Girls may have irregular menses caused by polycystic ovarian syndrome (see Chapter 6).

Despite these clues pointing to type 2, the two types of diabetes can be confused for several reasons. Type 1 diabetic children may be overweight. Type 2 children may have ketones in their urine, just as type 1 patients do. The glucose level at diagnosis in some type 1 children is not very elevated. And the overall occurrence of type 2 is still low enough that the doctor may not think of the possibility.

An important thing to remember is that type 2 diabetes responds to treatment with insulin much more rapidly than type 1, and the child may not need insulin at all after a proper diet and exercise are established. No child with type 1 diabetes can live without insulin except possibly during the brief honeymoon period described above.

If you have an overweight child — one who is more than 120 percent of his or her ideal weight for height — you should request that your doctor screen him or her for diabetes every two years by using a fasting blood glucose test.

The treatment of type 2 diabetes, both in children and adults, starts with lifestyle change. You, the parent, must make the commitment to exercise with your child every day. You should meet with a dietitian and discuss a diet for the whole family that provides sufficient nutrition for the growing child while allowing for weight loss. If these two things are accomplished, no more will be necessary. That means limiting TV and computer time so the child is active rather than passive. You might consider getting a pedometer for your child and encouraging him or her to build up the number of steps taken each day, with prizes for reaching goals.

Fad diets are not recommended for children with type 2 diabetes. Treatment requires adopting a lifelong program of healthy eating and exercise. A diet that emphasizes reduction in calories, especially fats, is far more likely to be followed over the years than one that drastically changes what the child is used to eating. Good nutrition can even be found in fast food restaurants (see my book *Diabetes Cookbook For Dummies, 2nd Edition* published by Wiley).

When diet and exercise do not return the blood glucose to normal, oral hypo-glycemic agents (see Chapter 10) are used. Although these medications are not approved by the FDA for children, most experts agree that they are acceptable, with metformin being the first drug used and the sulfonylureas added as needed. If oral agents fail, insulin is given.

Your Adolescent Has Diabetes

If an adolescent or young adult has type 2 diabetes, the information in the previous section applies, because the goal remains the same no matter what the age: normalize the child's weight and increase exercise in order to achieve normal blood glucose levels. Therefore, I focus my attention in this and the next section on type 1 diabetes.

Your adolescent or teenager with type 1 diabetes will provide some of your biggest challenges. This is the time period when most childhood diabetes begins. The Diabetes Control and Complications Trial (see Chapter 3) showed that tight glucose control can be accomplished beginning at age 13, and that this control can prevent complications. The higher frequency of severe hypoglycemia that accompanies tighter control was not found to be damaging to the brain of a child at this age. However, children at this age do not think in terms of long-term blood glucose control and prevention of com-plications. So they're not willing to do many of the tasks required to control their diabetes on a regular basis.

The goal of treatment at this stage is a hemoglobin A1c between 7 and 9 percent (see Chapter 7). A value above 11 percent indicates poor control. This is not true for smaller children, who are allowed to have a higher hemoglobin A1c.

This stage is when your child is most eager to become independent. You don't want to give up all control at this time for several reasons:

- ✔ Your child actually does better if he or she has limits that are clearly stated and enforced.
- ✔ The "shame" of diabetes may cause the child to skip shots and food, especially around friends.
- ✔ The problem of eating disorders (see Chapter 8) may pop up at this time, especially among girls trying to maintain a slim body image. Girls with diabetes know that if they skip their injections, they lose weight. They may ignore the high blood glucose that results.
- ✔ Teenagers with diabetes may still be unable to translate levels of blood glucose into appropriate action.

The hormonal changes that occur in puberty are often associated with insulin resistance. This may be a source of loss of control rather than any failure of your child to follow the diabetic treatment plan. Upward adjustment of the insulin may overcome this problem.

Strenuous exercise may play an even greater role in the life of your child at this age. The result will be a significant reduction in the amount of insulin required after exercise. Your blood glucose measurements will help you to define your child's need for insulin. If your child plays a team sport, the coach and teammates must be aware of the diabetes and permit your child to eat, go to the bathroom, and take insulin as required. Type 1 diabetes is no reason to prohibit strenuous exercise.

Make sure that your child snacks regularly; keep snacks readily available no matter where your child may be.

Your Young Adult Child Has Diabetes

When your child becomes a young adult, you definitely want to give up the control that has helped your child to thrive up to this point. Your child should be doing his or her own testing. He or she is ready to leave the pediatric level and begin to work with doctors who care for adults. This means that you are probably out of the loop. Your child should now have the skill to choose appropriate insulin treatment based upon blood glucose levels and calories of carbohydrate consumed (see Chapter 10).

Your child now has new challenges, including finding work, going to college, finding a future mate, and finding a place to live independently. At the same time, the reluctance to admit to diabetes and the desire for a thin body continue to complicate care.

Diabetes care must be intensive at this point (see Chapter 10). Multiple shots of intermediate and short-acting insulin are taken. Your child must follow a diabetic diet (see Chapter 8), and an exercise program is essential (see Chapter 9). The rest of this book really has to do with the tasks that your young adult child with diabetes faces.

Off to College

When your child leaves for college, he or she has all the responsibility for the diabetes. Your job is simply to make sure that all the equipment for testing the blood glucose and administering insulin is available to your child. You should also make the college aware of your child's medical condition. Encourage your child to find one or more people at the college, such as a roommate or sports teammate, who are prepared to help your child when necessary.

Two issues are particularly important to discuss before the student leaves for school: alcohol use and sexual activity. Alcohol use may significantly increase in college, which means that your child may consume many empty calories and run the risk of severe hypoglycemia if he or she fails to eat properly. Discuss concerns about making a girl pregnant with your son, and discuss the risk of pregnancy when diabetes is not in control with your daughter. (See Chapter 6 for information that can fuel both discussions.) Young adults of both sexes should know how to prevent sexually transmitted diseases.

College, like the rest of your child's life, can be experienced just as it would be if diabetes were not present. The key is planning.

Obesity and Type 2 Diabetes in Children

The epidemic of obesity, which has spread to children in the United States in the past few decades, has led to a much higher prevalence of type 2 diabetes in children than was ever seen before. Overweight or obesity is present in as many as 25 percent of all children. Only a fraction of these children go on to develop diabetes.

There are a number of conditions that can cause obesity in children but they represent probably 1 percent of the causes. Most of them can be diagnosed during the course of a good physical examination by your child's pediatrician. By far the major reason for obesity in children is too many calories in and too few burned up by exercise.

Even without diabetes, obesity is a burden for children. The obese child faces severe psychological and social consequences:

- ✔ Lower respect from peers than other disabled children get
- ✔ Less comfortable family interactions
- ✔ Poor body image
- ✔ Low self-esteem

Defining obesity in children

The definition of obesity in children age 2 to 19 is based on the body mass index, BMI (see Chapter 7). A child is obese or overweight if his BMI is at the 95th percentile or greater for his age and sex. He is at risk for overweight if the BMI is between the 85th and 95th percentile. The growth charts that indicate the percentiles for BMI can be found at: www.brightfutures.org/bf2/pdf/pdf/GrowthCharts.pdf.

Obesity is not just responsible for type 2 diabetes. It can also provoke a number of other dangerous medical conditions in children. These include:

- Metabolic syndrome, discussed in Chapter 5, leading to an increased tendency for heart attacks and strokes
- Polycystic ovarian syndrome, also discussed in Chapter 5, leading to infertility, abnormal menstrual periods and hairiness in girls
- Heart disease due to the increased work of the heart
- High blood pressure, which can damage the heart and the kidneys
- Sleep disorders like obstructive sleep apnea with snoring and increased blood pressure
- Fatty liver with abnormal liver enzymes in the blood
- Gallbladder disease
- Bone and joint diseases due to the weight on the bones
- Skin abnormalities like acanthosis nigricans, black velvety patches on the joints and under the arms
- Nervous system diseases such as increased pressure in the brain with headache and visual disturbances

Preventing obesity in children

Prevention of obesity is much preferred over treating the damage that it does. There are a number of things that you can do to prevent obesity in your child:

- Try to have a normal weight before you become pregnant.
- Exercise throughout your pregnancy.
- Breast feed for at least three months.
- Eat meals together as a family.
- Avoid sugary drinks and fatty foods.
- Restrict time for sedentary activities like TV or computers.
- Eliminate fundraisers that sell candy and cookies.
- Insist on exercise daily and do it with your child.

Dealing with type 2 diabetes

Adding type 2 diabetes into this mix can be devastating. The consequences of the preceding problems may lead to failure to manage the diabetes because the child wants to avoid any activity that makes him or her even more different from his or her peers.

It is important to separate type 1 diabetes from type 2 because the child with type 2 diabetes has a milder condition and can be treated with pills or diet and exercise alone. However, because children do not appreciate long-term consequences of their actions, you often have the problem of compliance.

You must help your obese child to lose weight because most obese children become obese adults. With the assistance of a dietitian, you can figure out the food that your child can eat to maintain growth and development without gaining more weight. One of the most helpful techniques is to take the child into the supermarket and point out the difference between empty calories and nourishing calories. Another is never to make high-calorie food, such as cake and candy, a reward. Finally, if you keep problem foods out of the house, there is much less likelihood that your child will eat them.

Once type 2 diabetes develops, treatment should begin as early as possible to minimize the development of complications. Depending upon the severity of the diabetes, the treatment can utilize any or all of the following approaches:

- ✔ **Lifestyle changes:** Parents must set an example of good dietary and exercise habits. Some studies suggest that if parents go first, children will follow. The best diet is one that emphasizes a variety of vegetables, some fruits and small amounts of protein with minimal processed carbohydrates like candy and pastries. The best exercise is what you will continue to do regularly.

- ✔ **Drugs:** The currently available drugs are either not recommended for children under 16 years of age or not useful for long-term treatment.

- ✔ **Surgery:** Children with extreme obesity with BMIs of 35 and greater may require bypass surgery or gastric banding. This has been successful but has complications like infection, deficiency of certain nutrients like vitamins and calcium, pneumonia and hernia. It should be used especially in children with other risk factors like a strong family history of heart disease, sleep apnea or high blood pressure. This surgery should only be performed in medical centers with large experience in children.

Sick Day Solutions

The comments in this section apply primarily to a child with type 1 diabetes, because children with type 2 diabetes do not lose diabetic control to nearly the same extent.

Any child is susceptible to all the usual childhood illnesses, but diabetes complicates your child's care. An illness can affect diabetes in opposite ways.

An infection may increase the level of insulin resistance so that the usual dose of insulin is not adequate. Or it may cause nausea and vomiting so that no food or drink can stay down, and the insulin may cause hypoglycemia. For this reason, you need to measure the blood glucose in your sick child every two to four hours. If the glucose is over 250 mg/dl (13.9 mmol/l), you need to give extra short-acting insulin (see Chapter 10). If it's under 250, you give more carbohydrate-containing nutrients.

You also need to test ketones in your child's urine or blood once or twice a day (see Chapter 7), especially if the glucose is over 300 mg/dl. If the ketones become elevated, you need to discuss the situation with your doctor.

You should probably feed your child with clear liquids like tea and soda during the sick days. Don't offer your child milk, because it upsets the stomach. As long as your child can hold down clear liquids, you can continue to take care of him or her. If clear liquids cannot be held down, you must contact your doctor and bring your child to the hospital.

While the blood glucose remains over 250 mg/dl, use tea, water, and diet soda so as not to add calories of carbohydrate. When the blood glucose is less than 250 mg/dl, you can use regular soda or glucose drinks.

Thyroid Disease in Type 1 Children

Because type 1 diabetes is an autoimmune disease (see Chapter 2), it is not surprising that children with type 1 have other autoimmune diseases more commonly than unaffected children. The disease that is found most commonly in association with type 1 diabetes is *autoimmune thyroiditis*. This condition is discovered by obtaining a blood test that shows an abnormal increase in proteins in the blood called *thyroid autoantibodies*. In a study of 58 patients with type 1 diabetes (*Diabetes Care,* April 2003), 19 were found to have autoimmune thyroiditis.

Autoimmune thyroiditis usually results in no symptoms, but occasionally it causes low thyroid function (*hypothyroidism*), and even more rarely it causes high thyroid function (*hyperthyroidism*). Autoimmune thyroiditis is found mostly in girls between 10 and 20 years of age. This condition is easily treated, as I explain in my book *Thyroid For Dummies, 2nd Edition* (Wiley).

Autoimmune thyroiditis is so common in type 1 diabetes that type 1 patients are recommended to be screened yearly for thyroid disease with a simple blood test that checks the level of thyroid stimulating hormone (TSH).

The Extra Value of Team Care

When your child is first diagnosed with diabetes, the stress can be overwhelming. The guilt that comes with this diagnosis may leave you unable to help your child much at first and certainly unable to learn all that you need to know to master the areas of importance to the health of your child. That is why you must depend upon the help of a diabetes care team throughout the duration of his or her childhood, and especially when the diagnosis is first made.

Who are your teammates, and what can they do for you?

- ✔ The pediatrician can show you how to administer insulin and test the blood glucose. This doctor can also explain how to use the information to determine an insulin dose.

- ✔ The dietitian can show you how many calories of which foods are needed for growth and development.

- ✔ The diabetes educator can explain the short- and long-term complications of diabetes and how your child can avoid them.

- ✔ The mental health worker can help you deal with the psychological issues at each stage of your child's development.

- ✔ One of these professionals can also help you with an exercise program for your child.

Another resource that can be tremendously valuable for you and your child is a diabetes summer camp. These camps are located all over the country and provide a safe, well-managed place where your child can go and be in the majority. He or she can learn a great deal about diabetes while enjoying all the pleasures of a summer camp environment. (Certainly not a minor benefit is the opportunity for you to have time off for perhaps the first time in years.)

You can find an extensive list of camps for diabetic children throughout the United States by going to the Web site www.childrenwithdiabetes.com/camps/index.htm. This is one of the many services of the Web site "Children with Diabetes."

In Chapter 11, I compare diabetes to a stage play. There, the person with diabetes was the author, the producer, the director, and the star. When you have a child with diabetes, he or she is the star, but you take on the roles of author, producer, and director. You obviously have a great responsibility but one that I feel certain you can handle. Just don't try to do it alone. Use your medical experts as well as your family and friends to make it manageable.

Chapter 14

Diabetes and the Elderly

- -

In This Chapter

▶ Diagnosing and managing diabetes in the elderly

▶ Minimizing the risk of heart disease

▶ Eating and taking medications properly

▶ Focusing on unique eye problems of the elderly

▶ Anticipating urinary and sexual problems

▶ Individualizing treatment considerations

▶ Understanding Medicare coverage

- -

Everyone wants to live a long time, but no one wants to get old. Nevertheless, getting old is better than the alternative. Woody Allen says the one advantage of dying is that you don't have to do jury duty. I think I would rather do jury duty.

The first issue I have to tackle in this chapter is defining *elderly*. Every year my definition seems to change, but I think it's fair to talk about the age of 70 as the beginning of being elderly. Using that definition, by the year 2020, more than 20 percent of the U.S. population will be elderly. As much as one-fifth of that elderly population will have diabetes.

Elderly people with diabetes have special problems. Because of those special problems, they're hospitalized at a rate that is 70 percent higher than the general elderly population. In this chapter, you find out about those problems and the way to handle them.

Diagnosing Diabetes in the Elderly

The incidence of diabetes in the elderly (which is almost always type 2 diabetes) is higher for many reasons, but the main culprit seems to be increasing insulin resistance with aging, even if the elderly person with diabetes is not particularly obese or sedentary. Doctors do not yet understand why insulin resistance increases. When they look at the pancreas, it seems to be able to make insulin at the usual rate. The fasting blood glucose actually rises very slowly as you get older. The glucose after meals, however, rises much quicker and leads to the diagnosis.

Because the fasting blood glucose is usually normal, some doctors recommend using the hemoglobin A1c (see Chapter 7) to help to make the diagnosis in the elderly population. A hemoglobin A1c that is 1½ percent higher than the upper limit of normal for that lab is considered diagnostic of diabetes. Because most labs have a normal of up to 5.4 percent, a value of 7 percent or greater is probably diabetes. Results that fall between normal and that value are in a gray zone that probably indicates impaired glucose tolerance (see Chapter 2).

Elderly people with diabetes often do not complain of any symptoms. When they do, the symptoms may not be the ones usually associated with type 2 diabetes, or they may be confusing. Elderly people with diabetes may complain of loss of appetite or weakness, and they may lose weight rather than becoming obese. They may have incontinence of urine, which is usually thought of as a prostate problem in elderly men or a urinary tract infection in older women. Elderly people with diabetes may not complain of thirst because their ability to feel thirst is altered.

Evaluating Intellectual Functioning

You need to evaluate the intellectual function of an elderly person with diabetes because managing the disease requires a fairly high level of mental functioning. The patient has to follow a diabetic diet, administer medications properly, and test the blood glucose. Studies have shown that elderly people with diabetes have a higher incidence of *dementia* (loss of mental functioning) and Alzheimer's disease than nondiabetics, making it much harder for them to perform these tasks.

The patient can take *cognitive screening tests* to determine his or her level of function. Testing makes it easier to tell whether the patient can be self-sufficient or will need help. Many older people who are living alone with no assistance really require an assisted-living situation or even a nursing home.

Considering Heart Disease

The major cause of death in the elderly person with diabetes is a heart attack. Strokes and loss of blood flow in the feet are also much more common in diabetics than nondiabetics. Usually, elderly diabetics suffer not only from diabetes but also have high blood pressure and high cholesterol, are overweight or obese, and do little exercise.

Although many of these patients have had a diagnosis of diabetes for a relatively short time, they have actually suffered from the metabolic syndrome for many years. This is the reason for their high frequency of vascular diseases in the heart, brain, and legs. I discuss both the metabolic syndrome and vascular diseases in Chapter 5.

After the diagnosis is made, it is too late for diabetes prevention, but a major effort should be made to control the glucose, the blood pressure, and the cholesterol in order to postpone the onset of vascular disease.

Aspirin has been shown to protect against blood clots in the heart and in the vessels that provide blood to the legs and brain. If there is no other drug being used that prevents clotting like Plavix or heparin, aspirin should be used in all elderly people with diabetes. Low dose aspirin, 75 to 162 mg/day is as effective as higher doses. Check with your doctor before you start it!

If you have been smoking for decades, although you can't do much about cancer or emphysema, you can prevent the sudden death associated with cigarette smoking. That complication of smoking disappears in a few days of no cigarettes.

Diabetics are at the same high risk of having a first heart attack as nondiabetics are of having a second heart attack. Blood pressure drugs called *beta blockers* have been shown to reduce second heart attacks in nondiabetics. Along with aspirin, beta blockers should be considered as standard treatment for diabetics before a heart attack ever occurs. Talk to your doctor about getting on these drugs.

Preparing a Proper Diet

Diet and exercise are the foundations of good diabetic care for the elderly just as they are in the younger population.

In addition to sometimes lacking the intellectual function required to understand and prepare a proper diabetic diet, the elderly have other problems when it comes to proper nutrition:

- ✔ They may have poor vision and be unable to see to read or cook.
- ✔ They may have low income and be unable to purchase the foods that they require.

> ✔ Their taste and smell may be decreased, so they lose interest in food.
>
> ✔ They often have a loss of appetite.
>
> ✔ They may have arthritis or a tremor that prevents cooking.
>
> ✔ They may have poor teeth or a dry mouth.

Any one of these problems may be enough to prevent proper eating by the elderly person, with the result that the diabetes is poorly controlled.

Anyone over the age of 65 who has Medicare part B insurance coverage is covered for the services of a dietitian for *medical nutrition therapy*. Be sure to take advantage of this benefit. The dietitian can analyze the elderly person's current intake and make recommendations to insure a balanced diet that will help with control of the blood glucose.

Avoiding Hypoglycemia

The elderly, who are already somewhat frail, are especially hard-hit by the consequences of hypoglycemia and are especially prone to it because of several factors:

> ✔ Their food intake may be uncertain.
>
> ✔ They may be taking multiple medications.
>
> ✔ They may sometimes skip medications.
>
> ✔ They often live alone.

In addition, their mental state may not permit them to recognize when they are becoming hypoglycemic.

Intensive diabetes treatment may not be possible when hypoglycemia is a frequent problem. Using medications properly, as I discuss in the next section, is essential to helping avoid hypoglycemia.

The hemoglobin A1c goal for healthy elderly adults is 7 percent. However, if the life expectancy is less than 5 years, the elderly person is frail or the risks of intensive therapy outweigh the benefits, the goal is 8 percent. This decreased level of control will help to avoid hypoglycemia.

Using Medications

Medications that may lower blood glucose to abnormally low levels, such as the sulfonylureas and insulin, are not the drugs of first choice in the elderly.

As I explain in the previous section, hypoglycemia hits elderly patients particularly hard and should be avoided if at all possible. With that goal in mind, I explain the proper order of drug usage for elderly diabetics below. Each of these medications is discussed in detail in Chapter 10.

Elderly people are often on several medications, and the monthly expense for drugs may be great enough to cause them to skip doses or not buy the drug. As I explain many times in this book, compliance with your treatment routine is essential to good health. If you are not taking your diabetes medication(s) as prescribed, you must let your doctor know.

✔ Metformin is probably the first drug to try because it does not increase insulin secretion (which can lead to hypoglycemia) and because it is inexpensive. Kidney function, which is decreased in the elderly, must be checked when using this drug. The doctor should measure the level of creatinine in the blood. If it is greater than 1.4 mg/dl in women or 1.5 mg/dl in men, it should not be used. The drug should be started at a low dose of 500 mg and gradually raised over several weeks to avoid stomach and intestinal problems.

✔ Actos also lowers blood glucose but not to hypoglycemic levels. When metformin does not give enough control, Actos can be added. It does tend to cause water retention, which is not good for an elderly person with some heart or liver disease. It can be used at a low dose or taken every two days to avoid this problem.

✔ Sulfonylureas are added when a third drug is needed. However, sulfonylureas can cause hypoglycemia — especially the older drug chlorpropamide. The newer drugs in this category, such as glyburide and glipizide, are preferred; glipizide may not cause hypoglycemia as often. Your doctor should start you on half the usual dose and raise it slowly over a number of weeks.

The newer sulfonylurea-like drugs called the *meglitinides* (repaglinide and nateglinide) may have an advantage in the elderly because they do not last as long. However, they cost a lot more than the others.

Drugs like acarbose have a very limited effect on the blood glucose and a lot of intestinal side effects. I do not recommend their use in the elderly.

If pills fail to provide reasonable control of the blood glucose so that the hemoglobin A1c is lower than 9, the patient must use insulin. A shot of glargine at bedtime, combined with taking a pill during the day, often accomplishes the desired level of control. In the worst cases, nighttime glargine and daytime short-acting insulin before meals may be necessary, but this is extremely rare. The infirmities of the elderly make insulin usage much more difficult. They may not be able to see the dose or have the hand–eye coordination to draw up the medication. Help from friends or family members becomes essential if the elderly diabetic doesn't live in a nursing facility. Premixed insulins and prefilled insulin pens may make taking insulin a lot easier for these patients.

A new drug that may have a role in diabetes in the elderly is Byetta (see Chapter 10). Two daily injections or the new once-a-week preparation may be very helpful in achieving some weight loss and lowering of the blood glucose.

Dealing with Eye Problems

Elderly people with diabetes are at risk for the eye problems brought on by the disease, and these problems can affect all aspects of proper diabetes care. Older patients often get cataracts, macular degeneration, and open angle glaucoma in addition to diabetic retinopathy (see Chapter 5).

Fortunately, the risk of developing eye diseases associated with diabetes has been found to decrease as people get older, at every level of hemoglobin A1c. For example, a 70-year-old with a hemoglobin A1c of 11 is at much lower risk than a 60-year-old with the same hemoglobin A1c. The blood glucose of the 70-year-old does not need to be controlled as strictly.

An annual eye examination is recommended. One of the biggest failures in diabetes care is that as many as one-third of the elderly never have an eye examination at all. If no examination is done, how can disease be found when it is early enough to treat? When problems are detected, they can be treated, and the patient's vision can be saved.

Coping with Urinary and Sexual Problems

Urinary and sexual problems are very common in elderly people with diabetes and greatly affect quality of life. An older person with diabetes may experience paralysis of the bladder muscle so that urine is retained; when the bladder fills, overflow incontinence is the result. Also, an older person may be unable to get to the bathroom fast enough. Or, spasms in the bladder muscle may lead to incontinence. The result may be frequent urinary tract infections. A urologist may be able to help manage these difficulties.

Almost 60 percent of all men over the age of 70 are impotent, and 50 percent have no *libido* (the desire to have sex). The percentages are even higher for diabetic men. These problems can have many causes (see Chapter 6), but older men are especially likely to have blockage of blood vessels with poor flow into the penis. The elderly take an average of seven medications daily, many of which affect sexual function.

To have sex at any age, you need sexual desire and the physical ability to perform, you need a willing partner, and you need a safe, private place. Any or all of these may be missing for the elderly.

It is not always necessary to treat sexual dysfunction if the male and his partner are okay with the situation. If they aren't, Chapter 6 points out a number of treatments for potency problems.

Considering Treatment Approaches

When deciding upon treatment for an elderly patient with diabetes, you first have to consider the individual. Does this person have a low life expectancy? Or is this person physiologically young, with the possibility of living for 15 or 20 more years? If the patient is only 65 years old and in relatively good health, he or she has a life expectancy of at least 18 more years — plenty of time to develop complications of diabetes, especially macrovascular disease, eye disease, kidney disease, and nervous system disease (see Chapter 5). That person may require more intensive diabetes care than someone who is older and has worse overall health.

The level of care provided to an elderly patient may be basic or intensive:

- **Basic care** is meant to prevent the acute problems of diabetes like excessive urination and thirst. You can accomplish this goal by keeping the blood glucose under 200 mg/dl (11.1 mmol/L). Basic care is used for an elderly person with diabetes who is not expected to live very long, either because of the diabetes or other illnesses.

- **Intensive care** is meant to prevent diabetic complications in an elderly person expected to live long enough to have them. The goal here is to keep the blood glucose under 140 mg/dl (7.7 mmol/L) and the hemoglobin A1c as close to normal as possible while avoiding frequent hypoglycemia.

The benefits in terms of preventing complications of diabetes are much greater when the hemoglobin A1c is lowered from 11 to 9 than when it is lowered from 9 to 7. The goal of treatment for many elderly people can be set higher in order to avoid hypoglycemia in these more fragile patients.

Treatment always starts with diet and exercise. Education about both can be of great value, especially if the patient's spouse is also involved. I discuss diet in the section "Preparing a Proper Diet," earlier in this chapter, and in Chapter 8.

Exercise may be limited in the elderly person with diabetes. Recent studies have shown that exercise is helpful even in the very old, because it reduces the blood glucose and the hemoglobin A1c. However, because elderly patients have more coronary artery disease, arthritis, eye disease, neuropathy, and peripheral vascular disease, exercise just may not be possible. (See Chapter 9 for more on exercise.)

If an elderly patient can't walk at all, he or she may still be able to do resistance exercises sitting in a chair. These exercises increase strength and lower the blood glucose.

When diet and exercise are inadequate to control an elderly patient's diabetes, medications must be added. I discuss medications in the section "Using Medications," earlier in this chapter, and in Chapter 10.

Understanding the Medicare Law

In 1998, the federal government began to offer benefits for the 4.2 million people with diabetes who are eligible for Medicare (over age 65). Under the policy, all people with diabetes enrolled in Medicare part B or Medicare managed care are eligible to receive coverage of glucose monitors, test strips, and lancets. It does not matter which method they use to control their disease.

If you're enrolled in Medicare, you can get these benefits by having your physician prescribe the supplies and document how often you use them.

The Health Care Financing Administration, which administers Medicare, has also passed regulations that permit people with diabetes to get reimbursed for education programs. In addition, if you have Medicare insurance and have type 1 diabetes, you are eligible for Medicare to pay for your insulin pump.

To find out more about Medicare, call the Medicare Hotline at 800-633-4227. The government provides a hotline for the hearing-impaired at 877-486-2048.

Chapter 15

Occupational and Insurance Problems

*A*fter we got his diabetes under control, one of my patients wrote to his mother, "Dear Mom, I'm not working, but my pancreas is." Most people need to work, and some people even want to work. People need to work for the same reason that a certain man did not turn in his brother-in-law who thought he was a chicken. We need the eggs (though not too many).

As a person with diabetes, when you try to get a job, you may run into various forms of discrimination. Part of the problem is the fear that the company will have to pay higher insurance premiums if it hires a person with a chronic illness. Part of the problem is a lack of understanding of the great strides that have been made in diabetes care so that a person with diabetes often has a better record of coming to work than a nondiabetic.

In this chapter, you find out what you need to know when you apply for work, health insurance, and life insurance. You discover how to work the health care system so that you derive the greatest benefits possible at the lowest cost.

Traveling with Diabetes

Whether you travel for your job or for pleasure, if you need insulin injections and must carry syringes and needles, you have to follow the rules of the Transportation Security Administration (TSA) if you fly within the 50 United

States. Airlines outside the U.S. may have different rules; check with your airline before you travel overseas.

The TSA instructs that you should "make sure injectable medications are properly labeled (professionally printed label identifying the medication or a manufacturer's name or pharmaceutical label). Notify the screener if you are carrying a hazardous waste container, refuse container, or a sharps disposable container in your carry-on baggage used to transport used syringes, lancets, etc." Updated information is available at the TSA Web site, `www.tsa.gov/public/display?theme=1`. You can also call the TSA call center at 866-289-9673.

The TSA permits prescription liquid medications and other liquids needed by persons with disabilities and medical conditions. This includes:

- ✔ All prescription and over-the-counter medications (liquids, gels, and aerosols) including KY jelly, eye drops, and saline solution for medical purposes

- ✔ Liquids including water, juice, or liquid nutrition or gels for passengers with a disability or medical condition

- ✔ Life-support and life-sustaining liquids such as bone marrow, blood products, and transplant organs

- ✔ Items used to augment the body for medical or cosmetic reasons such as mastectomy products, prosthetic breasts, bras or shells containing gels, saline solution, or other liquids

- ✔ Gels or frozen liquids needed to cool disability or medically related items used by persons with disabilities or medical conditions

If the liquid medications are in volumes larger than 3 ounces each, they may not be placed in the quart-size bag used for personal liquids of less than 3 ounces and must be declared to the Transportation Security Officer.

Specifically with respect to medications for diabetes, notify the Security Officer that you have diabetes and are carrying your supplies with you. The following diabetes-related supplies and equipment are allowed through the checkpoint after they have been screened:

- ✔ Insulin and insulin loaded dispensing products (vials or box of individual vials, jet injectors, biojectors, epipens, infusers, and preloaded syringes

- ✔ Unlimited number of unused syringes when accompanied by insulin or other injectable medication

- ✔ Lancets, blood glucose meters, blood glucose meter test strips, alcohol swabs, meter-testing solutions

- ✔ Insulin pump and insulin pump supplies (cleaning agents, batteries, plastic tubing, infusion kit, catheter, and needle; nsulin pumps and supplies must be accompanied by insulin)

   ✔ Glucagon emergency kit

   ✔ Urine ketone test strips

   ✔ Unlimited number of used syringes when transported in sharps disposal container or other similar hard-surface container

   ✔ Sharps disposal containers or similar hard-surface disposal container for storing used syringes and test strips

Knowing Where You Can't Work

You may have grown up watching Eliot Ness on television and had your heart set on being a member of the Federal Bureau of Investigation. If you require insulin, forget it. The FBI has a policy called a *blanket ban* on hiring certain groups of people, including people with diabetes who take insulin. A blanket ban does not take into account the condition of the individual, the past employment history, the way the person manages his or her diabetes, or the responsibilities of the position. It simply says, in effect, "You've got the disease, so you can't work here." This policy is a throwback to the days before 1980, when a person with diabetes could never be sure what his blood glucose was doing.

Another important institution that has a blanket ban in place is the United States military. If you have any kind of diabetes, you are not eligible to serve. If you develop diabetes after you've been in the military, you will probably be given a discharge. This does not make a lot of sense because many countries have people with diabetes in their military forces and have no difficulty with them. And so it goes.

But fortunately, blanket bans are falling faster than Alex Rodriquez home runs. For example, the Department of the Treasury lifted a blanket ban on becoming a member of the Bureau of Alcohol, Tobacco, and Firearms if you have insulin-requiring diabetes. Recently, several states lifted a ban on hiring people with diabetes to be school bus drivers. This action resulted from lawsuits against several school districts that fired drivers with spotless driving records just because they had diabetes. (This does not mean that no safeguards against risky drivers exist. Drivers are being evaluated on a case-by-case basis before they are accepted to drive children. This is fair.)

Previously commercial drivers could drive within a state but could not cross state lines. Now the Department of Transportation (DOT) looks at people with diabetes on a case-by-case basis to determine if it is safe for them to drive commercially from state to state. As long as there is no history of hypoglycemia with unconsciousness, the DOT grants an exemption that permits the individual to drive between states with reconsideration taking place every two years.

At one time, people with diabetes who took insulin were banned from becoming firefighters. Now they, too, are permitted to serve in this work on a case-by-case basis. However the rule says they must have a hemoglobin A1c of less than 8 percent. This needs to be changed since people function perfectly well at higher levels of hemoglobin A1c, even 10 or 11 percent.

Another blanket ban that is falling is the ban on piloting airplanes. For 37 years, a person who took insulin could not fly a plane. In 1996, the Federal Aviation Administration (FAA) reconsidered its ban based upon the great advances in controlling diabetes. The FAA decided to permit people to fly privately but not for commercial airlines. Even if they have a private license, however, they can't use it outside the airspace of the United States. Applications for a pilot's license are evaluated on a case-by-case basis.

Is there ever a justification for a blanket ban? The answer is no, and it has been proved in a number of studies. In one study of accidents of all kinds, people with diabetes actually had fewer accidents, including automobile accidents, than groups of people without diabetes. In another study of people over age 65 with diabetes, the rate of automobile accidents was no greater than that of the nondiabetic groups.

Becoming Familiar with Workplace Law

A number of laws protect you in the workplace, but the most important is probably the Americans with Disabilities Act (ADA) of 1990. This act states,

The determination that an individual poses a 'direct threat' shall be based on an individualized assessment of the individual's present ability to safely perform the essential functions of the job.

Flying a plane: It's not easy, but it's worth it

Getting a pilot's license is not easy but is well worth the effort for the person who loves to fly. To be successful, you must have no other disqualifying conditions, such as arteriosclerotic disease of the heart or brain, diabetic eye disease, or severe kidney disease (see Chapter 5). You must have had no more than one hypoglycemic reaction with loss of consciousness in the last five years and at least a year of stability after that. You must be evaluated by a specialist every three months after you get the license and measure your blood glucose multiple times a day. You must carry a glucose meter and meter supplies in flight, along with supplies for rapid treatment of hypoglycemia. Your blood glucose must be between 100 and 300 mg/dl (5.5 to 16.6 mmol/L) a half hour before takeoff, every hour of the flight, and a half hour before landing. However, you're not expected to measure your blood glucose in flight if doing so interferes with properly flying the plane. Phew! If Lindbergh were diabetic, he never would have made it to Paris.

In 1998, the U.S. Court of Appeals ruled that the ADA protects Americans with diabetes. The act applies to employers with 15 or more employees. What the ADA means is that you are qualified for a particular job if you can perform the essential functions of the job as determined by the employer, with or without reasonable accommodation. That means you can't be discriminated against in hiring, firing, promotion, training, pay, or any other aspect of employment because you have diabetes. Your boss cannot ask whether you have diabetes but can expect you to pass a physical examination to verify that you are well enough to do the job.

The Federal Rehabilitation Act of 1973 is an important law that protects you when you apply for a federal job or a job in a company that receives federal assistance. A person with diabetes is specifically protected under this law. The most important provision states:

> *No otherwise qualified handicapped individual in the United States shall, solely by reason of his handicap, be excluded from the participation in, be denied the benefits of, or be subjected to discrimination under any program or activity conducted by the Executive agency. . . .*

Federal agencies have to prove that you will not be able to perform safely if given the job. That is hard to do and puts the burden on them, not you. They must decide on a case-by-case basis. As I note earlier in the chapter, the FBI and the military are exempt from this law.

What can you do if you run into discrimination on the job due to your diabetes? You can contact the U.S. Equal Employment Opportunity Commission (EEOC). You can find the nearest EEOC office on the Web at www.eeoc.gov/offices.html or call 800-669-4000. You may have only 180 days from the alleged discriminatory act to file the charge.

Navigating the Health Insurance System

You can get insurance for your medical care several ways. This section describes the most common forms.

Private insurance

If you or your child has diabetes, you can count on several things being true when you interact with the medical insurance system in the United States. You will pay more out-of-pocket than families without diabetes even when you have coverage. And you may be denied coverage more often.

If you are an older adult with diabetes, you can expect to spend one and a half times as much for medical care as a person without diabetes, although Medicare pays for much of it. You want to be sure that you are not medically shortchanged in an effort to save money.

The good news is that you can get health insurance just as often as the person who does not have diabetes, although you may be turned down more often. And the type of insurance you will have is the same as the nondiabetic population: Blue Cross/Blue Shield, Health Maintenance Organizations (HMOs), CHAMPUS, and so on.

Currently, there are two major forms of payment for medical care — fee-for-service and capitated payment — with a lot of hybrids in between. The old *fee-for-service* method pays the medical provider — whether a physician, a lab, or a hospital — based on the number of services provided. More services and procedures mean more profit for the provider. So the incentive is to do more in order to make more money. (Not that providers would ever do more than is necessary for the money.)

The other main method of reimbursement is *capitation.* Here the provider gets a fixed amount of money for each patient. The risk is divided among many patients so that if one costs more, ideally another will cost less. This is the basis of the Health Maintenance Organization (HMO), which hires physicians to provide the care. HMOs look to enroll people who cost as little as possible for their medical care. The incentive is to do less in order to save money, which is then kept by the provider. (Not that providers would ever do less than is necessary for the money.)

Because they seem to end up costing less money overall, capitation plans are growing while fee-for-service plans are declining. The government is even encouraging HMOs to enroll Medicare recipients in order to reduce costs. At the same time, the government requires HMOs to enroll people who cost more, like most people with diabetes.

As a healthcare consumer, you want to look for a large group because such a group can spread out your extra expenses among many people who don't consume as much medical care. Before you sign up, ask several questions:

- ✔ What is your total annual cost, and how often is a payment required?

- ✔ Is there a *deductible,* meaning that you have to pay the first so many dollars before the insurance starts paying?

- ✔ Is there a *co-payment,* meaning that every time you use a provider, you have to pay some dollars?

- ✔ Does your plan pay for durable medical equipment like an insulin pump (see Chapter 10), which can be very expensive? (You want to ask this even if, when you sign up, you may not foresee a need for it.)

✔ Will your plan pay for your diabetes medication and diabetes supplies, and to what extent?

✔ Can your physician order any medications you need, or is he or she restricted to certain medications?

✔ How often will you need to travel to the pharmacy to pick up medications? (Some plans make you go back every 30 days.)

✔ Are you covered for specialists, particularly eye doctors and foot doctors?

✔ Are you limited to certain hospitals, certain physicians, and certain laboratories? (If so, this may be much more inconvenient for you, not to mention possibly requiring you to change from a physician with whom you are very comfortable.)

✔ Is home health care included in the plan, and to what extent?

 Each state has its own laws concerning the way medical insurance is offered in that state. Some states allow *medical underwriting,* where a company can refuse to insure a person with a particular medical condition. Other states forbid this. To learn the rules and regulations in your state, go to the site of the Georgetown University Health Policy Institute at www.healthinsurance info.net/. Here you can enter your state and find out the latest rules. You can also get a copy of its publication "A Consumer Guide For Getting and Keeping Health Insurance." Don't even think about health insurance without going here.

 After you sign up for a plan, you need to be vigilant to be sure you are getting what you paid for. You and your physician may need to make many phone calls to get what you need, but if you persist you can often come away with a "Yes." Even goods and services that are excluded in your original contract may be provided by the insurance company if you are persistent.

Insurance for low income patients

If your income falls below certain levels that are listed at the government Web site: www.cms.hhs.gov/home/medicaid.asp.

you may be eligible for health insurance for low income patients called Medicaid. Each state sets its own guidelines and administers the program for itself. You obtain a card that shows you are eligible and take it to your doctor, lab or hospital.

 Because the reimbursement under Medicaid is generally so low, many doctors will not accept patients whose only source of insurance is Medicaid. Inform the receptionist when you make the appointment that you have this insurance in order to avoid an unnecessary trip.

High-risk pools

About 60 percent of the US population gets its health insurance through their employer in a group health program. Another 27 percent gets its insurance through government programs like Medicare, Medicaid, military health care and native American care. The rest are self-employed or work for a small company that does not provide insurance. They can get insurance at a high premium, usually, but there are some who have had a chronic medical condition and can't find insurance at any price.

For those people about 34 states have formed pools of clients who can't get insurance anywhere else. The premium is usually higher than private insurance but at least they can get insurance.

To find out if you qualify and where the locations of the state high-risk pools are on the Internet, go to the Health Insurance Research Center at: `www.health insurance.org/riskpoolinfo.lasso`.

Changing or Losing a Job

One of the major reasons people with diabetes used to stay in jobs they did not care for was their fear of losing their health insurance. This does not have to stop you in today's job market. Several laws protect you from the loss of health insurance if you change or lose your job.

The *Consolidated Omnibus Budget Reconciliation Act* (COBRA) stipulates that your employer must keep you on your current health insurance for as long as 18 months after your job ends and longer if you are disabled. If your child is at the age when he or she is no longer covered under your policy, the child's coverage can continue for up to three years. You, rather than your employer, have to pay the premiums for this continued insurance.

If you are leaving work because of retirement at age 65, sign up for Medicare without fail. It is a generous program (which you supported while you were working) that recognizes the specific needs of people with diabetes. Since 1998, Medicare has expanded its coverage to include blood glucose monitors and test strips once your physician certifies the need. It also offers payment for specific types of outpatient diabetes education programs, as long as they are considered necessary by your physician. And recently it has begun to pay for nutrition counseling and eye examinations. The program is not entirely enlightened, however, because while it will pay for an insulin pump, it still does not cover insulin and syringes. To find out more about Medicare, call the Medicare Hotline at 800-633-227. The government provides a hotline for the hearing-impaired at877-486-2048.

Some employers have conversion policies that allow you to stay with your insurance company if you leave work, but with individual rather than group coverage. These policies can be pretty expensive.

Some states offer "Pooled Risk" health insurance for people who have lived in the state a certain number of months but can't get group or individual coverage. Check with your state insurance office.

Considering Long-Term Care Insurance

We are living longer and longer, especially those of us with diabetes, and we are going to need a way to pay for our care when we can no longer pay health insurance premiums. When you are 90, your 88-year-old wife will most likely not be in a position to pay for your insurance, nor will your 65-year-old daughter. Medicare does not cover most of your long-term care expenses. Medicaid does cover some long-term care, but not everything you may need. This is where long-term insurance may help, if you can afford it.

If you have plenty of money and want to protect it from the financial hit of a long-term illness, long-term insurance is for you. If you have little money, the years of premiums are going to wipe out your savings, and you may end up needing to drop the policy before you even use it.

One big problem is that many companies that sell long-term insurance will not cover a person with diabetes. If you can get this type of insurance coverage while you are still working, you may be able to get into a large group where your particular illness is not considered and the premiums may be relatively low. However, you'll obviously be paying those premiums for a longer time than if you start coverage when you are older.

Before you buy, you should check several important features of a long-term care insurance policy:

- ✔ What are the *benefit triggers,* the physical limitations that trigger coverage? To make this determination, generally insurance companies look at activities of daily living, such as the ability to bathe yourself, dress yourself, eat without help, go to the bathroom, and get out of bed. When you can't perform one or more of these, benefits begin.

- ✔ How much of the cost of care will the insurance pay, some or all?

- ✔ What levels of care does the policy provide? Your policy may offer coverage only for adult day care services or may cover anything up to and including living in a nursing facility.

✔ Is a waiver of premiums built in so that you don't have to pay premiums when you are disabled?

✔ Is the policy guaranteed renewable so you can renew no matter whether you use it, although the premiums will be higher?

Whatever you do, if you buy long-term care insurance, make sure you take good care of yourself so you live long enough to get some benefit from it.

Shopping for Life Insurance

As you might expect, the situation with life insurance and the person with diabetes is in a state of flux. Insurance companies like to calculate your chance of dying and charge you (or turn you down) based upon those calculations. Many companies are using calculations based on the life span of people with diabetes in 1980 or before. Using those statistics, diabetics clearly died earlier than their nondiabetic friends. Thus, the cost of life insurance is greater for people with diabetes than nondiabetics.

As new studies are done, they should indicate that the life spans of people with diabetes and nondiabetics are approaching equality. In some cases, people with diabetes, who take better care of themselves than people without a chronic illness, are living even longer. So the situation is improving, and insurance companies will catch up sooner or later. Can you imagine the surprise if insurance companies were ever to charge people with diabetes less than others because of their good habits?

Insurance companies look at levels of blood glucose and the hemoglobin A1c. Try to get yourself in excellent control before you apply. You could save a bundle or get your insurance much more easily.

With the Internet, you can quickly find and compare the cost of insurance at numerous companies based on your age; your habits (warning: if you smoke, you pay through the nose); and the presence of conditions such as diabetes, high blood pressure, and high cholesterol. Many companies will take a standard rate for a healthy person with no diseases and add 50 percent more if you have diabetes. Of course, your actual cost is dependent on your specific circumstances, including your age when you first buy the insurance.

Chapter 16

What's New in Diabetes Care

*I*n previous editions of *Diabetes For Dummies,* I have enthusiastically spoken about the great efforts of pharmaceutical companies to provide you with the best drugs to lower your glucose, reduce your blood pressure and lower your cholesterol. In this edition I have the sad responsibility to warn you about these same pharmaceutical companies.

As a consequence of my skepticism, I am not going to talk about new drugs in this chapter, only about old drugs that have potential new uses and new products that might make it easier for you to manage your disease. In addition, you will learn about the role of surgery in type 2 diabetes and major efforts to get cells that don't usually make insulin to turn into the insulin-producing beta cells. The Internet can help you to control your diabetes as well and I tell you about that below.

Protecting Yourself from the Dangers of New Drugs

In an effort to instantly gratify their stockholders and find the next "billion dollar drug," drug companies seem to have lost sight of their major goal, which is to find drugs that are both effective and safe for the treatment of diabetes. Although some drug companies continue to pursue this goal, many of them are guilty of:

✔ Withholding studies that they have paid for that show that their drug is not as effective as they claim. A study in the *New England Journal of Medicine* in January 2008 showed that the companies that make antidepressants allowed 94 percent of positive studies to be printed but only 14 percent of negative studies. Even the positive studies, if carefully evaluated, were not nearly as positive as the companies claimed. This behavior is not limited to companies that make antidepressants.

✔ Strongly advertising the one study that shows positive effects when many others show negative effects.

✔ Withholding studies that indicate their drug may have dangerous side effects.

✔ Promoting their drug for purposes that are not permitted by the FDA.

✔ Advertising their drug as though it is the best or only treatment when older and better treatments exist.

✔ Providing catered lunches and other goodies to doctors to convince them to use their drugs. There is a basic conflict of interest in the relationship of doctors and pharmaceutical companies.

✔ Paying large sums of money to private doctors to do "studies" of their drugs, studies that rarely find negative things about the drugs.

✔ Paying rebates to private doctors to use their drugs, whether or not it is the best choice for the patient.

These problems are not limited to doctors and the pharmaceutical industry. Any time "advisors" are also salespeople, they will advise the purchase of what they sell. But just because it takes place in every industry does not make it right. And in the medical industry it is often a matter of life or death.

What steps can you take to avoid the dangers I outline above? Here are a few suggestions:

✔ Do not ask your doctor to prescribe new drugs that are heavily promoted by advertising. Too few people have used them and too little time has passed to truly know the potential of these new drugs.

✔ Don't take samples from your doctor. Drug companies use samples to get you and your doctor "hooked" on their drug.

✔ Don't ask for a drug just because a key organization like the American Heart Association, the American Diabetes Association, the Endocrine Society or many others promotes the drug. These organizations have become big and fat from the money provided by those drug companies.

✔ The easiest and best policy is to wait several years before trying a new drug. The drugs that are currently available are more than adequate to control your blood glucose, your blood pressure and your cholesterol *if you take them as prescribed.*

Avoiding Diabetic Complications with DHEADHEA or dehydroepiandrosterone is a substance that is found normally in the human body as a byproduct of the production of certain hormones. A recent study in *Diabetes Care* in November 2007 suggests that DHEA may have an important role in prevention of complications of diabetes. Earlier in the book (see Chapter 5) I indicated that production of advanced glycation end products (AGE) may play a role in the complications of diabetes including eye disease, kidney disease and nerve disease (neuropathy).

The authors of this article found that in recently diagnosed patients with T2DM who were controlled with diet alone and did not have complications there was evidence of significant AGE production. Giving DHEA produced a 50 percent reduction in markers of AGE production.

DHEA levels were restored to the levels found in young adults and the development of complications was presumably reduced. This may be a promising new treatment for both prevention of complications and progression of those that have already developed.

Surgery and Not Conventional Therapy Cures T2DMIn Chapter 8 I discussed bariatric surgery as a last ditch treatment for the heavy patient with T2DM. Recent evidence suggests that this should be considered much earlier in the disease and in patients who are not nearly as heavy.

In a study in the *Journal of the American Medical Association* in January 2008 the authors compared the results of laparoscopic gastric banding with conventional weight loss therapy for the treatment of T2DM in recently diagnosed (less than 2 years) patients: 55 patients were divided into the two groups; 73 percent of the operated group but only 13 percent of the conventional group had a remission of T2DM with their treatment. The surgically treated patients lost 21 percent of their weight while the conventional patients lost only 5 percent. This is strong evidence for the early use of surgery to bring diabetes under control, even in patients who are not grossly obese.

Red Wine to Defy Aging

Red wine has been promoted as a way to avoid heart attacks. It was suggested that the French people have a lower rate of heart attacks than Americans because they drink red wine containing a chemical called resveratrol that is protective.

New evidence from two studies suggests that resveratrol can slow the aging process. In one from Harvard University, published in the *Journal of the American Medical Association,* middle-aged mice were fed a high-fat diet. Some were also given resveratrol while others were not. Those given resveratrol were less likely to die early.

Another study from a group in France, published in *Cell,* similarly showed that mice fed a high-fat diet and high doses of resveratrol were protected from the metabolic syndrome (see Chapter 5) and did not gain weight compared to mice not fed resveratrol.

Don't rush to your nearest wine shop, however. It has been calculated that a person would have to drink 750 bottles of wine a day to get the amount of resveratrol fed the animals in these studies. You better get an early start!

Resveratrol or something else in red wine probably protects your heart, but don't drink more than two glasses a day and a total of ten a week or your liver may be very unhappy.

Taking a Statin for All People With Diabetes

Some diabetes specialists suggest that all people with diabetes should be taking a cholesterol-lowering drug from the group of drugs known as statins. The drugs in this class include:

- ✔ Atorvastatin (brand name Lipitor)
- ✔ Lovastatin (brand name Mevacor)
- ✔ Pravastatin (brand name Pravachol)
- ✔ Simvastatin (brand name Zocor)

A study in the January 2008 issue of *The Lancet* would seem to put that question to rest. The authors looked at numerous studies of the effects of statin drugs on people with diabetes. 1,466 people with T1DM and 1,7220 people with T2DM were evaluated in these various studies. They were observed for a mean follow-up of 4.3 years. They found that:

- ✔ There were 3,247 major occlusions involving the arteries in these patients.
- ✔ For every millimole per liter reduction in LDL cholesterol there was a 9 percent reduction in deaths from any cause.
- ✔ For every millimole per liter reduction in LDL cholesterol there was a 21 percent reduction in major closures of arteries.
- ✔ There were reductions in heart attacks and deaths due to heart attacks, and strokes due to closure of the arteries to the brain.
- ✔ After five years fewer people with diabetes who had taken a statin had had a major closure of blood vessel.

The authors' conclusion was that all people with diabetes should be on a statin to protect against a blood vessel closure. I agree and have all my patients with diabetes take one of the statin drugs.

Correcting the Cause of Complications

When the Diabetes Control and Complications Trial (DCCT) was published in the *New England Journal of Medicine* in September 1993, the study showed that people with type 1 diabetes could be controlled "intensively" with multiple daily shots of insulin. The better control resulted in a very significant reduction in complications of diabetes like eye disease, kidney disease, and nerve disease (see Chapter 5).

Some of the intensively treated patients did not achieve the lowering of hemoglobin A1c to 7 percent, Yet the patients who were intensively treated and still had a hemoglobin A1c of 9 percent had fewer complications than the conventionally treated patients who had a hemoglobin A1c of 9 percent. The explanation was that the conventionally treated patients had much wider swings in their blood glucose levels from low to high. It was suggested that wider swings led to more complications than narrower swings in blood glucose. For 15 years this has been thought to be the case.

Recently I attended the 55th Postgraduate Course of the American Diabetes Association in San Francisco. At that course two doctors debated whether it was true that wide swings in blood glucose caused more complications than more narrow swings. After the debate, the original statistician for the DCCT spoke and said that in the near future a medical journal would be publishing the information that the original statistics were incorrect. In fact, there is no difference in the complication rate whether the blood glucose swings widely or more narrowly, if the mean blood glucose is the same in both cases.

If you find that your blood glucose tends to swing widely, as long as your mean blood glucose or hemoglobin A1c is 7 percent or less, you need not worry that you are developing complications.

Using the Internet to Control Your DiabetesThe Internet is an amazing, information-gathering tool where you can find just about any information you want, if you know how to look. It also provides a way to interact with experts from a distance. A number of companies are using this faculty to help people to lose weight (see Chapter 12). Now a company called Entra Health Systems at: `http://www.entrahealthsystems.com/index.html` is using the interactive nature of the Internet to help people with diabetes and their doctors to control their blood glucose. Evaluation of the program is taking place in the United Kingdom, where the basics of the program may be found at `http://myglucohealth.co.uk`.

The program starts with a glucose meter that can upload the blood glucose tests to its Internet site either via a cellphone connection or by connecting the meter to your computer and uploading the results from there. The blood glucose readings are managed by a data management system that allows you or your doctor to see the trends in your glucose. When you can see what time of day your glucose tends to be higher or lower, you can correct the abnormalities by adjusting your medication, diet, and/or exercise.

The program goes further. You can set high and low levels for the blood glucose as well as appropriate frequencies of testing. When the levels are too high or too low a certain number of times in a certain number of days, both of which your doctor can set, the program notifies you and your doctor to take corrective action. Additionally, when you are not testing enough to manage your diabetes correctly, the program notifies you and your doctor of that.

The site allows you to build an online medical record that can be examined by any doctor to whom you give permission. You can add information about your diet, exercise, hypoglycemic reactions, and so forth.

Once it is available in the United States, this program may allow you and your doctor to make much better use of all the tests that you do in a much more timely fashion. It also permits secure communication between you and your physician.

Getting Cells to Make Insulin

Dr. Lijun Yang, an associate professor at the University of Florida College of Medicine, has come up with a unique and promising way to produce insulin-secreting cells. She has been able to synthesize a protein called recombinant Pdx1. This protein has the ability to regenerate beta cells in the pancreas and turn liver cells into insulin-producing beta cells. So far the protein has worked successfully in mice. Mice with T1DM given this protein began to produce insulin for the first time. The mice no longer have diabetes after receiving this protein. It has caused no adverse effects in the mice.

Dr. Yang has been able to synthesize the human form of this protein. She is about to undertake a study of humans with T1DM to see if she can regenerate sufficient cells in them to allow them to be free of insulin injections. If it works and the body does not reject these insulin-producing cells as it did the beta cells, this could be a cure for T1DM.

Understanding the Importance of the ACCORD Study

The ACCORD study is a study of 10,250 people who have had T2DM and are at high risk to have a heart attack. The average hemoglobin A1c was 8.2 percent, which is higher than the average patient with T2DM. The patients were randomized into two treatment arms, a standard treatment arm that had a goal of an A1c target between 7 and 7.9 percent and an intensive treatment arm that had a goal of an A1c target less than 6 percent.

All patients already had known heart disease and at least two other risk factors besides diabetes including:

- ✔ High blood pressure
- ✔ High cholesterol
- ✔ Obesity
- ✔ Smoking

When patients with these characteristics are allowed to maintain their usual A1c of 8.2 percent, their death rate is 50 per 1000 patients per year.

The study was due to be completed in 2010, but in early February 2008, the researchers announced that they were closing the part of the study that attempted to get the A1c down to 6 percent because there was a higher death rate among the intensively treated patients than the other group. The results up to that point were:

- ✔ The intensive group had an average A1c of 6.4 percent.
- ✔ The standard group had an average A1c of 7.5 percent.
- ✔ The standard group had a death rate of 11 per 1,000 patients per year.
- ✔ The intensive group had a death rate of 14 per 1,000 patients per year.

Therefore, although the death rate for both groups was far below the level for these people with an A1c of 8.2 percent initially (11 or 14 versus 50 per 1,000), the intensively treated group that reached their goal had a slightly greater death rate than the standard group that reached their goal.

The moral of this story is *not that intensive treatment is dangerous in T2DM*, but that *intensive treatment in this population of high risk patients with heart disease already and more risk factors is dangerous.*

Note that the death rate for both groups is much lower than that of the poorly treated patients. These patients are so sick that the difficulties associated with trying to keep their blood glucose at a level of 100 mg/dl all the time may be too great.

The more you control your blood glucose early in diabetes, the less chance that you will get to the point of the patients in this study.

Clarifying the A1cThe hemoglobin A1c is a key test in the evaluation of the person with diabetes. It is based on the laboratory that did the A1c for the Diabetes Control and Complications Trials. All labs in the world are supposed to calibrate their testing machines to the results from that lab.

Unfortunately, that lab measured hemoglobins A1a, A1b, and A1c. And the units of measurement are a percent rather than an absolute number like the average blood glucose. It is unfortunate because it is much easier to think in terms of an absolute number than a percentage and people get an absolute number from their glucose meter, not a percentage.

Now at the beginning of 2008 the American Diabetes Association and other organizations have joined to use a new assay for the hemoglobin A1c that only measures the A1c subfraction of the hemoglobin As. The result will, therefore, be lower, but is a better measure of the A1c.

Beginning soon, the hemoglobin A1c will be expressed in three ways, the old hemoglobin A1c, the new, true hemoglobin A1c, and the average blood glucose to which it corresponds. You will get a much clearer picture of how you are doing over time.

But don't get upset if the average blood sugar that you get from your meter is very different from the measured average blood glucose. Remember that your few blood glucose levels represent a few dots on a large painting. With just that much information, you can hardly expect to know what the whole picture looks like.

Chapter 17

What Doesn't Work When You Treat Diabetes

. . . .

In This Chapter

▶ Recognizing the signs that a treatment won't work

▶ Identifying drugs, diets, and other treatments that don't work

. . . .

*E*veryone wants a quick and easy solution to their problems. For every problem, five people offer a quick and easy answer. Just send in the money. These cheats have got what it takes to take what you've got.

Being fooled by these claims may be a lot more serious for you than for the person who walked up to the man dressed as a polar bear who was promoting soft drinks in a shopping center. The first man said: "Don't you feel foolish, dressed like a bear?" The "bear" replied: "Me, foolish? You're the one talking to a bear."

This chapter tells you as much as I know about diabetes tests and treatments that don't work. Don't expect to find every "wonder cure" for diabetes that you've read or heard about. As soon as this book is published, new, more seductive claims will be made. I hope that you will remain skeptical, use the information in this chapter to test claims out, and check with your doctor before you try something that may do more harm than good.

Developing a Critical Eye

Many clues can alert you that a treatment may not work. Here are a few:

✔ **If a treatment is endorsed by a Hollywood star or a basketball player or other sports figure, be highly skeptical.** Always consider the source and make sure that it's reputable. In this case, the fame of the star is being used to convince you, not any special knowledge that he or she possesses.

✔ **If the treatment has been around for a long time but is not generally used, don't trust it.** If a treatment has been around for a while and really works, it will have been tried in an experimental study where some people take it and some don't. Doctors and medical texts recommend drugs that pass that test.

✔ **If it sounds too good to be true, it usually is.** An example would be the claims about chromium improving blood glucose levels. The study that "proved" it was done on chromium-deficient people, a situation that does not exist in the United States.

✔ **Anecdotes are not proof of the value of a treatment or test.** The favorable experiences of one or a few people are not a substitute for a scientific study. Perhaps those people did respond to the drug, but it may have been for entirely different reasons.

A lot of information about diabetes is available on the Web. In Appendix C, I provide the best resources currently available for diabetes from this amazing source. The same rules apply when you consider the validity of claims made on the Web, with a few extra rules thrown in:

✔ **Don't rely on search engines for validity.** Search engines do not check claims for validity.

✔ **Go to the site of the claim and see whether most of the information there makes sense.** If you find a lot of silly information, that should be a red flag. If you still feel the treatment might work, ask the Webmaster for references. If none are forthcoming, forget about the idea.

✔ **Go to sites that you know are reliable to see whether you can find the same recommendations.** The treatments discussed on sites like the American Diabetes Association (ADA) and The Diabetes Monitor (see Appendix C) can be relied upon. When a treatment's value is uncertain, these sites can usually tell you.

✔ **Go to medical conferences put on by reputable experts.** You will be given Web addresses that are reliable. Another reliable source for such addresses is a book by Warner V. Slack, *Cybermedicine: How Computing Empowers Doctors and Patients for Better Health Care.* Although the last edition was 2001, it remains an excellent resource for online medical information.

Identifying Drugs That Don't Work

In the past decade, so many drugs have been touted as the cure for diabetes that you would think everyone would be cured by now. The fact is, as I say again and again, you *do* have the tools right now to control diabetes, but the

How the ADA evaluates new drugs

The American Diabetes Association evaluates new therapies and places them in one of four categories:

✔ Clearly effective

✔ Somewhat/sometimes effective or effective for certain categories of patients

✔ Unknown/unproven but possibly promising

✔ Clearly ineffective

If you're about to try a new therapy that has not been recommended by your doctor and is not discussed in this book, you may want to contact the ADA and find out its position on the treatment. Of course, if you're involved in a clinical trial that is trying to determine the effectiveness of a therapy, no one will know whether it works or not.

solution is not as simple as taking a pill. If it were, this book would not be necessary. In this section, I tell you about some drugs that have received unwarranted hype because they "worked" in a few people.

If you participate in a clinical research study of a new drug, a system is in place to protect you. Make sure that the study has been approved by a review board in an institution that has been approved to do the research. Such institutions are usually accredited by an established organization like the Association for the Accreditation of Human Research.

See the sidebar "How the ADA evaluates new drugs" for information on how the American Diabetes Association evaluates new treatments.

Chromium

You can find articles singing the praises of chromium for controlling the symptoms of diabetes in all kinds of magazines and newspapers, and on the Internet. Should you take supplements of chromium?

The strongest case for chromium comes from a study of people with type 2 diabetes in China. They were given high doses of chromium and were found to improve their hemoglobin A1c, blood glucose, and cholesterol while reducing the amount of insulin they had to take. However, these people were chromium deficient in the first place. People in the United States and other countries where the diet is sufficient in chromium do not have this deficiency and do not show improvement in glucose tolerance when they take chromium. In addition, chromium is present in such small amounts normally that it is hard to measure even in people without chromium deficiency.

The exact amount of chromium you need in your diet is uncertain but is estimated to be 15 to 50 micrograms daily. People who take much more than that tend to accumulate it in their livers, where it can be toxic. Some studies suggest that chromium can cause cancer in high doses.

For now, the evidence does not support the use of chromium in diabetes except for people who are known to be chromium deficient.

Aspirin

People who take the sulfonylurea drugs (see Chapter 10) sometimes have a greater drop in blood glucose when they take aspirin. This is because aspirin competes with the other drug for binding sites on the proteins that carry sulfonylureas in the blood. When they're bound to protein, the sulfonylureas are not active; when they're free, they are. Aspirin knocks the sulfonylureas off so that they're free. As a result, aspirin has been recommended as a drug to lower blood glucose.

By itself, aspirin has little effect on blood glucose. Its effect with sulfonylureas is so inconsistent that it can't be reliably depended upon to lower the blood glucose.

Cinnamon

A number of articles in the medical literature since 2001 have suggested that cinnamon will lower the blood glucose in type 2 diabetes and improve fat levels as well. To verify these claims a study called a meta-analysis was done and published in *Diabetes Care* in January 2008. In a meta-analysis all studies that are randomized so that the subjects don't know if they are getting the drug or a placebo are analyzed to see if they confirm the hypothesis. In this case, none of five studies showed that cinnamon had a positive affect either on the blood glucose or blood fats. You may have noticed the same thing if you were taking a daily dose of a teaspoon of cinnamon. You can cease and desist!

Pancreas formula

Pancreas formula is sold on the Internet as a mixture of herbs, vitamins, and minerals that help diabetes. No clinical or experimental evidence shows that pancreas formula does anything of value in the human body. The claims that are made for this "treatment" are not supported by factual evidence.

The facts about aspartame

Many news sources report that aspartame (see Chapter 8) causes cancer. Because so many people eat and drink products that contain aspartame, I want to clarify.

Aspartame is an acceptable artificial sweetener with no known dangers to human beings. No evidence shows that aspartame causes cancer when used in normal amounts. The Food and Drug Administration has an acceptable daily intake for food additives, including a 100-fold safety factor. It is inconceivable that anyone would use more aspartame than that.

Fat Burner

You may hear and read a lot of advertising for the Fat Burner product in reputable newspapers and on reputable radio stations. Advertising claims that you can "burn fat without diet or exercise," and they will even throw in, ABSOLUTELY FREE, a bottle of Spirulina to enhance your Fat Burner weight control program. If you believe this is possible, I have a bridge I would like to sell you, *cheap*. In order to burn fat, you must exercise and stop taking in large amounts of carbohydrates or other sources of calories.

Ki-Sweet

The literature for Ki-Sweet offers another lesson in being skeptical. The creators of this "miracle" sweetener claim that it has a "special designation from the American Diabetes Association." The ADA denies the claim, but how many people will buy something when they see ADA approval and not bother to see whether it's true? No evidence exists that Ki-Sweet, made by squeezing the juice of kiwi, has any advantages over other sweeteners (which I discuss in Chapter 8).

Gymnema silvestre

Gymnema silvestre is a plant found in India and Africa that is promoted as a glucose-lowering agent as part of an alternative medical treatment called *Ayurvedic medicine*. Gymnema silvestre has never been tested in a controlled study in humans. One statement in its advertising is, "For most people, blood sugar lowers to normal levels." No evidence exists that this is the case.

Avoiding Illegal Drugs

Drugs like cocaine, heroin, speed, and marijuana are not just illegal; they are especially harmful for the person with diabetes for several reasons:

- ✔ Some make you excessively hungry, and you take in too many calories.

- ✔ All cause you to lose your awareness of hypoglycemia so you don't treat it.

- ✔ All cause a loss of judgment that results in the failure to take medications, eat properly, and exercise.

- ✔ Some cause a reduced insulin response to food so you become hyperglycemic.

- ✔ Some cause you to lose your appetite so you become hypoglycemic and malnourished with vitamin deficiencies.

Not a lot of valid information is available about each illegal drug's impact on diabetes, because we cannot do studies where these drugs are given to one group of diabetics while a control group takes a placebo. But we do know the following:

- ✔ Marijuana (grass, weed, bud, cannabis) causes increased appetite, which results in taking in too many calories.

- ✔ Amphetamine (speed, Dex, crank) and ecstasy (derived from amphetamine and also called MDMA, E, X, adam, bean, and roll) increase the body's metabolic rate, resulting in hypoglycemia because the user often does not eat properly and is unaware of the onset of low blood glucose.

- ✔ Cocaine (coke, snow, nose candy, dust, toot) and freebase cocaine (crack, rock) lead to food deprivation, increased metabolism and caloric needs, and vitamin deficiency.

- ✔ Heroin (dope, junk, smack) is similar to cocaine but has additional risks associated with injections, such as infection.

Do you need any more reason to get high on exercise rather than drugs?

Knowing the Dangers of Some Legal Drugs

Just because a drug is legal does not mean it has no undesirable side effects. Several classes of drugs need to be used with caution.

What about hypnosis?

As respected a source as the National Institutes of Health has listed hypnosis as a treatment for "stabilization of blood sugar in diabetes." Although it has a disclaimer that says that publishing this statement does not imply endorsement of the treatment, the fact that the statement comes from the NIH gives this treatment credibility. The only trouble is that no experimental evidence exists that proves the usefulness of hypnosis. So you have to be wary, even when the advice comes from the most respected of sources.

Antipsychotics

In an issue of *Diabetes Care* (February 2004), four major medical associations warned that second-generation antipsychotic drugs, used to treat a variety of severe mental illnesses, can cause rapid weight gain, most of which is fat, leading to prediabetes, diabetes, insulin resistance, and abnormal blood fats.

The drugs differ in their risks, but clozapine (Clozaril made by Novartis) and olanzapine (Zyprexa made by Eli Lilly) appear to be the worst offenders. Other drugs named include risperadone (Risperdol made by Johnson & Johnson), quetiapine (Seroquel made by AstraZeneca), ziprasidone (Geodon made by Pfizer), and aripiprazole (Abilify made by Bristol-Myers Squibb).

If you are taking one of these drugs, ask your doctor to screen and monitor you for evidence of weight gain and insulin resistance. The benefits of taking the drug may outweigh the risks. In the article, the panel suggests that baseline screening consisting of a medical history and physical examination along with fasting glucose and blood fats be done before using the drug.

If you are overweight or obese, you should receive nutritional and physical activity counseling if you take one of these drugs. If you are at risk of developing diabetes, your doctor should use the drug that is least associated with this problem.

AIDS medications

Certain drugs that control AIDS, called *protease inhibitors,* block the body's ability to store glucose so that people who use them may develop diabetes. More than 80 percent of the people who use them develop excess stomach fat, and half develop glucose intolerance. More than 10 percent develop diabetes. Table 17-1 shows the specific drugs with their brand names and manufacturers.

Table 17-1	Protease Inhibitors That Affect Glucose Metabolism	
Generic Name	*Brand Name*	*Manufacturer*
Saquinavir (hard gel)	Invirase	Hoffman–La Roche
Saquinavir (soft gel)	Fortovase	Hoffman–La Roche
Ritonavir	Norvir	Abbott Laboratories
Indinavir	Crixivan	Merck & Co
Nelfinavir	Viracept	Pfizer
Amprenavir	Agenerase	GlaxoSmithKline
Lopinavir and ritonavir	Keletra	Abbott Laboratories
Atazanavir	Reyataz	Bristol-Myers Squibb
Fosamprenavir	Levixa	GlaxoSmithKline

You should be screened before starting these drugs, and your doctor should monitor you carefully for weight gain and glucose intolerance. If diabetes does develop, the protease inhibitors are continued and the diabetes is treated. So far, none of the protease inhibitors stands out as more likely to cause diabetes.

Recognizing Diets That Don't Work

For the overweight person with type 2 diabetes, any diet that causes some weight loss helps for a time. But you have to ask yourself these questions:

✔ Am I prepared to stay on this diet indefinitely?

✔ Is this diet healthy for me in the long run?

✔ Does it combine all the features I need — namely weight loss, reduction of blood glucose, and reduction of blood fat levels — with palatability and reasonable cost?

If you can say yes to all these questions, the diet will probably work for you.

So how do you know which diets are healthy and effective, and which aren't? First, take a close look at Chapter 8, where I discuss diet in much more detail. Next, develop a discerning eye for defects in the latest diet fads.

When you walk into a reasonably large bookstore, you may be overwhelmed by the number of diet books. But the more books that are written about this subject, the less we seem to know for certain. Why would authors bother to write dozens of new books on dieting each year if the solution rested in some older book? You can bet that word of mouth would have made that book the all-time bestseller in any category.

The diet books in print these days are way too numerous to list here, but they can be grouped into a few categories:

- ✔ **Diets that promote a lot of protein with little carbohydrate:** The trouble with these diets is that they're not a healthy and balanced approach. Unless you use tofu as your source of protein, you will be getting a lot of fat in your diet, much of it saturated fat. That is not good for you. The diet is lacking in vitamins that a supplemental vitamin pill may or may not provide. Few people stay on such a diet for long. How many people can eat chicken for breakfast, lunch, and supper? The diet is also lacking in potassium, an essential mineral.

  People who do follow this kind of diet for a long time also find that they have problems with hair loss, cracking nails, and dry skin. Their breath and their urine smell of acetone because of all the fat breakdown. They become very dry and need to drink large quantities of beverages.

  I see a place for this diet as a starter. Some people with type 2 diabetes who have high blood glucose levels show rapid improvement when started on a diet like this. As the glucose comes under control, the diet can be changed to a more balanced one.

- ✔ **Diets that promote little or no fat:** The people who can follow a diet that is less than 20 percent fat deserve a new designation — *fatnatics* (fat fanatics). This kind of diet is extremely difficult to prepare and perhaps even more difficult to eat unless you're a squirrel. In order to make up the calories, people on this diet eat large amounts of carbohydrates. Chapter 8 makes it clear why this is not a good idea for people with diabetes.

  Like the protein diet, this diet may be lacking in essential vitamins and minerals, especially the fat-soluble vitamins. Rarely do people stay on such a diet after they leave the confines of a spa or other sanctuary where the diet is promoted. However, this approach may also be a good way to start a dietary program for a person with type 2 diabetes, as long as the total calories are not greater than the daily needs of that individual.

- ✔ **Very low calorie diets:** These diets require taking in food and drinks that contain less than 800 kilocalories daily (and generally do not taste very good). They are lacking in many essential nutrients and must be supplemented by vitamins and minerals. This approach cannot form the basis of a permanent diet because the dieter would eventually become emaciated. Most dieters who start this kind of program do not last on it and regain every ounce they have lost and then some. (There are always exceptions, of course.)

I do not like this kind of diet even as a starter diet because it is so unlike our usual eating habits that people rapidly find it to be intolerable. Eating is a basic part of our existence, and it's a source of great pleasure for human beings and other animals. A diet that takes away this fundamental activity cannot be tolerated for very long.

The transition from a very low calorie diet to a balanced diet is very difficult and rarely succeeds.

Part V
The Part of Tens

The 5th Wave   By Rich Tennant

"I'll have two lettuce filled, three carrot glazed, five celery frosted,..."

In this part . . .

The part of tens puts it all together and gives the most valuable techniques for thriving with diabetes. With just a little background from the other parts, you can use this section to really fine-tune your diabetes care. You find the ten commandments of excellent care, along with ten major myths about diabetes that you can discard. Finally, you find out how to utilize the skills and knowledge of the people around you, both the diabetes experts and your friends and family.

Chapter 18

Ten Ways to Prevent or Reverse the Effects of Diabetes

. . . .

In This Chapter

▶ Understanding the importance of monitoring, dieting, testing, and exercising

▶ Solidifying prevention with medication, the right attitude, and planning

. . . .

*W*hen I originally wrote this chapter, there were 20 things you had to do in order to prevent or reverse the effects of diabetes. I decided that was too much to ask of you, so I reduced it to ten. Surely you can do everything in this chapter when you consider that it is only half as difficult!

Can you pick and choose what you will do? No. Everything here is essential to living a long and high quality life with diabetes. You wouldn't want to save your sight and lose your kidneys. So read this chapter very carefully and practice every recommendation. And if you think I should have left any of the other ten behaviors in, let me know.

Major Monitoring

You have this incredibly compact and accurate glucose meter. Now you want to use it to find out how your blood glucose is doing at any time of day or night under any circumstances. You don't feel well. Is it low blood glucose or the beginning of a cold? Test! You just ate a large portion of pasta. Did it raise your blood glucose too much? Test!You can monitor your glucose in so many ways, almost without pain, that you have no excuse for not doing so. And you don't have to do it with a finger stick every time. Most meters allow you to do it in other parts of your body, your arm, leg or abdomen for example, especially when the blood glucose would not be expected to change rapidly as it would during or after exercise or after a meal. Those times you should only use your finger.

People with type 1 diabetes need to test at least before meals and at bedtime because their blood glucose level determines their dose of insulin. People who have stable type 2 diabetes may test once a day at different times or twice a day. If you're sick or about to start a long drive, you may want to test more often because you don't want to become hypoglycemic — or hyperglycemic for that matter. The beauty of the meter is that you can check your blood glucose in less than ten seconds any time you feel it's necessary.

Devout Dieting

If you are what you eat, then you have the choice of being controlled or uncontrolled depending upon what you put into your mouth. If you gain weight, you gain insulin resistance, but a small amount of weight loss can reverse the situation. The main point you should understand about a "diabetic diet" is that it's a healthy diet for anyone, whether they have diabetes or not. You should not feel like a social outcast because you're eating the right foods. You don't need special supplements; the diet is balanced and contains all the vitamins and minerals you require (although you want to be sure you're getting enough calcium).

You can follow a diabetic diet wherever you are, not just at home. Every menu has something on it that's appropriate for you. If you're invited to someone's home, let them know you have diabetes and that the amount of carbohydrate and fat that you can eat is limited. If that fails, limit the amount that you eat. (See Chapter 8 for more on your diet.)

A person with T2DM who follows a careful diet can reduce his hemoglobin A1c by 1 percent or more. This translates into a reduction in the occurrence of complications like eye disease, kidney disease and nerve disease of more than 25 percent. Is that worth your effort?

Tenacious Testing

The people who make smoke detectors recommend that you change the battery without fail each time you have a birthday. You should use the same simple device to remember your "complication detectors." Make sure that your doctor checks your urine for tiny amounts of protein and your feet for loss of sensation every year around the time of your birthday. It takes five to ten years to develop complications of diabetes. When you know the problem is present, you can do a lot to slow it down or even reverse it. Never has it been truer that "an ounce of prevention is worth a pound of cure." (For more on complications that may develop, see Chapters 4 and 5.)

I make it very easy for you to get the tests you need at the time you need them. The cheat sheet at the front of this book gives you the current testing recommendations. Make a copy for your doctor if he or she does not already have such a list. Demand that you get the tests when they are due. A doctor with a busy medical practice may forget whether you have had the tests you need, but you don't have an excuse for forgetting.

Enthusiastic Exercising

When you take insulin (as opposed to pills), controlling your diabetes is a little harder because you have to coordinate your food intake and the activity of the insulin. But I have patients who have had diabetes for decades and have little trouble balancing their food and insulin. They are the enthusiastic exercisers. They use exercise to burn up glucose in place of insulin. The result is a much more narrow range of blood glucose levels than is true of the insulin takers who do not exercise. They also have more leeway in their diet because the exercise makes up for slight excesses.

I am not talking about an hour of running each day or 50 miles on the bike. Moderate exercise like brisk walking can accomplish the same thing. The key is to exercise faithfully. (For more on exercise, see Chapter 9.) Thirty minutes of moderate exercise every day will not just improve your diabetes. It will reduce the possibility of a stroke, a heart attack, many cancers, and just keep you feeling generally good. Exercise can reduce your hemoglobin A1c by 1 percent or more just like diet.

Lifelong Learning

When I see a patient new to me who has had diabetes for some time, I am amazed at the lack of knowledge of many fundamental areas of their disease. You would think that they would want to know anything that might help them to live more comfortably and avoid complications.

So much is going on in the field of diabetes that I have trouble keeping up with it, and it's my specialty. How can you expect to know when doctors come up with the major advances that will cure your diabetes? The answer is lifelong learning. After you get past the shock of the diagnosis, you are ready to learn. This book contains a lot of basic stuff that you need to know. You can even take a good course in diabetes. Then you need to keep learning. Go to meetings of the local diabetes association. Become a member of the American Diabetes Association and get its terrific magazine called *Diabetes Forecast,* which usually contains the state of the art. Go to the Web sites that I discuss in Appendix C.

I assume you want to learn or you would not have bought this book. (You did buy it, didn't you? It should sit on your shelf right next to your dictionary and your encyclopedia.)

Remember that a lot of misinformation is available on the Web, so you must be careful to check out a recommendation before you start to follow it (see Chapter 17). Even information on reliable sites may not be right for your particular problem.

Above all, never stop learning! The next thing you learn may be the one that will cure you.

Meticulous Medicating

Compliance, which means treating your disease in accordance with your doctor's instructions, is a term that has special relevance for the patient with a chronic disease like diabetes who must take medications day in and day out. Sure, it's a pain (even if you could take insulin by mouth and not by injection). But the basic assumption is that you're taking your medication. Your doctor bases all his or her decisions on that assumption. Some very serious mistakes can be made if that assumption is false.

Check with your pharmacist to make sure that your pills don't interfere with one another. Some pills are taken with food; others are taken with no food for a period before and after that medication. Taking them correctly is just as important as taking them at all.

Every time a study is done on why patients' health conditions do not improve, compliance is high up or leads the list of reasons. Do you make a conscious decision to skip your pills, or do you forget? Whatever the reason, the best thing to do is to set up a system so that you're forced to remember. Keeping your pills in a dated container quickly shows you if you have taken them or not. You might even divide the pills by time of day.

Appropriate Attitude

Your approach to your disease can go a long way toward determining whether you will live in diabetes heaven or diabetes hell. If you have a positive attitude, treating diabetes as a challenge and an opportunity, not only is it easier for you to manage your disease, but your body actually produces chemicals that make it happen. A negative attitude, on the other hand, results in the kind of pessimism that leads to failure to diet, failure to exercise, and failure to take your medications. Plus, your body makes chemicals that are bad for you when you are depressed.

Diabetes is a challenge because you have to think about doing certain things that others never have to worry about. It brings out the quality of organization, which can then be transferred to other parts of your life. When you're organized, you accomplish much more in less time.

Diabetes is an opportunity because it forces you to make healthy choices for your diet as well as your exercise. You may end up a lot healthier than your neighbor without diabetes. As you make more and more healthy choices, you feel and test less and less like a person with diabetes.

Preventive Planning

Life is full of surprises. Like the sign on a display of "I Love You Only" Valentine cards: Available in Multipacks. You never know when you will get more than you bargained for. That is why having a plan to deal with the unexpected is so important. Say you're invited to someone's home, and they serve something that you know will raise your blood glucose significantly. What do you do? Or you go out to eat and are given a menu of incredible choices, many of which are just not for you. How do you handle that? You run into great stress at work or at home. Do you allow it to throw off your diet, your exercise, and your drug taking?

Does your mother make the wrong things when you go over to her house for a meal? Do you eat out a lot at fast food places and make poor choices. A little advance planning can overcome any eating challenge. Discuss good foods with your mother. Check out the calorie breakdown of the foods you eat at fast food places, usually available on the Internet. Go to the Web site of the particular restaurant and you will be directed to pages that show the calorie breakdown for all their foods. Make a diet for yourself and follow it.

The key to these situations is the realization that it's not possible for everything to go right all the time. In the case of the friend who cooked the wrong thing for you, you can at least eat a small portion to limit the damage. At the restaurant, you should come prepared with the food choices you know will keep you on your diet. It may be better not to look at the menu and simply discuss with your waiter what is available from your list of correct foods .

Fastidious Foot Care

A recent headline read: "Hospital sued by seven foot doctors." I would certainly not like to treat any doctor with seven feet or even a doctor who is seven feet tall. Whether you have two feet or seven feet, you must take good care of them. The problem occurs when you can't feel with your feet because of neuropathy (see Chapter 5). You can easily know when this problem exists just by checking with a 10-gram filament. If your feet cannot feel the filament, they will not feel burning hot water, a stone, a nail in your shoe, or an infected ulcer of your foot.

When you lose sensation in your feet, your eyes must replace the pain fibers that would otherwise tell you there is a problem. You need to carefully examine your feet every day, keep your toenails trimmed, and wear comfortable shoes. Your doctor should inspect your feet at every visit.

Diabetes is the primary source of foot amputations, but this drastic situation is entirely preventable if you pay attention to your feet. Test bath water by hand, shake your shoes out before you put them on, wear new shoes only a short while before checking for pressure spots, get a 10-gram filament and see whether you can feel it. If you smoke, you are especially at a high risk for an amputation of your toes or foot. The future of your feet is in your hands.

The other aspect of fastidious foot care is making sure the circulation in the blood vessels of your feet remains open. This is done by your doctor performing an ankle-brachial index (see Chapter 5). This test should be done once a year and quickly tells you and your doctor if you're experiencing a problem with your circulation.

Essential Eye Care

You're reading this book, which means you are seeing this book. So far, there are no plans to put out a Braille edition, so you had better take care of your eyes or you will miss out on the wonderful gems of information that brighten every page.

Caring for your eyes starts with a careful examination by an ophthalmologist or optometrist. You need to have an exam at least once a year (or more often if necessary). If you have controlled your diabetes meticulously, the doctor will find two normal eyes. If not, signs of diabetic eye disease may show up (see Chapter 5). At that point, you need to control your diabetes, which means controlling your blood glucose. You also want to control your blood pressure because high blood pressure contributes to worsening eye disease, as does high cholesterol.

Although the final word is not in on the effects of excessive alcohol on eye disease in diabetes, is it worth risking your sight for another glass of wine? Smoking has definitely been shown to raise the blood glucose in diabetes. Even at a late stage, you can stop the progression of the eye disease or reverse some of the damage if you stop smoking now.

Chapter 19

Ten Myths about Diabetes That You Can Forget

. . . .

In This Chapter

▶ Separating diabetes fact from fiction

▶ Being wise about your medical care

. . . .

Myths are a lot of fun. They're never completely true, but you can usually find a tiny bit of truth in a myth. The trouble is that some myths can hurt you if you allow them to determine your medical care. This chapter is about those kinds of myths — the ones that lead you to fail to take your medication or stay on your diet, or even lead you to take things that may not be good for you.

Perfect Treatment Yields Perfect Glucoses

Doctors are probably as responsible as their patients are for the myth that perfect treatment results in perfect glucose levels. For decades, doctors measured the urine glucose and told their patients that if they would just stay on their diet, take their medication, and get their exercise, the urine would be negative for glucose. Doctors failed to account for the many variables that could result in a positive test for glucose in the urine, plus the fact that even if the urine was negative, the patient could still be suffering diabetic damage. (The urine becomes negative at a blood glucose of 180 mg/dl [10 mmol/L] in most people, a level that still causes damage.)

The same thing is true for the blood glucose. Although you can achieve normal blood glucose levels most of the time if you treat your diabetes properly, you can still have times when, for no apparent reason, the glucose is not normal. So many factors determine the blood glucose level at any given time that this should hardly be a surprise. These factors include

- ✔ Your diet
- ✔ Your exercise
- ✔ Your medication
- ✔ Your mental state
- ✔ Other illnesses
- ✔ The day of your menstrual cycle

You Can Have Borderline Diabetes for Years

Borderline diabetes does not exist! Borderline diabetes does not exist any more than borderline pregnancy or borderline stealing. Either you have diabetes or you don't. You have it if your fasting blood glucose is greater than or equal to 126 mg/dl on more than one occasion or your glucose after eating is greater than or equal to 200 on more than one occasion.

Forget about this "borderline" stuff. Go ahead and lose some pounds and start an exercise program or increase it if you already do something, Not only will you prevent diabetes if you don't have it already or decrease the damage it does if you do, but your health in general will take a giant step in a positive direction.

Unorthodox Methods Can Cure Diabetes

In Chapter 17, I talk about some treatments that don't work. Those treatments are just the tip of the iceberg. Many treatments do not help you and may hurt you. Whenever a problem affects a huge number of people, others are eager to exploit this potential gold mine.

How can you know if what you read in your favorite magazine or see on the Internet is actually useful? Check it out with your physician, your diabetes educator, or other members of your team (see Chapter 11). They will know or can find out for you about any appropriate treatment. To date, diabetes has no simple cures. A book or organization that promises an easy cure is not doing you any favor.

You Can Tell the Level of Your Blood Glucose by How You Feel

Many of my patients have claimed that they can tell their blood glucose level by how they feel, and I have challenged them to prove it. Guess who wins every time with the exception of significant hypoglycemia? Sure, if your blood glucose is below 50 mg/dl and you are sweaty and have palpitations and a headache, you know that you are low — but even then, you don't know how low. Therefore, you don't know how much treatment to give yourself to bring it back up, but not too high.

Those who don't test and rely on the way they feel will suffer one or several of the short term and long term complications described in Chapters 4, 5 and 6.

Patients with high blood glucose rarely can tell within 50 mg/dl what their level is. Less than half of patients who guess come close to the correct answer.

Measure your glucose a couple of times daily if you have type 2 diabetes and before meals and at bedtime if you have type 1 diabetes. The more information you gather, the better will be your glucose control and the more likely you will be to minimize or avoid complications.

Hypoglycemia Kills Brain Cells

Hypoglycemia (see Chapter 4) often comes on fast and leaves you with a headache or a general feeling of weakness and sometimes confusion. Because of this, people have believed that low blood glucose, especially if it occurs repeatedly, may destroy mental functioning. People who have had repeated episodes of hypoglycemia have shown no loss of mental functioning. Children may have different results because their brains are still developing.

Fortunately, your body is supplied with hormones to reverse hypoglycemia. Some things you can do to prevent it include checking your blood glucose prior to heavy exercise and keeping a supply of rapidly absorbable glucose nearby. Also, let coworkers and loved ones know about your diabetes and how to recognize hypoglycemia. If you're prone to frequent low blood glucose, wear an ID bracelet.

If You Need Insulin, You're Doomed

Many people with type 2 diabetes believe that once they have to take insulin, they're on a rapid downhill course to death. This is not so. If you're using insulin, it probably means that your pancreas has pooped out and cannot produce enough insulin to control your blood glucose, even when stimulated by oral drugs. But taking insulin is no more a death sentence for you than it is for the person with type 1 diabetes.

Some people believe that insulin, itself, causes complications like impotence or other damage. There is no evidence for this. A recent study that was publicized but not yet published suggested that using insulin to lower the blood glucose so the hemoglobin A1c was less than 6 percent caused more deaths than lowering it to a more modest level like 7 percent.

These were patients who had already had a heart attack and were quite sick when the study began. Even so, the doctors could not get their hemoglobin A1c to the level they wanted with insulin. The goal was set too low. It does not take lowering to 6 percent to prevent complications in new patients with diabetes; 6.5 percent will accomplish this. First of all, using insulin is often a temporary measure for when you're very sick with some other illness that makes your oral drugs ineffective. When the illness is over, your insulin needs end.

Secondly, you may be on insulin because oral agents you tried failed to control your glucose. I see many people in this situation who can be taken off the insulin and given one of the newer oral agents, which actually control their glucose better than the insulin. One typical patient came to me on 60 units of insulin weighing 180 pounds with a hemoglobin A1c of 7.4. I gradually lowered his insulin as I added rosiglitazone (now I would add pioglitazone instead; see Chapter 10) to his treatment. He lost 22 pounds, came off insulin entirely, and now has a hemoglobin A1c of 6.

Thirdly, elderly people with diabetes may need insulin to keep their blood glucose at a reasonable level but do not need very tight control because their probable life span is shorter than the time it takes to develop complications. Their treatment can be kept very simple. The insulin is being used to keep them out of immediate trouble, not to prevent complications.

Finally, people with type 2 diabetes who truly need to be on insulin intensively need to check their blood glucose more often and live more like a person with type 1 diabetes. I hope you realize that with today's methods, this level of intensive treatment means a much higher quality of life than it used to.

People with Diabetes Shouldn't Exercise

If any myth is really damaging to people with diabetes, it is this one: People with diabetes shouldn't exercise. The truth is exactly the opposite. Exercise is a major component of good diabetes management — one that, unfortunately, all too often gets the least time and effort on the part of the patient as well as his or her care providers.

Sure, if you have certain complications, like hemorrhaging in your eye or severe neuropathy, you need to take precautions or not exercise at all for a time. Certainly, if you're older than 40 and have not exercised, you need to have an examination and start gradually. But except for these and a few other reasons (see Chapter 9), exercise ought to be done regularly by every person with diabetes.

And I'm not just talking about aerobic exercise where your heart is beating faster. Some form of muscle strengthening needs to be a part of your lifestyle. (See Chapter 9 to find out the benefits of muscle strengthening.) If you have a muscle that you can move, move it!

You Can't Get Life and Health Insurance

I devote Chapter 15 to showing you that you *can* get life and health insurance. As the insurance industry recognizes that people with diabetes take better care of themselves than the general population does, it is more and more willing to insure them. Some unenlightened insurance companies still exist, but most are seeing the light as the vital statistics of the diabetic population improve.

The old problem of a *preexisting condition* seems to be disappearing as well. Insurance companies are not being allowed to use this excuse to block you from getting new insurance when you change jobs.

One thing that is true is that the cost of medical care is significant and is not declining. You don't want to be without medical insurance for any length of time. You may have to look a little longer than the person without diabetes, but you can eventually get insurance, and the price will be no higher than anyone else is paying.

Most Diabetes Is Inherited

Although type 2 diabetes runs in families, type 1 diabetes more often occurs as an isolated event in a family rather than being handed down from parent to child. (Chapter 3 explains why this is the case.) Even type 2 diabetes does not come out in every family member. It depends on factors such as body weight and level of activity.

Parents should not feel guilty if their small child develops diabetes. Such feelings make it harder to perform the necessary functions that parents must do to help their child be healthy.

Diabetes Wrecks Your Sense of Humor

After the initial stages of accepting diabetes, your sense of humor should return. (See Chapter 1 for more on dealing with diabetes.) If your humor doesn't return, it's no laughing matter.

Dr. Joel Goodman, director of The HUMOR Project, pointed out in a lecture I attended that you "jest for the health of it." Numerous scientific studies have shown the health benefits of laughter.

The comedian Steve Allen pointed out in an interview performed by Dr. Goodman that there is humor in every aspect of life — you just have to look for it. The saying goes "Someday we'll laugh about this." The question is "Why wait?"

My diabetic patients have been the source of many funny stories, some of which I tell in this book. I want to give you the assignment of coming up with *at least* one funny story from your diabetic past. Send me an e-mail at drrubin@drrubin.com or write me a note about it. Remember that what you think is funny may not be funny to someone else. This is clearly shown by our individual preferences in comedians. Ask ten of your friends who their favorite comedian is and see if you don't come back with 12 answers.

Soak Your Feet Daily if You Have Diabetes

Here's an eleventh myth since you just gave me a standing ovation for writing this book. A standing ovation deserves a brief encore.

This myth causes more damage than it prevents. Soaking the feet tends to dry them. The skin can crack and infection can occur. This is, of course, the opposite of what you are trying to accomplish. Protect your skin by using a moisturizing lotion on a regular basis.

Make sure you inspect your feet every day, particularly if there is any question about your ability to feel abnormalities in your feet. Washing your feet with a good soap containing a moisturizing lotion is a good time to do that inspection.

Follow that up by applying a thick, not a thin watery moisturizing lotion to your feet. They will continue to give you good service for many years to come.

Chapter 20

Ten Ways to Get Others to Help You

Diabetes is a social disease. No, I don't mean that you catch it like herpes. I mean that you can't continue very long with diabetes without calling on the help and expertise of others. Asking for help is not such a bad thing. People who regularly interact with others seem to live longer and have a higher quality of life.

Diabetes has become so pervasive in the United States that practically everyone knows someone who has diabetes or has it himself. There is a huge, growing body of knowledge about all aspects of diabetes, but you have to be willing to share your diagnosis with others so they can help you. These days I even get new patients when people who know they have diabetes share their diagnosis and symptoms with someone else and that person realizes that he has diabetes as well.

In this chapter, you discover how to make use of the great resources that are available to people with diabetes. So many knowledgeable people are out there — it would be a shame not to utilize their information. (Why, even I use my colleagues' knowledge on very rare occasions!)

Explain Hypoglycemia

If you take either insulin or one of the sulfonylurea medications (see Chapter 10), you may become hypoglycemic. Occasionally, hypoglycemia can be so severe that you're unaware of the problem. At that point, someone in your environment needs to know the symptoms of hypoglycemia and how to treat it. Chapter 4 contains all that information.

You may want to make a list of the signs and symptoms of hypoglycemia and pass it around to your family and friends. You should keep that list and an emergency kit to treat hypoglycemia at home and at work. You may even want to wear a medical alert bracelet so someone can identify your problem when none of these people are around.

Follow the Standards of Care with Your Doctor

Decades of following diabetes patients, along with increasing scientific knowledge, has led to the establishment of "standards of care" for the person with diabetes. These recommendations usually appear in a supplement to the January issue of *Diabetes Care,* a journal of the American Diabetes Association. I outline these standards in Chapter 7 and on the Cheat Sheet at the front of this book. By following the standards of care, you have a good chance of avoiding the short- and long-term complications of diabetes. If these complications have already occurred, you have a good chance of having them diagnosed while they are still treatable.

You are the one who needs to make sure that you get an annual eye examination, get your urine tested for microalbumin and your nerves tested for sensation, and get all the other tests that must be done regularly and routinely. (See Chapter 7 for more on these tests.) You can't do these tests alone, however. You need your physician to order the tests and send you to the eye doctor. Don't expect your physician to remember all these details. Just as you have trouble keeping to a program of care over a lifetime, your physician does much better with acute illnesses than chronic ones.

Find an Exercise Partner

Few people (and I certainly count myself among this group) continue a regular exercise program completely on their own. However, when you know that someone is waiting for you, you tend to perform the exercise much more regularly. I have many patients who are regular exercisers because I emphasize exercise so much. All of them exercise with a partner.

If you belong to a club, finding an exercise partner is easy. First, you select the sport, and then you hang out in the place where the sport is played. If the sport is a racket sport, you will soon find others at about your level. If the sport is something like running, you have to be a little forward and ask whether you can join someone or a group about to run. The people you can keep up with are your natural exercise partners.

If you're not a member of a club, finding an exercise partner is a little more difficult. You may have to approach people with whom you work, or you may need your significant other to commit to exercising with you. Most people are happy to walk with you, and some will run and bike with you. Cyclists seem to like group activity, and you can usually find a bike group to ride with. Check out listings at a local bike shop or the Sunday newspaper in the activities section.

Use Your Foot Doctor

Your foot doctor is your first line of defense against lesions of the foot. He or she knows what the foot should look like and will notice problems very early when they're still reversible. Your doctor will usually have a foot doctor that he likes to work with.

One of the most useful things the foot doctor can do is to cut your nails. It is too easy to accidentally cut your skin when you try to cut your own nails. If you have diabetes, the consequences can be serious.

Should you notice an abnormality, you must get to the foot doctor immediately. This is a situation where you are much better off erring on the side of too much rather than too little medical care. In my practice, I ask the patients about their feet at every visit and examine the feet of those who have been found to have neuropathy (see Chapter 5) in the past. If I discover a foot problem, the foot doctor sees it that day.

Doctors recently performed the first hand transplantation, which seems to be going well, but as far as I know, no plans exist to do a foot transplantation. Take good care of your feet because they have to last a lifetime. Your foot doctor can be your major ally in this endeavor.

Enlist Help to Fight Food Temptation

Ever since Adam and Eve, the problem of temptation has been on the front burner. For a diabetic, the constant temptation is to eat foods that do not further your major diabetic goal, which is to control your blood glucose. The opportunities for screwing up your diet are boundless. Just like your exercise partner, your "food partner" — your significant other — can make staying on your diet a lot easier for you.

If your partner cooks most of the meals in your household, he or she has a responsibility to prepare the right kinds of foods. To do this, your partner must know what to make and what to avoid (see Chapter 8). If you go to the dietitian, take your partner along.

Numerous books of recipes and meals are written specifically for the person with diabetes. The first cookbook you should look at is *Diabetes Cookbook For Dummies, 2nd Edition* (Wiley), which I wrote with Alison Acerra. That book would not have been written if it didn't offer a special feature — the recipes of some of the finest chefs in the United States and Canada. You can also go on the Internet to find good recipes; see Appendix C for a list of great Web sites to check out.

I believe that the big problem in diabetes (as well as the nondiabetic obese population) is large portions of food. One of the simplest of diets is to eat the same foods but half as much. As I worked with the chefs in the various restaurants represented in Appendix A, again and again they remarked to me that Americans eat much more food in a portion than Europeans. Americans have learned to avoid fat, but they eat too much carbohydrate.

When it comes to eating out, your loved one can steer you to restaurants where you can choose foods that work for you. When you're in the restaurant, he or she can point out the healthy choices. The best way to direct you is to set an example of appropriate eating for you.

If you're asked to dinner in someone's home, your loved one can help by telling your host or hostess in advance that you have diabetes and need to avoid eating certain foods. It is unwise, however, to turn your loved one into a nag. Don't ask that you be reminded each time you stray from your diet. That will lead to hostility.

Expand Your Education with Diabetes Educators

The person who serves as your diabetes educator is the source of a huge amount of necessary and sometimes critical information. Every person with diabetes ought to go through a program of education after the initial shock of the diagnosis is past (see Chapter 1). Never hesitate to ask a question, no matter how basic you think it may be. You will be surprised by how many others want the same information.

Of course, every caregiver should be a diabetes educator as well. When you are past the formal diabetes education program, don't hesitate to ask questions of your physician, your dietitian, or any of the other people in your team (see Chapter 11).

Knowledge about diabetes is expanding so fast that great advances are arriving almost daily. Some of these advances may be just what you need.

Fit Your Favorite Foods into Your Diet with a Dietitian

Years ago when you got diabetes, it meant you had to make enormous changes in your diet. This was hard enough for people who ate the usual American diet, but much harder for people who came from another culture and had an entirely different diet. This situation has changed dramatically.

The dietitian's job is to come up with a diabetic diet plan based upon *your* food choices, not those of the dietitian. If you have special dietary needs because of your culture, a dietitian must be able to accommodate those needs if they are reasonable.

Members of your culture ate the foods that you like for generations without developing diabetes in large numbers. The main reasons they didn't develop diabetes in large numbers are that they did not eat the large portions you eat and they were much more physically active than you are. If you want to keep enjoying "your" foods, eat and exercise like your great-grandparents.

Do not be satisfied with a printed sheet of paper with the heading "Diabetic Diet." The key word in diabetic diets is *individualization*. You probably won't stay on a diet that you do not enjoy.

Seek Out Appropriate Specialists

The specialist who knows the most about diabetes is the *diabetologist,* a physician with advanced training in diabetes care who maintains his or her edge by attending diabetes meetings regularly and keeping up with the literature by reading the most important clinical diabetes journals. In addition, these days an up-to-date specialist has to be aware of what is on the Internet and how to differentiate reality from hype. This person can explain the latest advances in diabetes to you.

Not only do you want to find a diabetes specialist, but should you develop a complication of diabetes, you want to use a specialist in that area. At the first sign of kidney disease associated with diabetes, ask your doctor to refer you to a nephrologist. You should already be examined by an eye doctor on an annual basis. If there is any question of loss of sensation or abnormal muscle movements, see a neurologist. If there is any indication of heart trouble, get a referral to a cardiologist.

The pace of advances in diabetes is amazing. A general physician cannot keep up with it. The diabetes specialist concentrates on diabetes and the other specialists concentrate on their fields, and that is to your benefit.

Discuss Your Medications with the Pharmacist

One of your most valuable and least utilized resources is your pharmacist. He or she is loaded with information about drug actions, interactions, side effects, proper dosage and administration, and contraindications, as well as what to do in case of an overdosage. Every time you get a new medication, you can have your pharmacist run it against the medications you're already taking and see whether any problems might occur. Thanks to computers, this comparison should take only a few minutes. If you work with one drug store, you should be able to get a printout of your entire list of medications, which you can carry with you in case you ever need medical care.

The pharmacist can also save you money by recommending generic equivalents to the brands that your doctor prescribes. The doctor may have good reason to prescribe them so the pharmacist will check with him before giving you a different medication.

The information in the computer tends to be all-inclusive. If a drug has ever had a side effect, no matter how rare, it will probably be in the computer. The drug manufacturer wants to be able to say that it warned you about every possibility. If a side effect or drug interaction is serious, discuss it with your physician before you start the new medication.

Share This Book with Everyone

If you really want your friends and loved ones to understand what you're going through, why not give them a copy of this book and ask them to read it? You can select the chapters that are most important to you. Your family and friends will probably be delighted to have a resource they can understand, and you can expect a lot more help from them.

When I began writing this book, I did so because I saw a need for information that could be understood by most people without the benefit of a medical school education. At the same time, I wanted you to have a little fun because "a spoonful of sugar helps the medicine go down." But I did not want to trivialize diabetes and hope I have not done so. If you believe I have succeeded in what I set out to do, share this book with others.

Part VI
Appendixes

"Oooo, what's in here? Is that sun-dried eye of newt? How gourmet!"

In this part . . .

Appendix A is the *Diabetes For Dummies* Mini-Cookbook. Here you find some of the most delicious and satisfying recipes that you can make, proof that you can have diabetes and eat delicious food. If you don't feel like making them, you find the name of the restaurant that has provided the recipe in case you live near the restaurant.

Appendix B presents an introduction to the magnificent World Wide Web and the almost limitless resources about diabetes to be found there. You will be amazed at how much is given away for free on the Web. Just make sure the source is reliable. Appendix C is a glossary of terms you encounter as you read and hear about diabetes. In this glossary you should be able to find any diabetes-related term that you do not understand.

Appendix A

Mini-Cookbook

· ·

*T*his appendix should make it clear to you that you can have great food from every ethnic corner of the world and still stay within the requirements of a diabetic diet. In a short appendix like this, I could not include every possible type of food, but I tried to select foods that most people enjoy either at home or in a restaurant. I chose the restaurants from among the best in the country, with an emphasis on San Francisco because that is where I reside and (happily) get to try them. If you want even more variety, see my book *Diabetes Cookbook For Dummies* (Wiley).

Sometimes it was necessary to alter a recipe slightly to keep it appropriate for a diabetic diet, but this was never done without the approval of the chef who created it. These chefs and restaurants were a pleasure to work with and deserve great praise for their willingness to accommodate the needs of the diabetic patient.

Some recipes may take a little longer to prepare, but all are worth the time and the effort. In any case, you can go to the restaurant that provided the recipe, order that meal, and know that you are on your diabetic diet.

Keep in mind that all temperatures are in Fahrenheit.

Aqua

Situated in a grand post-1906 earthquake building on California Street, Aqua is located in the heart of San Francisco's bustling Financial District. At Aqua, owner Charles Condy and Executive Chef Michael Mina have joined forces to redefine dining and to pay elegant tribute to the flavors of the sea. The contemporary American design, combining a relaxed yet elegant ambiance, has set the stage for Chef Mina's imaginative menu.

Since becoming the Executive Chef of Aqua, Michael Mina's intensely flavorful and creative seafood cooking has earned him a reputation as one of the nation's most influential and respected chefs. Embracing a straightforward approach in coaxing lusty flavors from California's seasonal bounty, this young chef continues to capture hearts and palates of diners and critics. His culinary skills resulted in his designation as the James Beard Foundation's Rising Star Chef in 1997, and other prestigious awards have followed.

Aqua, 252 California Street, San Francisco, California. 415-956-9662.

Warm Asparagus and Morel Salad

This dish is perfect as the first or second course to any meal.

Preparation time: *1 hour*

Cooking time: *30 minutes*

Yield: *8 servings*

48 asparagus spears	*Salt and pepper to taste*
1 cup balsamic vinegar	*2 heads frisee*
8 ounces morel mushrooms	*1 to 2 tablespoons water*
1 tablespoon butter, plus 1 teaspoon to warm asparagus	*¼ cup olive oil*

1 Peel each piece of asparagus 2 inches from the top to the base (you won't need to do this if you're using young, thin asparagus). Cut each spear, leaving a 3- to 4-inch tip. Use remaining asparagus by slicing ¼-inch rounds. Do not use woody part of asparagus. Keep tips and rounds separate.

2 Boil water, adding salt to taste. Add asparagus tips to boiling water. Once tender but still firm, about 2 minutes, place the asparagus in ice cold water to cool. Proceed by blanching asparagus rounds another 2 to 3 minutes. Use same process to cool. Set the cooling tips and rounds aside, keeping them separate.

3 Over low heat, in a heavy-bottom saucepan, cook the vinegar for 20 to 30 minutes, never allowing it to reach a boil. Once the balsamic reaches a syrupy consistency, remove from heat. This process requires attention. It is quite easy to burn the balsamic.

4 Slice the morel mushrooms into ¼-inch rounds and place in warm water to remove excess dirt. Dry mushrooms to get rid of the moisture. In a medium sauté pan, heat the butter over medium heat. When bubbly, add the mushrooms. Cook, occasionally stirring gently, until soft, about 4 to 5 minutes. Season with salt and pepper to taste. Set aside.

5 Remove all outside leaves from the frisee, leaving only the inner white leaves. Separate the leaves from the stem, rinse under cold water, and spin or pat dry. Set aside.

6 To serve: Drizzle the balsamic glaze decoratively on each plate. In a medium sauté pan, warm the asparagus tips in the remaining butter mixed with 1 to 2 tablespoons water. Place the asparagus tips facing outward toward the rim of the plate. In the same sauté pan, heat the asparagus rounds with the morel slices. Then place the morels and asparagus rounds in a neat mound slightly overlapping the ends of the asparagus tips.

In a medium bowl, mix the frisee with the olive oil. Finally, top the mushrooms and asparagus with the frisee.

Nutrient analysis per serving: 133 calories; 3 grams protein, 13 grams carbohydrate, 9 grams fat, 2 grams saturated fat, 4 milligrams cholesterol, 3 grams fiber, 37 milligrams sodium.

Marinated Grilled Duck Breast

Although duck is higher in fat than other types of poultry, it still can be served as a dish for special occasions. Round out this meal with a cup of wild rice and sautéed vegetables.

Preparation time: *30 minutes*

Cooking time: *1 hour*

Yield: *4 servings*

1 cup balsamic vinegar	*½ bunch Italian parsley*
½ cup Worcestershire sauce	*½ bunch rosemary*
¼ cup honey	*½ bunch chives*
1 cup extra virgin olive oil	*4 duck breasts*
1 tablespoon chopped garlic	*Salt and pepper to taste*
½ tablespoon lemon juice	

1 *For marinade:* Place all ingredients, except for duck, in a large bowl and mix well. Score (make crisscross patterns with the tip of a sharp knife) skin side of the cleaned duck breast. Place the duck into the bowl, coat it with marinade, and cover the bowl. Refrigerate and marinate for 24 hours.

2 Preheat grill. Remove duck from marinade and pat dry with a clean towel. Season with salt and pepper. Grill for 10 minutes on skin side; turn, moving the breasts to cooler portions of the grill, and cook another 5 minutes, or until medium rare. (To sear duck rather than grilling, place 2 nonstick skillets over medium-high heat. When hot, add the duck breasts, skin side down. Cook for 10 minutes. Reduce the heat, turn breasts over, and cook another 5 minutes or until medium rare.) Slice just before serving.

Nutrient analysis per serving: 507 calories; 47 grams protein, 6 grams carbohydrate, 32 grams fat, 8 grams saturated fat, 177 milligrams cholesterol, 0 grams fiber, 300 milligrams sodium.

Grilled Swordfish with Worcestershire Vinaigrette and Roasted Vegetables

This dish is a delightful way to flavor both the fish and vegetables. It is a complete meal, but low enough in carbohydrate to include a couple slices of French bread.

Preparation time: *40 minutes*

Cooking time: *1 hour, 10 minutes*

Yield: *8 servings*

Vinaigrette

½ cup Worcestershire sauce

1 sprig rosemary, leaves only, chopped

⅛ cup chopped chives

1 clove garlic, minced

1 tablespoon balsamic vinegar

Juice of ¼ lemon

1 cup extra-virgin olive oil

Roasted Vegetables

8 new potatoes, cut in half

16 baby beets, well rinsed and ends trimmed

24 baby carrots, peeled

16 shiitake mushrooms, stems removed

16 shallots, unpeeled and cut in half

2 pounds red and yellow cherry tomatoes

3 tablespoons olive oil

8 swordfish, approximately 6 ounces each

Salt and pepper to taste

1 pound arugula

1 *For vinaigrette:* Mix all ingredients together. This vinaigrette should be made 24 hours in advance. The nutritional analysis reflects only 2 tablespoons.

2 *For roasted vegetables:* Heat oven to 375°. Place iron skillet in oven until hot. Keeping vegetables separate, in a large bowl, toss the potatoes, beets, carrots, mushrooms, shallots, tomatoes, 2 tablespoons olive oil, and salt and pepper, then transfer to hot skillet. Roast vegetables until tender, about 45 minutes. You can do this ahead of time and then reheat the vegetables when you're ready to cook the fish.

3 *To serve:* Reheat the vegetables in the oven if they're done ahead of time. Preheat the grill. Season the swordfish on both sides and cook until medium rare, about 3 minutes per side.

4 In a large sauté pan, heat the remaining olive oil over high heat. Add the arugula and cook, tossing or gently mixing with kitchen tongs, just until the greens start to wilt, about 1 minute. Mix greens with the hot vegetables and place in the center of the plate, dividing vegetables evenly.

5 Place swordfish on top of vegetables. Drizzle 2 tablespoons vinaigrette over each portion.

Nutrient analysis per serving: *519 calories; 48 grams protein, 36 grams carbohydrate, 22 grams fat, 3 grams saturated fat, 126 milligrams cholesterol, 3 grams fiber, 544 milligrams sodium.*

Miso Marinated Sea Bass

This unique marinade adds a tremendous amount of flavor without the use of fat. You can add a tossed green salad with your favorite vinaigrette. This dish is also low in carbohydrate, so you can complete the meal with a cup of rice.

Preparation time: *45 minutes*

Cooking time: *5 minutes*

Yield: *8 servings*

¼ pound brown sugar

¼ pound sugar

½ pound miso paste

¼ cup soy sauce

1 cup sake

1 cup rice wine vinegar

8 6-ounce portions Chilean sea bass

Vegetable oil

1 cup chicken consommé

1 cup snow peas

1 cup carrots, sliced thin and boiled in salted water 3 to 4 minutes

½ pound baby bok choy, boiled in salted water 1 to 2 minutes

5 assorted radishes, thinly sliced

1 cup shiitake mushrooms, sliced

1 8-ounce package enoki mushrooms

1 *For marinade:* In a large bowl, mix together the sugars, miso paste, soy sauce, sake, and rice wine vinegar. Place the fish into the bowl, coat it with marinade, and cover the bowl. Refrigerate and marinate for 24 hours.

2 Preheat the broiler. Rub a shallow roasting pan (large enough to fit the fish in 1 layer) lightly with vegetable oil. Remove the sea bass fillets from the marinade, place them on the roasting pan, and place under the broiler. Cook until the fish begins to brown, about 2 to 3 minutes. Transfer the pan to the oven and cook through, about 5 minutes, depending on the thickness of the fillets.

3 Combine the consommé with snow peas, carrots, bok choy, radishes, and shiitake and enoki mushrooms in a medium sauté pan. Simmer, covered, until vegetables are warm. Season to taste. Place a pile of vegetables in the center of each large serving bowl, set a sea bass fillet on top, and spoon the consommé around.

Nutrient analysis per serving: 295 calories; 37 grams protein, 26 grams carbohydrate, 4 grams fat, .5 grams saturated fat, 82 milligrams cholesterol, 2 grams fiber, 1,295 milligrams sodium.

Border Grill

Situated in Santa Monica, California, the critically acclaimed Border Grill Restaurant features the bold foods of Mexico. The original restaurant has been joined by another Border Grill, this time in Las Vegas, and by Ciudad in downtown Los Angeles, which emphasize the cooking of Central and South America, Spain, and the Caribbean.

The restaurants are the inspiration of two women who are chefs, restaurateurs, cookbook authors, and television and radio personalities: Mary Sue Milliken and Susan Feniger. They are hosts of the Food Network's popular series *Two Hot Tamales* and *Tamales World Tour*. They are natural teachers who share their passion for bold flavors and strong statements through many media. If you find, as I did, that their recipes make you hunger for more, look for their book *Mexican Cooking For Dummies* (Wiley).

Border Grill, 1445 4th St., Santa Monica, California. 310-451-1655.

Cinnamon-Brandy Chicken

Looking for a different way of cooking chicken? Here is a wonderful recipe brimming with flavor and easy to prepare. Serve with the rice pilaf and roasted vegetable dishes, later in this section.

Preparation time: *30 minutes*

Cooking time: *40 minutes*

Yield: *6 servings*

½ cup brandy	1 teaspoon salt
1 tablespoon cinnamon	½ teaspoon freshly ground black pepper
¼ cup honey	1 frying chicken, 2½ to 3 pounds, cut into pieces
½ cup lemon juice	
½ cup orange juice	2 tablespoons vegetable oil
4 garlic cloves, minced	

1 In a medium bowl, mix the brandy, cinnamon, honey, lemon and orange juices, garlic, salt, and pepper. Add the seasoned chicken and toss to evenly coat. Cover and marinate in the refrigerator 8 hours or overnight.

2 Preheat oven to 350°. Remove the chicken from the bowl, shaking off excess marinade. Pour the marinade into a small saucepan and bring to a boil. Boil until it begins to thicken and about 1 cup remains, 5 to 10 minutes.

3 Heat the oil in an ovenproof skillet over medium-high heat. Sear the chicken until golden on both sides. Pour the reduced marinade over the chicken and place in the oven. Bake about 20 minutes and serve.

Nutrient analysis per serving: 506 calories; 42 grams protein, 16 grams carbohydrate, 25 grams fat, 7 grams saturated fat, 134 milligrams cholesterol, 0 grams fiber, 502 milligrams sodium.

Green Rice Pilaf

This dish can accompany the chicken in the preceding recipe, or it can be served with meat or fish.

Preparation time: 40 minutes

Cooking time: 25 minutes

Yield: 6 servings

1½ tablespoons vegetable oil

1 small onion, finely diced

1 cup long-grain white rice

2 cups hot vegetable or chicken broth, preferably homemade

½ teaspoon salt

3 medium poblano chiles, roasted, peeled, seeded, and cut into strips

1 cup fresh or frozen peas

½ cup crumbled Mexican queso fresco or feta cheese

½ bunch Italian parsley leaves, finely chopped

½ bunch cilantro, finely chopped

1 Heat the oil in a heavy saucepan over medium heat. Add the rice and onion and cook, stirring frequently, about 7 minutes, until the onion is softened but not browned.

2 Add the hot broth, salt, and chiles and bring to a boil. Reduce to a simmer and cook, covered, about 10 minutes.

3 Add the peas and simmer 5 minutes longer. Remove from heat and let stand, covered, about 10 minutes.

4 Add the cheese, parsley, and cilantro, evenly mix, and fluff with a fork. Serve immediately.

Nutrient analysis per serving: 202 calories; 12 grams protein, 28 grams carbohydrate, 7 grams fat, 3 grams saturated fat, 1 milligram cholesterol, 2 grams fiber, 948 milligrams sodium.

Red Roasted Root Vegetables

You can substitute any of your favorite root vegetables in this dish. It is a great side dish for chicken, fish, or meat.

Preparation time: *35 minutes*

Cooking time: *40 minutes*

Yield: *6 servings*

½ pound turnips, peeled and cut into 1-inch chunks

½ pound beets, peeled and cut into 1-inch chunks

½ pound carrots, peeled and cut into 1-inch chunks

½ pound butternut or other firm squash, peeled and cut into 1-inch chunks

1 onion, coarsely chopped

2 garlic cloves, minced

½ bunch fresh oregano leaves, coarsely chopped

⅓ cup olive oil

1 teaspoon salt

½ teaspoon freshly ground pepper

1 Preheat oven to 450°. In a large bowl, toss together all the ingredients until well mixed.

2 Arrange in a single layer in an enameled cast-iron casserole or baking dish. Cover and roast 30 to 40 minutes, stirring every 10 minutes. The vegetables are done when golden, lightly caramelized on the edges, and easily pierced with the tip of a knife.

Nutrient analysis per serving: 171 calories; 2 grams protein, 15 grams carbohydrate, 11 grams fat, 2 grams saturated fat, 0 milligrams cholesterol, 4 grams fiber, 432 milligrams sodium.

Baked Apples

This dessert is a wonderful way to top off any meal. It is light, healthy, and low in calories.

Preparation time: *35 minutes*

Cooking time: *1 hour*

Yield: *6 servings*

1 cup plus 2 tablespoons apple juice

¼ cup raisins

¼ cup apple butter

¼ cup toasted chopped walnuts

2 tablespoons maple syrup

2 tablespoons brandy

6 medium apples, cored and the top third peeled

2 tablespoons unsalted butter

1 In a small saucepan, bring 2 tablespoons apple juice and the raisins to a simmer and remove from heat. Let sit for 10 minutes.

2 Preheat the oven to 350°. In a bowl, stir together the apple butter, walnuts, maple syrup, brandy, and raisins with their juice and mix well.

3 Stuff the apples with the raisin mixture. Place the apples in a small roasting pan and top each with a dab of butter. Pour the remaining cup of apple juice into the pan and bake 50 to 60 minutes, or until tender but not split or mushy.

Nutrient analysis per serving: 218 calories; 2 grams protein, 38 grams carbohydrate, 8 grams fat, 3 grams saturated fat, 11 milligrams cholesterol, 4 grams fiber, 2 milligrams sodium.

Charlie Trotter's

One of the most innovative restaurants in the country, Charlie Trotter's specializes in creative American cuisine with French and Asian overtones. It stresses the use of healthful, fresh foodstuffs. Naturally raised meats, game birds, organic fruits, and vegetables form the heart of Trotter's cooking.

Charlie Trotter's has won numerous awards and other recognition for the quality of its food, its décor, and its service. It received five stars from the *Mobil Travel Guide*, is listed in the very prestigious *Relais and Chateaux,* and was given the Grand Award by *Wine Spectator* as The Best Restaurant in the World for Wine and Food (1998).

Owner and chef Charlie Trotter began to cook professionally in 1982. He trained in Europe and America with Norman Van Aken, Bradley Ogden, and Gordon Sinclair.

The recipes provided by Charlie Trotter tend to take a little more time to prepare than some from the other restaurants, but the results more than make up for the time spent. (If you like the recipes, you may want to check out Charlie Trotter's book, *Gourmet Cooking For Dummies* [Wiley].)

Charlie Trotter's, 816 West Armitage, Chicago, Illinois. 773-248-6228.

Scallops with Barley, Wild Mushroom Ragout, and Chicken Stock Reduction

This meal is low in carbohydrate, which allows you to have a couple slices of bread or a serving of sherbet to round it out.

Preparation time: *1 hour*

Cooking time: *45 minutes*

Yield: *4 servings*

3 tablespoons chopped fennel

3 tablespoons canola oil

½ cup red wine

¼ cup peeled, seeded, and diced tomato

3 cups chicken stock

1¼ pounds mixed wild mushrooms (shiitake, cepe, portobello, and so on)

6 tablespoons Madeira

Salt and pepper

1 teaspoon chopped parsley

1 teaspoon tarragon leaves

20 medium sea scallops

2 cups cooked barley

1 *For the reduction:* In a medium sauté pan, cook the fennel in 1 tablespoon canola oil for 5 minutes or until thoroughly softened. Add the red wine and stir continuously until the wine is reduced to a glaze. Add the tomato and chicken stock and cook over medium-low heat for 30 minutes or until reduced to 1 cup.

2 *For mushrooms:* Cut the mushrooms into large pieces (smaller mushrooms can be used whole). In a medium nonstick sauté pan, heat 1 tablespoon canola oil over medium-low heat. Add the mushrooms and cook, tossing or stirring occasionally, for 10 minutes, or until mushrooms are tender and all the liquid is evaporated. Add the Madeira and cook until it is completely reduced. Season the mushrooms to taste with salt and pepper and add the parsley and tarragon. Set aside.

3 *For scallops:* Heat the remaining 1 tablespoon canola oil in a nonstick sauté pan over medium-high heat. Add the scallops and cook for 2 minutes, or until golden brown. Season the scallops with salt and pepper. Turn over the scallops and cook for 1 minute.

4 *To serve:* Place the cooked barley on each plate. Spoon some of the fennel sauce onto each plate, place a neat mound of mushrooms over the sauce, and surround with 5 scallops, leaning them against the mushrooms.

Nutrient analysis per serving: *398 calories; 27 grams protein, 36 grams carbohydrate, 20 grams fat, 5 grams saturated fat, 42 milligrams cholesterol, 2 grams fiber, 1,084 milligrams sodium.*

Steamed Whitefish with Haricotes Verts and Potato–Apple–Celery Puree

This dish allows for an extra serving of starch or fruit and 1 tablespoon fat. Why not share a dessert with your dinner companion?

Preparation time: 1 hour

Cooking time: 1 hour

Yield: 4 servings

1 cup chopped celery

2 cups chopped apples, preferably Granny Smith

1½ cups chopped potatoes, boiled

Salt and pepper to taste

2 cups celery juice

3 tablespoons plus 2 teaspoons butter

1½ cups haricots verts (French string beans)

6 tablespoons chopped fresh chives

2 tablespoons chopped fresh chervil

Canola oil

4 3-ounce pieces whitefish

1½ cups julienned Spanish onion

1 For puree: Place the celery and 1 cup apple in a medium saucepan, cover with water, and simmer over medium heat for 5 to 7 minutes, or until slightly soft. Drain and puree with the cooked potatoes, adding water as needed, until smooth. Place the puree in a nonstick pan and slowly dry over medium heat for 10 minutes, stirring continuously, until the puree has a thick consistency. Season to taste with salt and pepper. Set aside, covered, to maintain heat.

2 For sauce: Place the celery juice in a small saucepan with the remaining 1 cup apple and simmer over medium heat for 15 minutes. Strain through a fine-mesh sieve and season to taste with salt and pepper. Set aside.

3 For onion: In a small sauté pan, heat 2 teaspoons butter over medium-high heat and cook onion for 12 minutes, tossing or stirring often, until golden brown. Set aside.

4 For haricots verts: Blanche the haricots verts in boiling salted water for 2 minutes, drain, and season to taste with salt and pepper.

5 To finish the sauce: Heat the sauce until simmering. Remove from heat and whisk in 3 tablespoons butter, 3 tablespoons chives, and 1½ tablespoons chervil until frothy. Keep warm.

6 For fish: Lightly brush the whitefish with canola oil. Season both sides with salt and pepper. Crust the top with the remaining 3 tablespoons chives and ½ tablespoon chervil. Place on a rack in a steamer and steam for 3 minutes, or until just cooked.

7 To serve: Spoon some of the puree in the center of each shallow bowl and top with a piece of steamed fish. Spoon the haricots verts and julienned onions around the fish and ladle the sauce around the bowl.

Nutrient analysis per serving: *350 calories; 22 grams protein, 44 grams carbohydrate, 11 grams fat, 6 grams saturated fat, 56 milligrams cholesterol, 5 grams fiber, 768 milligrams sodium.*

Fringale

Fringale has been called the perfect French bistro. The owners, Gerald Hirigoyen and J. B. Lorda, consider it a California/Basque bistro. By whatever designation, the food is straightforward and flavorful, and the social atmosphere is full of character and energy. The high quality of the food is in contrast to the moderate prices of everything on the menu. Much of the menu can be enjoyed not only for taste but also for the healthful qualities of the food.

Partner Gerald Hirigoyen is also the chef. He trained in the Basque region of France and in Paris with some of the great names in French cuisine. He came to San Francisco in 1980 and ran the kitchens of several fine restaurants, but in 1991, he decided to go out on his own and start this restaurant. He has received numerous awards and much recognition for the quality of his food. *Food and Wine* called him one of 1994's "Best New Chefs in America."

Fringale Restaurant, 570 Fourth Street, San Francisco, CA. 415-543-0573.

Marinated Chicken in Red Wine with Braising Greens, Parsnips, and Cippolini Onions

This dish allows room for two additional servings of starches. You may want to include a couple servings of bread to soak up this wonderful sauce!

Preparation time: *30 minutes*

Cooking time: *1 hour, 20 minutes*

Yield: *4 servings*

4 chicken thighs, without skin	1 cup veal stock
4 chicken breasts, split, without skin	8 cippolini onions, peeled
2 cups red wine	8 baby carrots, peeled
1 small onion, chopped	2 medium parsnips, peeled and cut into large matchsticks
2 garlic cloves, chopped	
6 sprigs thyme	3 tablespoons unsalted butter
1 tablespoon whole black peppercorns	2 pounds braising greens, such as green chard, with stems removed and leaves torn into large pieces
Kosher salt and freshly ground black pepper to taste	
2 tablespoons olive oil	2 tablespoons finely chopped parsley

1 In a large bowl, combine the chicken thighs, breasts, red wine, onion, garlic, thyme, black peppercorns, and salt and pepper to season. Cover with plastic wrap and refrigerate for at least 6 hours, preferably overnight.

2 Preheat oven to 450°. Separate the chicken from the marinade and set both aside.

3 Warm 1 tablespoon olive oil in a large casserole. Add the 4 chicken thighs and sauté until browned, about 5 minutes. Pour the marinade into the casserole with the thighs, add the veal stock, and bring to a boil. Once it boils, reduce heat and let the ingredients simmer for 25 to 30 minutes.

4 Warm 1 tablespoon olive oil in a large sauté pan over high heat. Add breasts and sauté until browned, about 3 to 4 minutes. Season with salt and pepper to taste and place in the oven until cooked, about 10 minutes.

5 Place the cippolini onions in a small pan with enough water to cover, bring to a boil, and cook until soft and tender, about 20 minutes. Strain and set aside. Fill a saucepan two-thirds full of water, bring to a boil, add baby carrots, and cook until tender, about 6 to 8 minutes. Strain and set aside. Place parsnips in a saucepan with enough water to cover, bring to a boil, and cook until tender, about 10 to 12 minutes. Strain and set aside.

6 When the chicken thighs are done, separate them from the marinade and set aside. Using a fine meshed sieve, strain the marinade into a small saucepan and discard the vegetables.

7 Bring the marinade to a boil and reduce by half. Turn off the heat, swirl in 1 tablespoon butter in a steady motion until completely incorporated, and season with salt and pepper to taste.

8 To prepare braising greens, combine ⅓ cup water, 1 tablespoon butter, the braising greens, and salt and pepper to taste in a large saucepan. Cover and cook over high heat just until wilted, about 5 minutes.

9 In a separate sauté pan, warm 1 tablespoon butter and then add the onion mixture and salt and pepper to taste and sauté until nicely caramelized, about 6 minutes. Add the parsley and set aside.

10 To assemble the dish, using a slotted spoon, place a small bed of the braising greens in the center of each plate. Lay one chicken thigh and one breast on top of the greens. Evenly scatter the cippolini onions, carrots, and parsnips on top of the chicken and spoon the sauce on top of and around the edges of the dish.

Nutrient analysis per serving: 596 calories; 49 grams protein, 30 grams carbohydrate, 25 grams fat, 9 grams saturated fat, 195 milligrams cholesterol, 5 grams fiber, 936 milligrams sodium.

Onion Pie with Roquefort and Walnuts

This dish is a feast for the eyes as well as the tongue. Serve as a main course for lunch. A fresh fruit salad and French roll are perfect complements to this meal.

Preparation time: *1 hour*

Cooking time: *15 minutes*

Yield: *8 servings*

2 tablespoons olive oil

2 white onions, very thinly sliced

¼ cup water

3 ounces Roquefort cheese, crumbled into small pieces

Salt and freshly ground pepper to taste

½ cup walnuts, coarsely chopped

1 tablespoon melted butter

2 puff pastry sheets (11 x 15-inch sheets), fresh or thawed frozen

1 egg, lightly beaten

8 slices of prosciutto (about .5 ounce each)

Mixed greens to garnish

1 Place a baking sheet with sides in a freezer.

2 In a sauté pan over medium-high heat, warm the olive oil. Add the onions and sauté until golden brown (about 10 minutes). Add the water and continue to sauté until all the moisture evaporates, about 5 minutes longer. Reduce heat to medium-low. Add the Roquefort cheese and continue cooking, stirring occasionally, until melted, about 5 more minutes. Season only lightly with salt, if needed, and add pepper to taste. Stir in the walnuts and then spread the mixture out onto the chilled sheet pan. Place in the freezer until the onions cool down completely (about 10 minutes).

3 Preheat oven to 450° and evenly brush a sheet pan with melted butter.

4 Place the puff pastry on a cutting board. Using the rim of a small plate about 5 inches in diameter as a guide, cut the pastry into 8 rounds. Discard scraps.

5 Place the rounds onto the prepared baking sheet. Brush the outer rims and tops with the beaten egg. Evenly distribute the cooled onion mixture in the middle of each of the 8 rounds, leaving 1 inch uncovered all around the edges. Place 1 prosciutto slice on top of each mound of the onion mixture. Fold over the pastry round to create a half-moon shape. Pinch down firmly around the edges to seal in the filling. Brush the top of each pie with more of the beaten egg. Using a sharp knife, pierce the top of each pie with a small slit.

6 Bake until the pastry is pale golden and fully puffed, about 20 to 25 minutes.

Nutrient analysis per serving: *454 calories; 13 grams protein, 26 grams carbohydrate, 34 grams fat, 7 grams saturated fat, 47 milligrams cholesterol, 1 gram fiber, 562 milligrams sodium.*

Lemon Braised Sea Bass with Star Anise and Baby Spinach

This meal is low in total carbohydrate and total fat, so you can complete the meal with a couple servings of carbohydrate (such as a serving of French bread and rice) and a tossed green salad with vinaigrette dressing.

Preparation time: *30 minutes*

Cooking time: *15 minutes*

Yield: *4 servings*

4 sea bass fillets (about 4 ounces each)	*1½ cups water*
Salt and freshly ground pepper to taste	*⅓ cup finely diced cucumber*
1 teaspoon olive oil	*⅓ cup finely diced tomato*
¼ cup finely diced celery root	*⅛ cup finely diced apple*
⅓ cup finely diced fennel	*4 cups baby spinach leaves*
¼ cup finely diced carrot	*2 teaspoons extra-virgin olive oil*
3 garlic cloves, peeled and chopped	*Pinch mild cayenne powder*
4 star anise	*2 tablespoons fresh chopped chives*
¼ cup freshly squeezed lemon juice	*2 tablespoons fresh chopped parsley*

1 Preheat oven to 475°. Rub both sides of the sea bass fillets with salt and pepper and set aside.

2 Heat 1 teaspoon olive oil in a large sauté pan (preferably nonstick) over high heat. Add the celery root, fennel, carrot, garlic, and star anise and sauté until slightly caramelized, 4 to 5 minutes. Soften the caramel with the lemon juice and cook for 1 minute.

3 Lay the sea bass fillets on top of the sautéed vegetables, add the water, and cover the pan. Place the pan into the preheated oven just until the fish is cooked though (5 to 6 minutes). Remove the pan from oven and remove the fillets of fish and set them aside, covered to keep warm.

4 Add the cucumber, tomato, and apple to the sauté pan and place over high heat. Bring to a boil and cook for 1 to 2 minutes. Add the spinach, extra-virgin olive oil, mild cayenne, and salt and pepper to taste. Cook just until the spinach wilts (30 seconds to 1 minute).

5 *To serve:* In 4 shallow soup bowls, spread an even amount of the vegetables and juice from the pan. Lay a fillet on top of the vegetables in each bowl and place a star anise on top to garnish. Sprinkle the chives and parsley over the top of each dish and serve immediately.

Nutrient analysis per serving: *236 calories; 31 grams protein, 17 grams carbohydrate, 6 grams fat, 1 gram saturated fat, 77 milligrams cholesterol, 3 grams fiber, 240 milligrams sodium.*

Gaylord India Restaurant

A bit of India in San Francisco — Gaylord is synonymous with delicious and authentic Indian food, served with true Indian hospitality. Located atop world famous Ghirardelli Square in San Francisco, the setting is one of relaxed elegance, with magnificent views of San Francisco Bay and the Marin County Headlands. At Gaylord, master chefs specialize in North Indian cuisine including centuries-old techniques of tandoori cooking.

Head chef Santok Kaler has been at Gaylord for 19 years. He was trained in the Punjab in India, the home of North Indian cooking.

Gaylord India Restaurant, Ghirardelli Square, 900 North Point, San Francisco, California. 415-771-8822.

Seekh Kabab (Barbecued Lamb on Skewer)

Spices are a wonderful way of adding full flavor to a dish without using extra fats. This dish can be served as an entrée or as an appetizer. Combine this recipe with 1 cup rice to provide the necessary carbohydrate. Two servings of vegetables, one of which could be the Saag, the last recipe in this section, round out the meal.

Preparation time: *30 minutes*

Cooking time: *10 minutes*

Yield: *6 servings*

1 medium onion	*½ teaspoon coriander powder*
1-inch fresh ginger	*½ teaspoon cumin powder*
2 garlic cloves	*¾ teaspoon garam masala (available in Indian food stores)*
2 teaspoons water	
1 teaspoon salt	*1 pound lean ground lamb*
¼ teaspoon cayenne pepper	

1 In a blender or mini food processor, grind onion, ginger, and garlic with 2 teaspoons water. Transfer to a medium bowl and mix in salt, cayenne pepper, coriander powder, cumin powder, and garam masala.

2 Add the ground lamb and mix until thoroughly combined. Let stand for 20 to 30 minutes in the refrigerator.

3 Preheat oven to 375°. Divide the mixture into 6 equal portions. Lightly oil the skewers. Shape the lamb mixture into sausage shapes on the skewers, about 1 inch thick. Place skewers on a rack over a pan and bake for 15 to 20 minutes or until done. To broil, place skewers 3 to 4 inches from heat and cook approximately 7 minutes per side. Serve hot with lemon garnish.

Tip: *If using wood or bamboo skewers, soak them overnight in water and oil them lightly. This step prevents burning the skewers while cooking.*

Nutrient analysis per serving: 144 calories; 12.6 grams protein, 2 grams carbohydrate, 9 grams fat, 42 milligrams cholesterol, 0.2 grams fiber, 419 milligrams sodium.

Chicken Tikka Kabab (Barbecued Chicken Kebab)

Marinades can add great flavor to a meal without extra fat and/or sodium. Make this dish early in the day and grill right before serving. Combine this recipe with 1 cup rice to provide the necessary carbohydrate. Two servings of vegetables, one of which could be the Saag, the last recipe in this section, round out the meal.

Preparation time: *30 minutes*

Cooking time: *10 minutes*

Yield: *6 servings*

2 tablespoons chopped ginger	½ teaspoon red pepper
2 tablespoons chopped garlic	½ teaspoon ground turmeric
¼ cup nonfat yogurt	¼ cup lemon juice
½ teaspoon ground white pepper	2 teaspoons vegetable oil
½ teaspoon ground cumin	Salt to taste
¼ teaspoon ground nutmeg	3 whole chicken breasts, boned, skinned, and cut into 18 pieces
¼ teaspoon cardamom	

1 Combine the ginger, garlic, yogurt, white pepper, cumin, nutmeg, cardamom, red pepper, turmeric, and lemon juice in a blender or food processor. With the motor running, drizzle in the oil.

2 Add the chicken pieces to the marinade. Mix thoroughly to coat. Cover and let marinade for 3 to 4 hours in the refrigerator.

3 Preheat oven to 375°. Place chicken breasts on a skewer about 1 inch apart. Place skewers on a rack over a pan and bake for about 10 to 12 minutes or until cooked. To broil, place skewers 3 to 4 inches from the heat and broil approximately 5 minutes per side. Serve hot with lemon garnish.

Nutrient analysis per serving: 197 calories; 31.6 grams protein, 2.2 grams carbohydrate, 6 grams fat, 1.52 grams saturated fat, 14 milligrams cholesterol, .1 gram fiber, 8 milligrams sodium.

Saag (Spinach)

Here's a sure way of jazzing up a bland vegetable. This can provide one of the servings of vegetables in the previous lamb and chicken dishes.

Preparation time: *15 minutes*

Cooking time: *15 minutes*

Yield: *6 servings*

2 10-ounce bags of fresh spinach, trimmed and washed

2 teaspoons vegetable oil

½ teaspoon cumin seeds

10 garlic cloves sliced into ¼-inch slices

2 dried red chiles

Salt to taste

1 In a large saucepan of boiling salted water, blanch the spinach in batches for 30 seconds or until wilted. Drain and refresh in cold water. Squeeze the moisture from leaves and chop finely.

2 Heat the vegetable oil over medium heat in a nonstick pan. Add the cumin seeds and stir for 5 seconds. Add garlic and fry until soft, 2 to 3 minutes. Add the chiles and cook another minute. Add the spinach, toss well, and sauté until heated thoroughly and liquid in the pan has evaporated (approximately 2 to 3 minutes). Season with salt. Serve hot.

Nutrient analysis per serving: 34.2 calories; 2.7 grams protein, 3.4 grams carbohydrate, 1.5 grams fat, 0.2 gram saturated fat, 0 milligrams cholesterol, 2 grams fiber, 63 milligrams sodium.

Greens

When residents of the San Francisco Bay area think of great vegetarian food, Greens is the first name that comes to mind. Greens uses the freshest ingredients, many of which come from the Zen Center's Green Gulch Farm, across the Golden Gate Bridge in Marin County. This brief trip results in no loss of freshness for the fine seasonal organic produce.

Chef Annie Somerville came to Greens in 1981 and became Executive Chef in 1985. In her 23rd year of cooking at Greens, she continues to create outstanding dishes with a balance of colors, flavors, and contrast of textures. In addition to the Green Gulch and Start Route Farms in Marin County, she uses artisan cheeses from West Marin and Sonoma counties. She has authored the award-winning book *Field of Greens: New Vegetarian Recipes from the Celebrated Greens Restaurant.*

Greens, Fort Mason, San Francisco, California. 415-771-6222.

Romaine Hearts with Sourdough Croutons and Parmesan Cheese

This is a wonderful dish to begin any meal. Combine it with the next recipe for Summer Minestrone and a bowl of fresh fruit, and you will be in vegetarian heaven.

Preparation time: *10 minutes*

Cooking time: *10 minutes*

Yield: *4 servings*

4 small heads of Romaine lettuce

2 garlic cloves, finely chopped

6 tablespoons extra-virgin olive oil, divided

4 thick slices of sourdough bread, cut into ½-inch cubes, about 1½ cups

1¼ teaspoon minced lemon zest

¼ teaspoon salt

1½ tablespoons vinegar or lemon juice

8 Geata or Nicoise olives, pitted and coarsely chopped

1 ounce Parmesan cheese, grated, about ⅓ cup

Freshly ground pepper to taste

1 Discard the outer leaves of the Romaine and use the whole leaves and the hearts, which should be pale green or yellow and firm. Wash the leaves, dry them in a spinner, and wrap loosely in a damp towel and refrigerate.

2 Preheat the oven to 375°. Add 1 garlic clove to 1 tablespoon olive oil and toss with the cubed bread. Spread the cubes on a baking sheet and bake for 7 to 8 minutes, until golden brown. Set aside to cool.

3 Make the vinaigrette. Combine the lemon zest, salt, remaining garlic, and vinegar. Then whisk in 5 tablespoons olive oil.

4 When you're ready to serve the salad, place the lettuce in a large bowl. Add the olives and toss with the vinaigrette, coating all the leaves. Add the croutons and Parmesan; toss again. Sprinkle with freshly ground pepper and serve.

Nutrient analysis per serving: 355 calories; 9 grams protein, 31 grams carbohydrate, 23 grams fat, 4 grams saturated fat, 6 milligrams cholesterol, 3 grams fiber, 696 milligrams sodium.

Summer Minestrone

This soup can be a complete meal. Serve with some crusty, fresh French bread, the salad in the preceding recipe, and a bowl of strawberries and an ounce of cream.

Preparation time: *30 minutes*

Cooking time: *1 hour*

Yield: *6 servings*

½ cup dried red beans, about 3 ounces, sorted and soaked overnight

6 cups cold water

2 bay leaves

2 fresh sage leaves

1 fresh oregano sprig

1 tablespoon extra-virgin olive oil

1 medium red onion, diced, about 2 cups

½ teaspoon salt

¼ teaspoon dried basil

Pepper to taste

6 garlic cloves, finely chopped

1 small carrot, diced, about ¼ cup

1 small red bell pepper, diced, about ¾ cup

1 small zucchini, diced, about ¾ cup

¼ cup red wine

2 pounds fresh tomatoes, peeled, seeded, and coarsely chopped (about 3 cups), or one 28-ounce can tomatoes with juice, coarsely chopped

¼ cup small pasta, cooked al dente, drained, and rinsed

½ bunch of fresh spinach or chard, cut into thin ribbons and washed, about 2 cups packed

2 tablespoons chopped fresh basil

Grated Parmesan cheese

1 Drain and rinse beans. Place in a 2-quart saucepan with the water, 1 bay leaf, sage leaves, and oregano. Bring to a boil; reduce heat and simmer, uncovered, until the beans are tender, about 30 minutes. Remove the herbs.

2 While the beans are cooking, heat the oil in a soup pot. Add the onion, ½ teapoon salt, dried herbs, and a few pinches of pepper. Sauté the onion over medium heat until soft, 5 to 7 minutes. Add the garlic, carrots, peppers, and zucchini and sauté for 7 to 8 minutes, stirring often. Add the wine and cook for 1 to 2 minutes, until the pan is almost dry. Add the tomatoes and then add the pasta, spinach or chard, and beans with their broth. Season with salt and pepper to taste. Add the basil just before serving. Garnish each serving with a generous tablespoon of Parmesan cheese.

Nutrient analysis per serving: *98 calories; 4 grams protein, 17 grams carbohydrate, 2 grams fat, 0 grams saturated fat, 1 milligram cholesterol, 2 grams fiber, 652 milligrams sodium.*

Sweet Pepper and Basil Frittata

You can serve this dish right out of the oven as a main course or let it cool and serve as a light lunch. You can also refrigerate the dish and cut it into small squares to serve as an hors d'oeuvre.

Preparation time: *30 minutes*

Cooking time: *25 minutes*

Yield: *10 servings*

2 tablespoons light olive oil	*6 eggs*
1 medium yellow onion, thinly sliced, about 2 cups	*3 ounces Fontina cheese, grated, about 1½ cups*
¾ teaspoon salt and pepper	*2 ounces Parmesan cheese, grated, about ¾ cup*
4 medium sweet peppers, preferably a combination of red and yellow, thinly sliced, about 4 cups	*¼ cup fresh basil leaves, bundled and thinly sliced*
4 garlic cloves, finely chopped	*3 tablespoons balsamic vinegar*
1 bay leaf	

1 Preheat oven to 475°. Heat 1 tablespoon olive oil in a large skillet; add the onion, ½ teaspoon salt, and a few pinches of pepper. Sauté the onion over medium heat until it begins to soften, about 4 to 5 minutes. Add the sweet peppers, garlic, and bay leaf; stew the onion and peppers together for about 15 minutes, until the peppers are tender. Set the vegetables aside to cool. Remove the bay leaf.

2 Beat the eggs in a bowl and add the onion–pepper mixture, cheeses, and basil. Season with ¼ teaspoon salt and ⅛ teaspoon pepper.

3 In a 9-inch nonstick sauté pan with an ovenproof handle, heat the remaining tablespoon of olive oil until almost smoking. Swirl the oil around the side of the pan to coat. Turn the heat down to low and then immediately pour the frittata mixture into the pan. The pan should be hot enough so that the eggs sizzle when they touch the oil. Cook the frittata over low heat for 2 to 3 minutes, until the sides begin to set; transfer to the oven and bake, uncovered, for 6 to 8 minutes, until firm and the eggs are completely cooked.

4 Loosen the fritatta gently with a rubber spatula; the bottom will tend to stick to the pan. Place a plate over the pan, flip it over, and put it on a plate. Brush the bottom and sides with the vinegar and cut into wedges. Serve warm or at room temperature.

Nutrient analysis per serving: *149 calories; 9.6 grams protein, 45 grams carbohydrate, 10 grams fat, 4 grams saturated fat, 159 milligrams cholesterol, 1 gram fiber, 349 milligrams sodium.*

Rhubarb–Strawberry Cobbler

This wonderful dessert is a snap to make. You can make it with less sugar (⅛ cup) if you use strawberries alone. You need 3 baskets of berries, about 5 cups washed, hulled, and cut into halves or left whole if small. You can serve it warm topped with a touch of whipped cream.

Preparation time: *40 minutes*

Cooking time: *40 minutes*

Yield: *6 servings*

Cobbler filling

1¼ pounds rhubarb

1 pint basket of strawberries, about 1½ cups

Cobbler topping

1½ cups unbleached white flour

¼ teaspoon salt

1 tablespoon baking powder

¼ cup sugar

2 ½ tablespoons unbleached white flour

Zest of 1 small orange

2 tablespoons sugar

4 tablespoons unsalted butter

1 cup heavy cream

1 Preheat oven to 375°. Wash the rhubarb well, cutting off any brown spots or leaves still on the stalks. If the stalks are especially thick, cut them in half lengthwise before slicing ½-inch thick so that all the pieces are approximately the same size.

2 Wash the strawberries, pat dry, and hull them. Cut them into halves or leave whole if small.

3 Toss the fruit with the sugar, flour, and zest; place in an 8-inch square baking dish, a 9-inch round cake pan, or 6 to 8 individual ovenproof dishes.

4 Make the cobbler topping by combining the dry ingredients. Cut in the butter with a food processor, an electric mixer, a pastry blender, or 2 knives until it resembles coarse meal. Add the cream and mix lightly, just until the dry ingredients are moistened.

5 Cover the fruit with tablespoon-size dollops of cobbler topping, using all the topping. Bake for 25 to 30 minutes, until the topping is browned and cooked through and the fruit is bubbling. Individual cobblers take about 20 minutes.

Nutrient analysis per serving: 328 calories; 5 grams protein, 60 grams carbohydrate, 8 grams fat, 5 grams saturated fat, 21 milligrams cholesterol, 2 grams fiber, 425 milligrams sodium.

Harbor Village

Acclaimed by *Gourmet Magazine* as a "gold cup restaurant commanding the respect of Chinese gastronomics," Harbor Village was serving award-winning food in Hong Kong for many years before coming to San Francisco and later Los Angeles. In an environment reminiscent of the fine restaurants of Hong Kong, the Chinese chefs prepare dim sum that has been called the finest in the United States. The seafood is prepared fresh from their fish tanks. Dishes are made up of fresh local ingredients, yet the result is exotic delicacies such as abalone, shark's fin, and bird's nest soup. The service is just as good as the food.

Executive chef Andy Wai runs a kitchen staff of 40 in San Francisco. He learned his craft in the finest Hong Kong restaurants, finally cooking at Harbor Village's parent restaurant in Hong Kong, Tsui Hang Village. From there, he came to San Francisco in 1989 where he has been the recipient of numerous awards for his creativity.

Harbor Village, Four Embarcadero Center, Lobby Level, San Francisco, California. 415-781-8833.

Chicken Soup with Watercress and Tofu

You can serve this dish as the first course to any meal. Try serving it with any of the recipes later in this section.

Preparation time: *20 minutes*

Cooking time: *45 minutes*

Yield: *8 servings*

1 teaspoon vegetable oil	½ teaspoon chicken powder, or ½ bouillon cube
Chicken bones of 1 chicken, cut into quarters	2½ quarts water
Chicken pieces of 1 chicken, finely chopped	1 bunch watercress, cleaned and trimmed of stems
1 ounce fresh ginger	1 container tofu, drained and cut into ½-inch cubes
4 ounces pork, boneless shoulder, cut in strips	½ teaspoon salt
8 red dates, quartered	Pinch white pepper
8 pieces shiitake mushrooms	
1 small carrot, diced	

1 Heat the oil in a wok over high heat. Add the chicken bones and ginger. Stir-fry for about 2 minutes.

2 In a large pot, add the chicken, pork, red dates, shiitake mushrooms, carrots, chicken powder or bouillon, and water.

3 Bring soup to boil, reduce heat, and simmer for 30 minutes, skimming any foam from the top. Using a skimmer, carefully remove the chicken bones. Then add the watercress and tofu and simmer for 10 more minutes. Season with salt and pepper.

Nutrient analysis per serving: 103 calories; 8.4 grams protein, 6.6 grams carbohydrate, 5 grams fat, .7 gram saturated fat, 9 milligrams cholesterol, 1.4 grams fiber, 176 milligrams sodium.

Shiitake Mushrooms with Baby Bok Choy

This recipe makes a great vegetable side dish, for example with the steamed rock cod recipe that follows.

Preparation time: *30 minutes*

Cooking time: *15 minutes*

Yield: *4 servings*

½ piece of ginger root, peeled and smashed

Pinch of sugar

Pinch of salt

1 tablespoon plus 1 teaspoon vegetable oil

4 cups water

2 bunches baby bok choy

1 teaspoon minced ginger

Salt to season

1 cup chicken stock

1 tablespoon oyster sauce

1 tablespoon dark mushroom soy sauce

1 tablespoon sherry

1 teaspoon sugar

½ pound shiitake mushrooms, cleaned, stemmed, and poached until tender

1 tablespoon cornstarch mixed with ½ cup cold water

1 Place the smashed ginger root, a pinch of sugar and salt, 1 teaspoon vegetable oil, and water in a large pot and bring to a boil. After 1 minute, using a skimmer, remove the ginger. Set aside to cool slightly and then mince.

2 Add the baby bok choy to the simmering water and cook for 1 minute. Drain. Set aside.

3 Heat the remaining vegetable oil in a wok and add the baby bok choy and minced ginger. Season with salt and stir-fry for 1 minute. Arrange the baby bok choy on a platter.

4 Pour the chicken stock, oyster sauce, soy sauce, sherry, and 1 teaspoon sugar into a hot wok and bring to a boil. Add the shiitake and cook until they are heated through. Stir the corn starch–water mixture into the mushrooms in the wok, simmering 2 to 3 minutes, until thickened.

5 Pour the sauce over the baby bok choy on the platter and serve immediately.

Nutrient analysis per serving: 98 calories; 7.3 grams protein, 22 grams carbohydrate, 4.7 grams fat, 2.5 grams saturated fat, 0 milligrams cholesterol, 4 grams fiber, 1,294 milligrams sodium.

Steamed Rock Cod

This dish is a perfect complement to the soup and vegetable dish recipes, earlier in this section. Round the meal out with a bowl of rice or noodles.

Preparation time: *15 minutes*

Cooking time: *15 minutes*

Yield: *6 servings*

½ cup water	Pinch white pepper
2 tablespoons light soy sauce	3½ pounds fresh whole rock cod
4 teaspoons vegetable oil	1 quart water (for steaming)
1 teaspoon oyster sauce	1 slice fresh ginger
½ teaspoon sugar	Salt and pepper to taste
½ teaspoon chicken powder	2 ounces scallions, finely chopped
Sesame oil to taste	¼ cup chopped fresh cilantro

1 Mix ½ cup water, the soy sauce, 2 teaspoons vegetable oil, oyster sauce, sugar, chicken powder, sesame oil, and white pepper in a medium saucepan. Heat the sauce, but do not boil. Keep warm over low heat.

2 In a Chinese steamer or a large pot fitted with a colander and a tight-fitting lid, bring 1 quart water to a boil. Lightly brush the cod with the remaining vegetable oil and season with salt and pepper. Place the fish into the steamer or colander and place a slice of ginger over top. Steam for 12 to 15 minutes, until firm and opaque in the center.

3 Using a large spatula, carefully remove the fish from steamer; sprinkle with chopped scallions and cilantro; pour the warm sauce over the fish and serve immediately.

Nutrient analysis per serving: 340 calories; 55 grams protein, 2 grams carbohydrate, 11 grams fat, 2 grams saturated fat, 154 milligrams cholesterol, .5 gram fiber, 285 milligrams sodium.

Il Fornaio

Il Fornaio *(eel for-NIGH-oh)* means "the baker" in Italian. The company began as a baking school outside Milan, Italy, in 1972, created in response to the disappearing art of centuries-old Italian baking. In 1981, Il Fornaio came to the United States and has since grown to include some of the most successful restaurants and bakeries in America. Today, you can enjoy Il Fornaio's authentic Italian food and baked goods at any of 21 locations in California, Portland, Seattle, Las Vegas, Denver, and Atlanta. For more information, you can visit www.ilfornaio.com on the Web.

Head chef Edmondo Sarti comes from the Emilia-Romagna section of Italy, which includes the great cuisine of Bologna. He learned to cook at his Uncle Salvatore's knee, going on to culinary school in Cervia, Italy. He apprenticed in the finest Italian restaurants and was offered a position at Valentino Restaurant in Los Angeles, where he met his wife. Italy's loss became San Francisco's gain when he took a position as head chef at Il Fornaio.

Il Fornaio, 1265 Battery Street, San Francisco, California. 415-986-0100.

Scallopine Al Funghi (Veal with Mushrooms)

This recipe makes delicious use of veal, but you can substitute chicken breasts for the veal. Just marinate the chicken with chopped sage and rosemary. Try using different types of mushrooms, which gives the recipe a different taste: bottom mushrooms, shitake, chanterelle, or porcini. A half cup of any pasta (or, if you prefer, a slice of bread and a quarter cup of pasta) provides the necessary carbohydrate.

Preparation time: *25 minutes*

Cooking time: *15 minutes*

Yield: *4 servings*

8 2- to 3-ounce veal scallops	1 chopped garlic clove
Salt and pepper to taste	1 cup sliced mixed mushrooms
1 tablespoon flour	½ cup white wine
2 tablespoons butter	10 leaves Italian parsley
2 tablespoons olive oil	¼ cup vegetable stock

1 Place the veal scallops two at a time between sheets of plastic wrap and pound them with a meat mallet until ¼ inch thick. Season them with salt and pepper. Cover the veal scallops with flour, shaking off excess. Heat the butter in a sauté pan. Add the veal and cook for 2 minutes on each side. Transfer veal to a plate.

2 In the same pan add the oil, garlic, mushrooms, white wine, and parsley. Cook for a few minutes and add the veal and stock. Simmer for about 5 minutes.

3 Set veal on a plate and top with the mushroom sauce.

Nutrient analysis per serving: 442 calories; 49 grams protein, 2 grams carbohydrate, 22 grams fat, 7 grams saturated fat, 179 milligrams cholesterol, .5 gram fiber, 175 milligrams sodium.

Maniche Al Pollo (Elbow Pasta with Chicken)

This recipe is fairly concentrated in calories but is a delicious way to give chicken an Italian flavor. It's a complete meal as written, but you can eat less pasta and replace it with a piece of bread if you prefer.

Preparation time: *10 minutes*

Cooking time: *20 minutes*

Yield: *4 servings*

2 tablespoons olive oil

12 ounces skinless chicken breasts, diced

Salt and pepper to taste

4 garlic cloves, sliced

½ cup white wine

10 ounces elbow pasta

4 sundried tomatoes

4 cups fresh broccoli florets

4 tablespoons Parmesan cheese

1 Heat the oil in large sauté pan over high heat. Add the diced chicken and salt and pepper. Sauté 2 to 3 minutes, or until cooked through. Add the garlic and lightly brown. Add the wine and cook until sauce is reduced to 1 to 2 tablespoons.

2 Boil the pasta according to directions. Three minutes before the pasta is ready, add the sundried tomatoes and broccoli. Drain and toss with the chicken, sauce, and Parmesan cheese.

Nutrient analysis per serving: 561 calories; 41 grams protein, 66 grams carbohydrate, 24 grams fat, 3 grams saturated fat, 70 milligrams cholesterol, 2.5 grams fiber, 283 milligrams sodium.

Risotto Ai Vegetali (Italian Rice with Vegetables)

A serving of this recipe provides all the carbohydrates for a full meal. It contains the vegetables you need as well. It lacks protein, which you can make up with a few ounces of chicken or fish. Use whatever vegetable is in season, including zucchini, artichokes, asparagus, or mushrooms. Be aware of the number of servings you have when you make this dish. Overeating is easy if you're not careful!

Preparation time: *10 minutes*

Cooking time: *1 hour*

Yield: *10 servings*

3 tablespoons butter	*½ cup white wine*
1 large shallot, diced	*8 cups vegetable stock*
3 cups seasonal vegetables, diced	*½ tablespoon grated Parmesan cheese*
2 cups Italian Arborio rice	*Salt and pepper to taste*

1 In a 4- to 6-quart heavy-bottom saucepan, heat 1 tablespoon butter over low-medium heat. Stir in the shallots and cook slowly for 4 minutes or until onions are soft and clear, but not brown. Increase the heat to medium, add all the vegetables, and cook, stirring, for 1 to 2 minutes. Stir in the rice and cook, gently stirring, for 1 to 2 minutes. Pour in the white wine and cook until it is almost completely reduced. Add the stock, 1 cup at a time, and cook at a low boil, stirring often, until absorbed. Each cup must be absorbed before the next is added. After 15 minutes, taste a grain of rice — it should have a slight resistance to the bite. If it seems too hard, add a little bit more stock and continue cooking for a couple more minutes.

2 When rice is ready, remove from heat. Add remaining butter and Parmesan cheese. Add salt and pepper to taste and mix with a wooden spoon until creamy in texture.

Nutrient analysis per serving: *204 calories; 4.6 grams protein, 34 grams carbohydrate, 5 grams fat, 2.3 grams saturated fat, 9 milligrams cholesterol, 1.6 grams fiber, 625 milligrams sodium.*

Bavarese Bianca Con Frutta
(White Gelatin with Fruit)

This recipe is a dessert treat that should not be eaten too often, but it shows that you can enjoy such treats in moderation and still follow your diabetic diet. Because the recipe is mostly carbohydrate and fat, it replaces those energy sources in your meal. The meal itself should be a few ounces of meat, fish, or poultry with a couple servings of vegetables.

Preparation time: *20 minutes*

Cooking time: *None*

Yield: *4 servings*

1 envelope plain gelatin	*¼ cup sugar*
1½ cups 1 percent milk	*1 cup mixed berries*
½ cup cream	*4 mint leaves*

1 In a small bowl, mix together the gelatin and milk; let sit 5 minutes, until gelatin is dissolved. In a double boiler, bring the milk, cream, and sugar to a boil, stirring continuously to dissolve sugar. Remove from heat and allow to cool slightly.

2 Line four 3-ounce espresso cups with clear plastic wrap. Pour mixture into cups and refrigerate overnight or at least 6 hours.

3 Turn over the cups onto a plate. Remove plastic wrap and garnish with berries and mint leaves.

Nutrient analysis per 2 tablespoons: *259 calories; 6 grams protein, 28 grams carbohydrate, 13 grams fat, 9 grams saturated fat, 56 milligrams cholesterol, 1.3 grams fiber, 64 milligrams sodium.*

Appendix B

Dr. W.W. Web

• •

*I*n just a few years, the World Wide Web went from containing little or no information on diabetes to hosting more information than anyone can digest. This appendix presents the best sites for you to check. You should be able to get answers online to just about any questions that you have, but you must be cautious about the source of the advice. Do not make any major changes in your diabetes care without checking with your physician.

As I note in Chapter 19, to determine whether information you find on a Web site is really useful, you need to discuss it with your physician, your diabetes educator, or other members of your team (see Chapter 11). Any Web site I discuss in this appendix can be relied upon, but sometimes free advice is worth no more than you pay for it. Remember that the Web is constantly changing and growing, so these addresses are valid at least on the day I list them.

My Web Site

You can start your search for information at my Web page:

www.drrubin.com

You can find general information and advice about diabetes, daily tips, new developments, and answers to questions. You also find all of the sites listed in this appendix so that you need only click on them to see them for yourself.

General Sites

These sites tell you about diabetes from A to Z. The site sponsors run the gamut from well-known organizations to individual doctors who specialize in diabetes. Sometimes the sites get a little technical. That is when you need to return to this book for clarification.

The American Diabetes Association

This huge site has just about everything you need to know about diabetes and then some. It may be a little technical in places, but that's probably because you got into the professional section by mistake. You can order all the ADA's publications from here.

    www.diabetes.org

Online Diabetes Resources by Rick Mendosa

Rick Mendosa, who has diabetes himself, has cataloged just about everything there is on the Web concerning diabetes. This is a huge undertaking, and he manages to bring it off beautifully. He also has some excellent articles that he has written on various topics in diabetes.

    www.mendosa.com/diabetes.htm

National Diabetes Education Program

The federal government is sponsoring the National Diabetes Education Program to improve treatments and outcomes for people with diabetes, to promote early diagnosis, and to prevent the onset of diabetes. It is a vast undertaking.

    http://ndep.nih.gov

National Diabetes Education Initiative

The federal government is determined to teach physicians about the importance of meeting the standards of diabetes care and how to go about doing this. You can learn a lot by looking at its programs.

    www.ndei.org/website

Medscape Diabetes and Endocrinology Home Page

You can find numerous articles about diabetes from medical literature, as well as free access to the files of the National Library of Medicine.

```
http://www.medscape.com/diabetes-endocrinology
```

The Diabetes Monitor

The Diabetes Monitor is the creation of diabetes specialist Dr. William Quick. He discusses every aspect of diabetes, including the latest discoveries.

```
www.diabetesmonitor.com
```

Juvenile Diabetes Research Foundation

The JDRF prides itself on its contribution to research in diabetes, and this site reflects that. You can find what you want to know about the latest government programs that emphasize finding a cure for diabetes.

```
www.jdf.org
```

Children with Diabetes

This site is the creation of a father of a diabetic child and has an enormous database of information for the parents of children with diabetes.

```
http://www.childrenwithdiabetes.com/index_cwd.htm
```

Joslin Diabetes Center

The Joslin Diabetes Center has been one of the world's leading pioneers in diabetes care, and the information on this site reflects that fact. The site also tells you how you can join Joslin, do research, or go to diabetes camp.

```
www.joslin.org
```

Canadian Diabetes Association

If you're Canadian, you want to visit this site because a lot of its information (obviously) pertains to the special needs of the Canadian with diabetes. However, much of the information is general and of use to everyone. A major benefit is that the information is in French as well as English.

        www.diabetes.ca

The International Diabetes Federation

This organization, representing more than 100 countries, meets every three years and can be a source for knowledgeable diabetes experts around the world.

        www.idf.org

Ask NOAH About Diabetes

This site provides a large amount of information in both English and Spanish. It comes from the New York Online Access to Health, a partnership of New York institutions.

        www.noah-health.org

Companies That Make Diabetes Products

This section helps you find the companies that make the products you need to control your diabetes. If you have questions about the proper use of a drug or a device, you can usually find answers here. But keep in mind that the companies are very limited (by the FDA) with respect to the uses of their products. Often doctors use drugs in ways that have proven to be successful but have not yet received FDA approval.

Glucose meters

The following companies make the meters used by the largest number of people with diabetes. You can expect that these companies will still be around when you start having problems with your meter after a year or two of use.

- ✔ **Abbott Laboratories:** www.abbott.com
- ✔ **Bayer:** bayercarediabetes.com
- ✔ **Home Diagnostics, Inc.:** thesmartchoice.com
- ✔ **LifeScan:** www.lifescan.com
- ✔ **Roche:** www.roche.com/home.html

Lancing devices

A company that has a very large share of the market for lancing devices is **Owen Mumford,** which you can find at www.owenmumford.com/en/.

Insulin pumps

Six companies dominate the market for insulin pump devices. They are

- ✔ **AccuChek Spirit Insulin Pump System:** www.disetronic-usa.com/dstrnc_us
- ✔ **Animas:** www.animascorp.com
- ✔ **CozMore Insulin Technology System:** www.cozmore.com
- ✔ **DANA Diabecare USA:** www.theinsulinpump.com
- ✔ **Medtronic MiniMed:** www.minimed.com
- ✔ **OmniPod Insulin Management System:** www.myomnipod.com

Insulin

Three companies dominate the insulin market in the United States.

- ✔ **Aventis:** www.aventis.com
- ✔ **Eli Lilly and Company:** www.lilly.com
- ✔ **Novo Nordisk:** www.novo-nordisk.com

Insulin syringes

If you want to find the major company for syringes, go to **Becton, Dickinson and Company** at www.bd.com/diabetes.

Insulin jet injection devices

Jet injection devices provide "painless" insulin injection. A number of companies are trying to monopolize this market, including

- **Activa Brand Products:** www.advantajet.com/mainsite.htm
- **Antares Pharma (formerly Medi-Ject Corporation):** www.mediject.com
- **Bioject Medical Technologies, Inc.:** www.bioject.com

Oral medications

This list contains only five companies at present, but the market for oral medications is heating up, so we'll most likely add several more in the not-too-distant future.

- **Aventis (Amaryl):** www.aventis.com
- **Bristol-Myers Squibb (Glucophage, Glucovance, Glucophage XR):** www.bms.com/landing/data
- **Eli Lilly/Takeda (Actos):** www.lilly.com
- **GlaxoSmithKline (Avandia):** www.gsk.com
- **Pfizer Inc. (Glucotrol):** www.pfizer.com

Diabetic Exercise and Sports Association

The Diabetes Exercise and Sports Association is a place where you can find out about many different kinds of exercise, how much you can and should do, and whether there are any limitations because of the diabetes. You can also find others who share your interests.

www.diabetes-exercise.org

Government Web Sites

These sites provide lots of authoritative information in their many online publications about diabetes. They also tell you about the latest government programs to eradicate the disease.

National Institute of Diabetes and Digestive and Kidney Disease

This site is loaded with great publications about diabetes.

```
http://diabetes.niddk.nih.gov
```

Centers for Disease Control

If you want to know all the latest statistics about every aspect of diabetes, go to this site.

```
http://www.cdc.gov/doc.do/id/0900f3ec802723eb
```

Healthfinder Web site

Healthfinder is a service of the U.S. Department of Health and Human Services. It has information about many important diseases and has a large section about diabetes.

```
www.healthfinder.gov
```

PubMed Search Service of the National Library of Medicine

This is where you go to use the National Library of Medicine. The site is easy to use and gives you (for free) a large number of the latest scientific papers on any medical topic of interest.

```
www.ncbi.nlm.nih.gov/PubMed
```

Nongovernment Web site for searching the National Library

MedFetch is an excellent site for creating repeated searches on a topic like diabetes over time. The information arrives by e-mail, and the results are delivered in one of six languages: English, Spanish, French, Italian, German, or Portuguese.

```
www.medfetch.com
```

Diabetes Information in Other Languages

Believe it or not, not everyone speaks and reads English. At this site, you find diabetes educational information in numerous languages.

```
http://multiculturalhealth.org/index/Health_Handouts
```

Sites for the Visually Impaired

Diabetes has a major impact on vision when the disease is not controlled (see Chapter 5). You can find huge quantities of information on every issue relating to visual impairment at the sites listed in this section.

American Foundation for the Blind

The American Foundation for the Blind has resources, information, reports, talking books, and limitless other facts and wisdom about dealing with visual impairment.

```
www.afb.org
```

Blindness Resource Center

This site points you in the right direction for information on every aspect of blindness. It is a guide to other sites about visual impairment.

```
www.nyise.org/text/blindness.htm
```

The Diabetes Action Network (National Federation of the Blind)

This national organization is another major source of information about every aspect of blindness.

        www.nfb.org/diabetes.htm

Animals with Diabetes

Yes, your dog and cat and many other animals can get diabetes, and Web sites exist that can help.

Dogs and other pets

This site tells you everything you need to know to manage your canine with diabetes.

        www.petdiabetes.org

Cats

This site is packed with helpful information for the pet owner who has a diabetic cat.

        www.felinediabetes.com

Recipes for People with Diabetes

You can find a number of excellent recipes on the Web, but approach them with caution. While you can generally count on the recipes in books to contain the nutrients they list, when you find a recipe on the Web, you need to evaluate its source to be sure the listed nutrients are accurate.

You can trust the sites that I list here. These are the best of the currently available Web sites that provide recipes appropriate for a person with diabetes. Things change so frequently on the Web that it's difficult to keep up to date, so check back often.

- ✔ The nutrition section of the American Diabetes Association Web site begins at www.diabetes.org/nutrition. Here you find discussions of nutrition, as well as lots of recipes.

- ✔ "Children with Diabetes" includes a large amount of information on meal planning, sugar substitutes, and the food guide pyramid, as well as many recipes, at www.childrenwithdiabetes.com/d_08_000.htm.

- ✔ The Joslin Diabetes Center points out that "There is no such thing as a diabetic diet." That's one of many statements about nutrition you can find at www.joslin.org/education/library.

- ✔ "Ask NOAH About Diabetes" supplies links to many important articles about diabetic nutrition, as well as diabetic recipes, at www.noah-health.org.

- ✔ "3 Fat Chicks on a Diet" has complete calorie counts for most fast food restaurants at www.3fatchicks.com.

- ✔ The Vegetarian Resource Group maintains a large site filled with information for vegetarians who have developed diabetes at http://www.vrg.org/.

- ✔ *Diabetic Gourmet Magazine* offers a valuable site that contains information about diagnosis and treatment, as well as numerous recipes that you can use, at diabeticgourmet.com.

Appendix C

Glossary

Acarbose: An oral agent that lowers blood glucose by blocking the breakdown of carbohydrates in the intestine.

ACE inhibitor: A drug that lowers blood pressure but is especially useful when diabetes affects the kidneys.

Acetone: A breakdown product of fat formed when fat rather than glucose is being used for energy.

Actos: An oral agent that lowers glucose by reducing insulin resistance.

Advanced glycated end products (AGEs): Combinations of glucose and other substances in the body. Too much may damage various organs.

Alpha cells: Cells in the Islets of Langerhans within the pancreas that make glucagon, which raises blood glucose.

Algorithm: In diabetes care, a step-by-step plan for determining how much insulin to use for the blood level of glucose and the intake of carbohydrates.

Amaryl: An oral agent that lowers glucose by raising insulin levels.

Amino acids: Compounds that link together to form proteins.

Amyotrophy: A form of diabetic neuropathy causing muscle wasting and weakness.

Angiography: Using a dye to take pictures of blood vessels to detect disease. In diabetes, angiography is often used in the eyes.

Antibodies: Substances formed when the body detects something foreign, such as bacteria.

Antigens: Substances against which the antibody forms.

Artificial pancreas: A large machine that can measure blood glucose and release appropriate insulin.

Atherosclerosis: Narrowing of arteries due to deposits of cholesterol and other factors.

Autoimmune disorder: Disease in which the body mistakenly attacks its own tissues.

Autonomic neuropathy: Diseases of nerves that affect organs not under conscious control, such as the heart, lungs, and intestines.

Avandia: One of a class of oral antidiabetic agents that lowers glucose by reducing insulin resistance. Not recommended.

Background retinopathy: An early stage of diabetic eye involvement that does not reduce vision.

Beta cells: Cells in the Islets of Langerhans in the pancreas that make the key hormone insulin.

Blood urea nitrogen (BUN): A substance in blood that reflects kidney function.

Body mass index (BMI): A number derived by dividing your weight (in kilograms) by your height (in meters), and dividing that number by your height (in meters) again. Your BMI is an indicator of your appropriate weight for your height.

Borderline diabetes: A term formerly used to mean mild or early diabetes; it is no longer used.

Carbohydrate: One of the three major energy sources — the one usually found in grain, fruits, and vegetables, and the one most responsible for raising the blood glucose.

Carbohydrate counting: Estimating the amount of carbohydrate in food in order to determine insulin needs.

Cataract: A clouding of the lens of the eye often found earlier and more commonly in people with diabetes.

Charcot's foot: Destruction of joints and soft tissue in the foot leading to an unusable foot as a result of diabetic neuropathy.

Cholesterol: A form of fat that is needed in the body for production of certain hormones. It can lead to atherosclerosis if present in excessive levels. Butter and egg yolks are high in cholesterol.

Conventional diabetes treatment: Usually refers to treatment in type 1 diabetes where only one or two shots of insulin are given daily.

Continuous subcutaneous insulin infusion (CSII): Continuous delivery of insulin under the skin, usually by an insulin pump, to mimic the way the body provides insulin.

Creatinine: A substance in blood that is measured to reflect the level of kidney function.

Dawn phenomenon: The tendency for blood glucose to rise early in the morning due to secretion of hormones that counteract insulin.

Diabetes Control and Complications Trial (DCCT): The decisive study of type 1 diabetes that showed that intensive control of blood glucose would prevent or delay complications of diabetes.

Diabetic ketoacidosis: An acute loss of control of diabetes with high blood glucose levels and breakdown of fat leading to acidification of the blood. Symptoms are nausea, vomiting, and dehydration. This condition can lead to coma and death.

Diabetologist: A physician who specializes in diabetes treatment.

Dialysis: Artificial cleaning of the blood when the kidneys are not working.

Endocrinologist: A physician who specializes in diseases of the glands, including the adrenal glands, the thyroid, the pituitary, the parathyroid glands, the ovaries, the testicles, and the pancreas.

Euglycemia: A state in which the blood glucose remains in the normal range.

Exchange plan: A dietary plan where foods that are similar in type are grouped together so that a diet can substitute any one for any other within that group. The seven groups are *starches and breads, meats and meat substitutes, fruits, milks, vegetables, fats,* and *other carbohydrates.*

Fiber: A substance in plants that can't be digested. It provides no energy but can lower fat and blood glucose if it dissolves in water and is absorbed, or it can help prevent constipation if it does not dissolve in water and remains in the intestine.

Fructose: The sugar found in fruits, vegetables, and honey. It has calories but is more slowly absorbed than glucose.

Gastroparesis: A form of autonomic neuropathy involving nerves to the stomach so that food is held in the stomach.

Gestational diabetes mellitus: Diabetes that occurs during a pregnancy, usually ending at delivery.

Glimeperide: *See Amaryl.*

Glucagon: A hormone made in the alpha cell of the pancreas that raises glucose and can be injected in severe hypoglycemia.

Glucose: The body's main source of energy in the blood and cells.

Glucophage: An oral agent for diabetes that lowers glucose by blocking release from the liver.

Glycemic index: The extent to which a given food raises blood glucose usually compared to white bread. Low glycemic index foods are preferred in diabetes.

Glycogen: The storage form of glucose in the liver and muscles.

Glycosuria: Glucose in the urine.

Glycosylated hemoglobin: *See Hemoglobin A1c.*

Glyset: An oral hypoglycemic drug that lowers blood glucose by blocking breakdown of complex sugars and starches.

Hemoglobin A1c: A measurement of blood glucose control reflecting the average blood glucose for the last 60 to 90 days.

High density lipoprotein (HDL): A particle in blood that carries cholesterol and helps reduce atherosclerosis.

Honeymoon phase: A period of variable duration, usually less than a year, after a diagnosis of type 1 diabetes when the need for injections of insulin is reduced or eliminated.

Humalog insulin: *See Lispro insulin.*

Hyperglycemia: Levels of blood glucose greater than 100 mg/dl fasting or 140 mg/dl in the fed state.

Hyperinsulinemia: More insulin than normal in the blood; often found early in type 2 diabetes.

Hyperlipidemia: Elevated levels of fat in the blood.

Hyperosmolar syndrome: Very high glucose in type 2 diabetes associated with severe dehydration but not excessive fat breakdown and acidosis. It can lead to coma and death.

Hypoglycemia: Levels of blood glucose lower than normal, usually less than 60 mg/dl.

Impaired glucose tolerance (IGT): Levels of glucose between 140 and 200 mg/dl after eating — not normal but not quite high enough for a diagnosis of diabetes.

Impotence: Loss of the ability to have or sustain an erection of the penis.

Insulin: The key hormone that permits glucose to enter cells.

Insulin dependent diabetes: Former name for type 1 diabetes.

Insulin glargine: *See Lantus.*

Insulin pump: Device that slowly pushes insulin through a catheter under the skin but can also be used to give a large dose before meals.

Insulin reaction: Hypoglycemia as a consequence of too much injected insulin for the amount of food or exercise.

Insulin resistance: Decreased response to insulin; found early in type 2 diabetes.

Intensive diabetes treatment: Using three or four daily insulin injections based upon measurement of blood glucose, along with very careful diet and exercise, to approximate the normal range of glucose.

Islet cells: The cells in the pancreas that make insulin, glucagon, and other hormones.

Juvenile diabetes mellitus: Previous term for type 1 diabetes.

Ketones or ketone bodies: The breakdown products of fat metabolism.

Ketonuria: Finding ketones in the urine with a test strip.

Lancet: A sharp needle to prick the skin for a blood glucose test.

Lantus: An insulin that provides a constant basal level 24 hours a day.

Laser treatment: Using a device that burns the back of the eye to prevent worsening of retinopathy.

Lente insulin: An intermediate-acting insulin that works in 4 to 6 hours and is gone by 12 hours.

Lipoatrophy: Indented areas where insulin is constantly injected.

Lipohypertrophy: Nodular swelling of the skin where insulin is constantly injected.

Lispro insulin: A very rapid-acting form of insulin, active within 15 minutes of injection.

Low density lipoprotein (LDL): A particle in the blood containing cholesterol and thought to be responsible for atherosclerosis.

Macrosomia: The condition of a large baby born when the mother's diabetes is not controlled.

Macrovascular complications: Heart attack, stroke, or diminished blood flow to the legs in diabetes.

Metabolic syndrome: A combination of hypertension, increased visceral fat, high triglycerides, low HDL cholesterol, often obesity, and high uric acid associated with increased heart attacks.

Metformin: *See Glucophage.*

Microalbuminuria: Loss of small but abnormal amounts of protein in the urine.

Microvascular complications: Eye disease, nerve disease, or kidney disease in diabetes.

Miglitol: *See Glyset.*

Monounsaturated fat: One form of fat from vegetable sources like olives and nuts that does not raise cholesterol.

Morbidity rate: The rate at which sickness occurs compared with those who remain well.

Mortality rate: The rate at which death occurs compared with the total population.

Nateglinide: *See Starlix.*

Neovascularization: Formation of new vessels, especially from the retina of the eye.

Nephropathy: Damage to the kidneys.

Neuropathic ulcer: An infected area, usually on the leg or foot, resulting from damage that was not felt.

Neuropathy: Damage to parts of the nervous system.

Noninsulin dependent diabetes: Former name for type 2 diabetes.

NPH insulin: An intermediate-acting insulin, which starts to work in 4 to 6 hours and ends by 12 hours.

Ophthalmologist: A doctor who specializes in diseases of the eyes.

Oral hypoglycemic agent: A glucose-lowering drug taken by mouth.

Pancreas: The organ behind the stomach that contains the Islets of Langerhans where insulin is produced.

Periodontal disease: Gum damage, which is more common in uncontrolled diabetes.

Peripheral neuropathy: Pain, numbness, and tingling, usually in the legs and feet.

Pioglitazone: *See Actos.*

Podiatrist: A person who specializes in treating the feet.

Polydipsia: Excessive intake of water.

Polyunsaturated fat: A form of fat from vegetables that may not raise cholesterol but lowers HDL.

Polyuria: Excessive urination.

Postprandial: After eating.

Prandin: An oral drug that lowers glucose by causing insulin secretion.

Precose: *See Acarbose.*

Proliferative retinopathy: Undesirable production of blood vessels in front of the retina.

Protein: A source of energy for the body made up of amino acids and found in meat, fish, poultry, and beans.

Proteinuria: Abnormal loss of protein from the body into the urine.

Receptors: Places on cells that bind to a substance like insulin to permit the substance to do its job.

Regular insulin: A fast-acting form of insulin, active in one to two hours and gone by four to six hours.

Repaglinide: *See Prandin.*

Retina: The part of the eye that senses light.

Retinopathy: Disease of the retina.

Rezulin: The first of the class of glucose-lowering agents that reverses insulin resistance. Liver problems have caused its removal from the drug market.

Rosiglitazone: *See Avandia.*

Saturated fat: A form of fat from animals that raises cholesterol.

Secondary diabetes: Diabetes caused by some other disease, which raises glucose or blocks insulin.

Somogyi effect: A rapid increase in blood glucose in response to hypoglycemia.

Starlix: A drug similar to Prandin that is given before a meal to stimulate insulin for that meal.

Sulfonylureas: The earliest class of glucose-lowering agents, which work by stimulating insulin secretion.

Synthetic: Produced by artificial means.

Triglycerides: The main form of fat in animals.

Troglitazone: *See Rezulin.*

Ultralente insulin: A long-acting insulin that lasts for 24 to 36 hours.

Visceral fat: The fat accumulation that results in increased waist measurement.

Vitrectomy: Removal of the gel in the center of the eyeball because there has been leakage of blood and formation of scar tissue.

VLDL: The main particle in the blood that carries triglyceride.

Index

• *S* •

SPORTS, FITNESS, PARENTING, RELIGION & SPIRITUALITY

0-471-76871-5

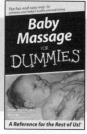

0-7645-7841-3

Also available:
- Catholicism For Dummies
  0-7645-5391-7
- Exercise Balls For Dummies
  0-7645-5623-1
- Fitness For Dummies
  0-7645-7851-0
- Football For Dummies
  0-7645-3936-1
- Judaism For Dummies
  0-7645-5299-6
- Potty Training For Dummies
  0-7645-5417-4
- Buddhism For Dummies
  0-7645-5359-3

- Pregnancy For Dummies
  0-7645-4483-7 †
- Ten Minute Tone-Ups For Dummies
  0-7645-7207-5
- NASCAR For Dummies
  0-7645-7681-X
- Religion For Dummies
  0-7645-5264-3
- Soccer For Dummies
  0-7645-5229-5
- Women in the Bible For Dummies
  0-7645-8475-8

TRAVEL

0-7645-7749-2

0-7645-6945-7

Also available:
- Alaska For Dummies
  0-7645-7746-8
- Cruise Vacations For Dummies
  0-7645-6941-4
- England For Dummies
  0-7645-4276-1
- Europe For Dummies
  0-7645-7529-5
- Germany For Dummies
  0-7645-7823-5
- Hawaii For Dummies
  0-7645-7402-7

- Italy For Dummies
  0-7645-7386-1
- Las Vegas For Dummies
  0-7645-7382-9
- London For Dummies
  0-7645-4277-X
- Paris For Dummies
  0-7645-7630-5
- RV Vacations For Dummies
  0-7645-4442-X
- Walt Disney World & Orlando
  For Dummies
  0-7645-9660-8

GRAPHICS, DESIGN & WEB DEVELOPMENT

0-7645-8815-X

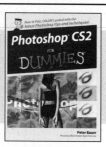

0-7645-9571-7

Also available:
- 3D Game Animation For Dummies
  0-7645-8789-7
- AutoCAD 2006 For Dummies
  0-7645-8925-3
- Building a Web Site For Dummies
  0-7645-7144-3
- Creating Web Pages For Dummies
  0-470-08030-2
- Creating Web Pages All-in-One Desk
  Reference For Dummies
  0-7645-4345-8
- Dreamweaver 8 For Dummies
  0-7645-9649-7

- InDesign CS2 For Dummies
  0-7645-9572-5
- Macromedia Flash 8 For Dummies
  0-7645-9691-8
- Photoshop CS2 and Digital
  Photography For Dummies
  0-7645-9580-6
- Photoshop Elements 4 For Dummies
  0-471-77483-9
- Syndicating Web Sites with RSS Feeds
  For Dummies
  0-7645-8848-6
- Yahoo! SiteBuilder For Dummies
  0-7645-9800-7

NETWORKING, SECURITY, PROGRAMMING & DATABASES

0-7645-7728-X

0-471-74940-0

Also available:
- Access 2007 For Dummies
  0-470-04612-0
- ASP.NET 2 For Dummies
  0-7645-7907-X
- C# 2005 For Dummies
  0-7645-9704-3
- Hacking For Dummies
  0-470-05235-X
- Hacking Wireless Networks
  For Dummies
  0-7645-9730-2
- Java For Dummies
  0-470-08716-1

- Microsoft SQL Server 2005 For Dummies
  0-7645-7755-7
- Networking All-in-One Desk Reference
  For Dummies
  0-7645-9939-9
- Preventing Identity Theft For Dummies
  0-7645-7336-5
- Telecom For Dummies
  0-471-77085-X
- Visual Studio 2005 All-in-One Desk
  Reference For Dummies
  0-7645-9775-2
- XML For Dummies
  0-7645-8845-1

HEALTH & SELF-HELP

0-7645-8450-2

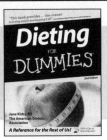

0-7645-4149-8

Also available:

- Bipolar Disorder For Dummies
  0-7645-8451-0
- Chemotherapy and Radiation
  For Dummies
  0-7645-7832-4
- Controlling Cholesterol For Dummies
  0-7645-5440-9
- Diabetes For Dummies
  0-7645-6820-5* †
- Divorce For Dummies
  0-7645-8417-0 †

- Fibromyalgia For Dummies
  0-7645-5441-7
- Low-Calorie Dieting For Dummies
  0-7645-9905-4
- Meditation For Dummies
  0-471-77774-9
- Osteoporosis For Dummies
  0-7645-7621-6
- Overcoming Anxiety For Dummies
  0-7645-5447-6
- Reiki For Dummies
  0-7645-9907-0
- Stress Management For Dummies
  0-7645-5144-2

EDUCATION, HISTORY, REFERENCE & TEST PREPARATION

0-7645-8381-6

0-7645-9554-7

Also available:

- The ACT For Dummies
  0-7645-9652-7
- Algebra For Dummies
  0-7645-5325-9
- Algebra Workbook For Dummies
  0-7645-8467-7
- Astronomy For Dummies
  0-7645-8465-0
- Calculus For Dummies
  0-7645-2498-4
- Chemistry For Dummies
  0-7645-5430-1
- Forensics For Dummies
  0-7645-5580-4

- Freemasons For Dummies
  0-7645-9796-5
- French For Dummies
  0-7645-5193-0
- Geometry For Dummies
  0-7645-5324-0
- Organic Chemistry I For Dummies
  0-7645-6902-3
- The SAT I For Dummies
  0-7645-7193-1
- Spanish For Dummies
  0-7645-5194-9
- Statistics For Dummies
  0-7645-5423-9

Get smart @ dummies.com®

- **Find a full list of Dummies titles**
- **Look into loads of FREE on-site articles**
- **Sign up for FREE eTips e-mailed to you weekly**
- **See what other products carry the Dummies name**
- **Shop directly from the Dummies bookstore**
- **Enter to win new prizes every month!**

* Separate Canadian edition also available
† Separate U.K. edition also available

Available wherever books are sold. For more information or to order direct: U.S. customers visit www.dummies.com or call 1-877-762-2974.
U.K. customers visit www.wileyeurope.com or call 0800 243407. Canadian customers visit www.wiley.ca or call 1-800-567-4797.

Do More with Dummies

Tickle my ribs!

Grilling FOR DUMMIES

12" x 12" kit
Scrapbooking Basics FOR DUMMIES

Quilting Notions FOR DUMMIES

Cocktail Kit FOR DUMMIES

Poker FOR DUMMIES

Golf FOR DUMMIES

Pilates Workout FOR DUMMIES

'80s Pop Music FOR DUMMIES

'70s Soul Music FOR DUMMIES

Wall & Ceiling Repair Kit FOR DUMMIES

Tarot Deck & Book Set FOR DUMMIES
Tarot for the Rest of Us!

Sudoku FOR DUMMIES The Game

Texas Hold 'em FOR DUMMIES
A Card Game for the Rest of Us!

**Instructional DVDs • Music Compilations
Games & Novelties • Culinary Kits
Crafts & Sewing Patterns
Home Improvement/DIY Kits • and more!**

MAY 1 9 2009

Check out the Dummies Specialty Shop at www.dummies.com for more information!

WILEY